Dying in an Institution

Dying in an Institution
Nurse/Patient Perspectives

Mary Reardon Castles, Ph.D., R.N.
Professor
College of Nursing
Wayne State University
Detroit, Michigan

Ruth Beckmann Murray, R.N., M.S.N.
Professor
School of Nursing
St. Louis University
St. Louis, Missouri

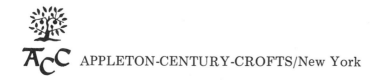 APPLETON-CENTURY-CROFTS/New York

79 80 81 82 83 / 10 9 8 7 6 5 4 3 2 1

Prentice-Hall International, Inc., London
Prentice-Hall of Australia, Pty. Ltd., Sydney
Prentice-Hall of India Private Limited, New Delhi
Prentice-Hall of Japan, Inc., Tokyo
Prentice-Hall of Southeast Asia (Pte.) Ltd., Singapore
Whitehall Books Ltd., Wellington, New Zealand

Library of Congress Cataloging in Publication Data

Castles, Mary Reardon and Murray, Ruth Beckmann
    Dying in an institution.

    Includes index.
    1. Nurse and patient. 2. Terminal care.
3. Death—Psychological aspects. I. Murray,
Ruth, joint author. II. Title.
RT86.C37 1979   610.73'069   79-15262

ISBN 0-8385-1846-X

Cover design: Susan Rich

PRINTED IN THE UNITED STATES OF AMERICA

To F.M. Reardon and J.M. Reardon Monro,
colleagues and kin

Contents

Preface

This book is addressed to registered nurses, licensed practical nurses, and nursing attendants who are caring for dying patients. With no power to say who will be part of their case loads, they are required to provide intimate care where and when it is needed. The excitement of the intensive-care unit and the prestige of membership on the life-saving team is not part of their professional lives; they have instead the drudgery of daily care to a bitter end. They are to be commended for the difficult tasks they perform, and it is the authors' hope that the discussion of death juxtaposed with the discussion of organizations will be useful in their daily practice.

We also wish to acknowledge our debts. We are exceedingly grateful to those nursing colleagues who agreed to answer the uncomfortable questions asked by an ivory-tower resident without patient-care responsibilities, and to the patients who were not deceived by tactful avoidance of the subject of dying. Academic colleagues and students discussed the data and worked with them. We wish also to acknowledge the support provided by the St. Louis University School of Nursing and the St. Louis University School of Medicine Cancer Committee.

Families, as always, were supportive; they know what is owed by us to them, and no more need be said. Last mentioned — but not least deserving of gratitude — is Mary Staels, who dealt without dismay with the handwriting of the senior author and the content of the interviews, and typed furiously to meet a publisher's deadline.

Mary Reardon Castles
Ruth Beckmann Murray

Chapter 1

Dying: An Overview of Attitudes

Nursing literature suggests that nurses are willing and able to identify and evaluate the psychological state of the terminal patient and provide support and care based on perception of psychological as well as physiological needs of patients. However, the constraints on nursing time and nurses' behavior imposed by organization policy and health system power hierarchies are not realistically addressed in nursing literature. While the nursing function certainly requires command of psychosocial and managerial as well as technical skills, it is somewhat less than all encompassing. There is no doubt that nurses have responsibilities to and for the dying patient which are not always met, but those responsibilities may not differ greatly from their responsibilities to all patients in their care.

Clinical observations lead to questions about certain statements in the literature related to dying patients. Although authors are likely to stress the strong influence exerted by the institutional structure on the behavior of patients, there is some indication that once a reasonable physical comfort is assured, families and religious beliefs are likely to be more important to the terminal patient than any support the institution is able to provide. This is in agreement with Hinton (1967), who suggests that the institution is most important to the patient when the care is very bad. Complaints expressed by patients in the study on which this book is based generally center on physical needs and not on a desire for closer relationships with the staff—a majority of patients conceive of nursing from the point of view of physical tasks requiring training and motor skills; they do not expect emotional support and reassurance from nurses.

Two general concepts of death behavior can be identified in the social science studies concerned with death. One group of behavioral scientists suggests that the style of dying is inherent in the style of living, and attitudes toward

1

death are based on whatever systems of belief and emotional strengths are brought to the task of dying. The other group presents the institution as being of primary importance to dying patients, with dying behavior based on the quality of the patients' interactions with environmental factors and institutional personnel. These concepts are not mutually exclusive, and may be considered as dominant factors rather than sole conceptual frameworks.

Many authors report studies of attitudes toward dying and the variables related to differences in these attitudes. Healthy respondents perceive death and dying as fearful and not to be discussed. Feelings of guilt and shame are associated with the death of significant others. Regression, anxiety, depression, and finally, acceptance are emotional states likely to be associated with dying. Interactions between the patients and the staff and the effect dying patients have on organizational patterns are also addressed.

The literature is explicit in indicating that terminal patients are likely to fear death, but want information concerning when and how they probably will die. Although a few writers question the therapeutic value of openly discussing death with patients, most authors agree that terminal patients would prefer to have the opportunity to discuss dying and death with institutional personnel and want some kind of personalized supportive relationship from them. Medical and paramedical personnel are described as being unwilling to tell a patient he is dying, and as coping with their own fears of death and dying by developing an impersonal attitude, and evolving strategies to force patients and families into behaviors with which the caretaking staff is comfortable.

Implicit in the literature is the assumption that some ways to die are more appropriate than others; proper behavior is equated with calm, dignity, and lack of fear. Staff expects certain kinds of death behavior which can be identified to some extent: patients should not manifest fear and not be troublesome. They are expected to die properly, that is, to be cheerful and dignified, and to continue to participate to some extent in family and ward life.

Unfortunately, patients may die from diseases considered by doctors and nurses to be uninteresting, and except for the cadre formed by the private physician and the supervisory nursing staff, they are faced with frequent changes in personnel giving care. Roommates are also likely to come and go. Considering the circumstance of job mobility and flexible staffing patterns, impersonal staff attitudes may be safer for the patient than a truncated personal relationship. It is not likely that the average hospital or nursing home is able to provide the kind of extended contact between the patients and personnel which Kübler-Ross (1973) established, or which medical researchers may be able to maintain with the patients they study; however, nursing writers perceive such contact to be necessary for the therapeutic use of the self in nursing. Personnel are not likely to have either the time or the qualifications for such relationships. Also, it is possible that those authors who point out nursing shortcomings in the area of emotional support may be mistaken in attributing the significance they do to the patient-personnel relationship.

Although the literature is unanimous in expecting nurses to provide emotional support to the patient who is dying in an institution, as well as in citing the apparent reluctance of nurses to assume that responsibility, it is less unanimous and not particularly explicit concerning appropriate nurse behaviors. Open communication with terminal patients is presented as a general good, with little discussion of the skills necessary for communicating with a withdrawn or hostile patient, and no apparent consideration of the time demanded for implementing the skills.

Although there is much discussion in nursing literature of the "individual patient care plan" and "nursing the whole person," even cursory observation of the activities on a nursing unit indicates that nursing and medical care are provided to patients at the times and in the ways which meet the requirements of the givers rather than the recipients of the care. The denigrating Parsonian "sick role" is pervasive, and those patients who endeavour to maintain their decision-making powers are labeled as hostile, demanding, and complaining. Their requests for information, particularly for information concerning either the results of, or the possible alternatives to, the prescribed therapies, are met in one of two ways: with blunt statements of physiological "fact," meaningless without further explanation of possible consequences and the willingness to repeat and re-explain; or the patronizing and paralyzing "now don't *you* worry, we are doing the best we can for you." These equally inappropriate responses frequently are to be found when the patient population is one in which cure is no longer expected by personnel.

The study upon which this book is based was designed to identify incongruence of perception between nurses and patients concerning relevant parameters of care when patients are institutionalized. The focus of the book is upon what the *patient* perceives as preferred nurse behaviors, and upon nursing intervention planned around patients' perceptions of patient needs.

The authors explicitly assume that in order for health personnel and patients to establish together an environment in which patients can achieve maximum health potential, the patients' perceptions of what care is needed must be considered equally with the requirements of the therapy and of the system. They espouse a care framework in which the "sick role" gives way to decision making by patients (and/or families), nurses, and doctors, and medical and nursing therapeutic endeavors are negotiated rather than imposed. It is further assumed that nurses are not and need not be qualified to meet all of the needs identified for patients by other health personnel.

Nurses possess professional skills which allow them to do much for patients of which patients are unaware. In the utilization of these professional skills, acceptance of patient perceptions as of equal importance with nurse and physician perceptions of patient needs can only improve both the care given and the nursing image.

People are sent to institutions to die, and while they are dying they are cared for by strangers who are paid to provide the care. This is stressful both for the patients and the caregivers, who must perform difficult, tedious, and poorly rewarded tasks in the institutional setting. Patients and personnel are expected by persons outside the institution to conform to certain amorphous standards of behavior, which institutional and professional constraints prevent them from meeting. Professional rewards are lacking, since these are to be found in acute-care curative settings.

Nurses are frequently confused and guilty because they do not find it possible to behave in expected ways. One facet of the confusion may be related to their ignorance of the power structures of the organization. This book is intended to provide information about organization theory and the requirements of institutional membership which may dispel the confusion and alleviate the guilt. It is a frank polemic, defending nursing from those who attack without knowledge of all relevant data, and suggesting to practicing nurses the need to move into the power structures in institutional settings.

EARLY INSTITUTIONS

Pre-Christian Greek and Roman establishments for the care of the sick were constructed near the sites of waters or woods, which were considered to have curative or therapeutic properties. These places of healing were temples: priest-healers worked under the aegis of the gods, providing an ambiance of peace and support for people who were of enough consequence to the community to be brought to the temples. Common persons who could not afford the temple fees utilized the services of local wise women with a knowledge of healing and lethal herbs when their own family lore was insufficient. The family rather than the community assumed (or did not assume) responsibility for its weaker members.

The advent of Christianity — with its separation of spirit and body and its emphasis on spiritual as opposed to physical needs — gave rise to a set of beliefs regarding the physical body that militated against all but the most cursory attempts at healing. Christian scripture was interpreted in such a way that dissection was forbidden by the Church, so that knowledge of the anatomy and physiology of the human body was lost for many years. While prayer remained a recognized strategy for healing, the healing arts moved from the province of the priesthood into the hands of secular groups that depended mainly on purgatives, bleeding, and miracles for cure. Care of the sick, however, remained a religious duty and became the focus of many religious communities. Under the auspices of various orders, the hospices of Western Europe — initially shelters for wayfarers who could not command a place as a guest in a private home — became shelters for sick wayfarers and finally developed into establishments for the care of the sick poor. These hospices were the earliest and the best of the institutions established by communities to accommodate the human debris of cities. Because contemplation of such a dreary existence was not pleasing to stronger and more fortunate persons, it is not surprising that these institutions were built away from the community and were run as economically as possible — generally for the benefit of the caretakers rather than the inmates. Although a few individuals, out of some feeling for humanity, for the brotherhood of man, or for the fatherhood of God, undertook to work for the good of the institutionalized, it is only in the last decades — when states began to consider the civil rights of conquered groups, of racial minorities, of old people, of prisoners, of children, and of women — that administration of institutions for the benefit of (and in line with the wishes of) the inmates began to be seriously discussed.

Furthermore, aside from the establishment of pesthouses for control of diseases considered dangerous to the community, required institutionalization of the sick did not occur until the tools of modern medicine advanced to a point at which it became immediately obvious (at least to the practitioners) that patients would be better off in institutions than they were at home. Nobody, not even the patients, considered it necessary to administer the institutions for the comfort of the patients, who were expected to be grateful and to cooperate with hospital requirements.

Beginning with the last two decades, however, there appears to be a trend toward closing institutions and developing other means of caring for weak and deviant community members. Orphanages are being replaced by foster homes. Patients having mental and emotional problems are dealt with on an out-patient basis using drugs and/or counseling, and the asylum is a short-term or last-resort strategy for the care of persons diagnosed as mentally ill. Alcatraz is a tourist attraction, and while prisons are still filled to overflowing, there is animated community discussion as to whether crime can be controlled by the institutionalization of captured criminals.

However, if there is a trend to close most institutions, it does not appear to hold for the care of the physically ill. These people continue to be housed in massive and expensive establishments, but for shorter and shorter periods of time. The expense to the community of maintaining a patient in an acute-care hospital is such that therapists are no longer finding it feasible to provide comprehensive care there. When the acute phase of the disease is over, patients are likely to become out-patients. If the disease is such that cure is impossible, and treatment is such that it is not considered appropriate to discharge patients to their homes, people are transferred to institutions that are less expensive to maintain. That is, they finish their dying in a more economical setting.

The fact that over two-thirds of the people dying in the United States are dying in institutions means that the responsibility for the care of such persons rests with institutional personnel rather than families. There is evidence that personnel do not relish the task, and that the following staff behaviors can be observed when patients begin to die (Glaser and Strauss 1968).

1. There is an immediate, pronounced decrease in patient contact by both doctors and nurses, although good physical care is likely to be stressed.

2. Staff tends to reinforce gentle, accepting behavior in dying patients.

3. Staff maintains a detached regard for the event of death if the patients have certain characteristics. For instance, nurses go on with their tasks in the presence of death of the elderly, or of the very poor, or of persons assessed as having lived morally exemplary lives. However, efficiency is likely to suffer when the death involves a child; a successful, middle-aged, middle-class person; or someone considered to be deviant in some way (e.g., suicides, alcoholics, prostitutes, drug abusers).

4. Staff prefers anticipated deaths; routine is likely to break down when sudden or unexpected deaths occur.

There is really very little in medical or nursing curricula related to how to cope with the difficulties of caring for dying patients, although nurses are beginning to develop such literature (Benoliel 1972; Epstein 1975). Also, with more exciting, successful, and equipment-oriented care taking precedence in both education and service facilities, caring for the dying patient is not likely to be rewarded in either medicine or nursing. Finally, *time* to establish supportive relationships with patients is not provided by hospital budgets — even for patients who are not dying. All of this can perhaps be understood in the light of cultural and professional inputs into professional behavior. Almost all writers on the subject hasten to point out that ours is a death-denying, death-defying culture; it is not surprising that staff who are a part of such a culture, and are also educated in professions with an explicit commitment to life, find it difficult to assume responsibility for the care of patients who cannot live.

What do such patients need from their custodians? At a fairly abstract level, there is some agreement as to general needs and how they can be met. Staff can help patients maintain social relationships and contacts, promoting the value of each day's existence. They can support the dignity of the individual by not being embarrassed by or contemptuous of uncontrolled behavior; they can facilitate the dropping of role facades in an effort to support conflict resolution. The mechanics of these interventions are less well described. There is agreement among practitioners that dying patients need frequent contact with healthy others, and need to be allowed to talk about their fears. Permitting this discussion of concerns and needs is time consuming (therefore expensive), possibly stressful to both patients and staff, and requires a fairly explicit personal philosophy of life and death. Those who have no place in their personal and professional thinking for the fact of death do not find it easy to remain with the dying.

THE MEANING OF DEATH

Certainly the meaning of death to both patients and personnel is neither simple nor uniform; in fact, there is no universally shared meaning, although it is conceded that probably there is no such thing as a "natural" death. All men must die, but for any one individual *his* death is an accident and an unjustifiable violation (DeBeavoir 1973).

Historical View

Aries (1974) provides a history of changing attitudes toward death. In the past, from the 10th century onward, literature tells how a person was forewarned that he would soon die, either from doing battle or from injury or illness that could not be treated. Warning came through natural signs or an inner conviction, and the person made no attempt to flee or deny. Knowing that the end was near, the dying person would prepare for death, going through certain rituals, such as lying on his back with his head facing east, spreading his arms to form a cross, or lying with his hands crossed on his breast (the funerary position that comes to us from the 12th century). Certain other tasks were done: sorrow and a few fears were expressed over the end of life; companions and helpers were pardoned and their forgiveness for any unintentional wrongs was sought; God's blessing was asked for close survivors, and prayers to God (asking for forgiveness and life eternal) were said. After his last prayer, the person waited in silence for death. Death was a ritual organized by the dying person himself: he presided over it and knew its protocol. It was a Christian and public ceremony; many of the close survivors would form a procession into the sickroom. Only at the end of the 18th century did physicians begin to complain about the crowd in the sick room causing unhygienic conditions. Children were originally included in the deathbed scene, and the rituals were carried out simply and matter-of-factly, with no great show of emotion. This attitude — in which death was familiar and near, evoking no great fear or awe — offers a contrast to current attitudes in which death is frightful and taboo.

However, the ancients reacted differently. For instance, they feared keeping the dead with them. Ancient funeral cults had as their purpose preventing the dead from returning to disturb the living. In old Rome, no cemeteries were inside the city.

Christians began burying their dead within the churches, or building monks' basilicas near extraurban cemeteries. The motivation was to be buried near the early martyrs and saints, and eventually church and cemetery would be built together. The poor were simply enshrouded and thrown into a ditch several yards wide and deep, which was covered when it was full. Bones were eventually unearthed and used to decorate portions of the church. At this time the destination of the bones was unimportant, as long as they remained near the church. Only later were the dead put into a box: a house of their own.

Attitudes about death began to change, having more dramatic and personal meaning, as shown by art forms and literature. Early Christians felt that believers would be saved on the Day of Judgment, without individual responsibility, and nonbelievers would be abandoned. In about the 12th century, resurrection and separation of the just and the damned were portrayed artistically. In the 13th century, justice was emphasized along with the weighing of souls, with intercession of the Virgin and St. John. By the beginning of the 16th century, each person was thought to have an account book of his good and bad deeds. Humankind believed in an existence after death that did not necessarily continue for eternity, but which was an extension between death and the end of the world. The Christian Last Judgment is linked with the individual on the last day of the world, not at the hour of death.

Later art forms show that the old death-bed rituals were still carried out, but that the Last Judgment had become a part of the deathbed scene. The forces of good and evil battle for the dying man's soul; God watches to see how the man conducts himself during this trial. The man is tested with final temptations that will determine his eternal fate. His deathbed attitude will either erase his sins or wipe out his good deeds.

An increasingly close relationship had formed between death and personal biography by the 15th century, and this persisted until the 19th century. The popular belief was that it was not necessary to take pains to live virtuously, since a good death redeemed everything. But that idea was being refuted by spiritual writers as early as the 17th and 18th centuries, and was finally cast off in the 20th century.

In the Middle Ages, dying was the time when a man reached his greatest awareness and control of self. Now, dying is seen as the time when a person is least aware and least in control.

Art of the 14th to 16th centuries often portrayed death in the form of a mummy, a partly decomposed cadaver. In the 17th century death was portrayed as a skeleton. Today the horror of death is a sign of love of life, but during the Middle Ages death was not seen as horrible but rather as peaceful. The man of the Middle Ages was acutely aware of the brevity of life; death was always present. He loved life and felt no failure. Now, although life is longer, there is an existential pessimism and depression about not accomplishing aspirations. The certainty of death and the frailty of life is little considered.

In Western civilized areas in the first five centuries A. D. graves were often marked, often with a portrait of the dead. Later the dead person was given over to the Church, which watched over his person until the Resurrection, and cemeteries had anonymous graves. In about the 13th to 14th centuries, important persons had their tombs engraved; in later practice use of an effigy reappeared, although this was not a true portrait. Death masks were produced in the 14th century. Funeral art forms became increasingly personal and lifelike until the early 14th century; tombs became monumental in size to preserve identity after death.

Beginning with the 18th century, man in Western societies tended to give death new meaning: he exalted it, dramatized it, thought of it as disquieting and greedy. He was less concerned with his own death, and more concerned with memorials to others. Loss and memory of others inspired new cults of tombs and cemeteries and romantic, rhetorical treatment of death. Death and love became intertwined.

Death came to be seen as a rupture rather than a familiarity — something beautiful, though not desirable. In the 19th century, death, being viewed as a break, was no longer accepted. However, emotion was high (crying, prayers, and gestures) and the sorrow of the survivors was expressed passionately: the idea of death moved people to manifest distress.

Change also came in the relationship between the dying person and his family. Until the 18th century, death was a concern only for the dying person. It was up to each person to express his ideas, feelings, and wishes through his last will and testament. This was not only a statement about disposing of property but also of religious faith, attachments to possessions and people, decisions made to ensure salvation of the soul, and to oblige the church to carry out wishes. The will revealed a distrust of surviving family and even of the church.

In the last half of the 18th century, a change occurred in wills; they were reduced to legal documents similar to those of today (distributing property). This secularization of wills is considered to be one sign of the de-Christianization of society. Mourning became more spontaneous and open, lasted longer, and was demonstrated in specific ceremonies. Survivors accepted the death of another with greater difficulty than in the past. Now the death of a loved one was to be feared more than the death of self.

By the 19th century, burial in churches was unacceptable, and a return to tombs and cemeteries is noted. Public-health ideas also spoke against common graves and having the bones of the dead in areas where the living congregated. The church was reproached for having cared for the souls but not the bodies of the dead. The tombs began to show the survivors' unwillingness to part with the deceased, and an effort to bestow a kind of immortality of stone. Often the person would be buried on family land, so the dead could remain at home. Cemeteries were planned to look like parks so that people could visit their dead and maintain their memories. Cemeteries were again placed in the city.

In the United States, particularly, the 20th century has witnessed a revolution in traditional ideas and feelings. Death — so omnipresent and familiar in the past — disappears, or becomes shameful and forbidden. The beginning lies in a sentiment already expressed: those surrounding the dying person have a tendency to spare him and hide from him the gravity of his condition. Motivation for the lie was the desire to spare the sick person and assume the burden of his ordeal. That sentiment became a different one: to avoid (for society's sake and the sake of the survivors) the disturbance and overly strong emotion caused by death. The idea was that life should always seem happy. Hushing up had begun.

Between 1930 and 1950 this evolution accelerated as the person no longer died at home with the family, but in the hospital, alone.

The person dies in the hospital because it has become the place to receive care that can no longer be given at home. Death in the hospital is no occasion of ritual ceremony over which the dying person presides with his loved ones around. Now death is a technical phenomenon, obtained by cessation of care. The dying person usually loses consciousness, and it is hard to know the real moment of death. No one waits at the bedside for the weeks it may take, and the initiative for care is passed from the family to the doctor and the hospital team who are the masters of death. An acceptable death has become one which is tolerable for the patient. Survivors do not have the right to become emotional, except in private. Funeral rights are modified. The manifestation of too much sorrow is a sign of instability or bad manners. In the family, little emotion is expressed for fear of upsetting the children, and a solitary and shame-ridden mourning is the only recourse. The tomb is no longer visited, especially since cremation has become more popular and ashes are dispersed. Death has replaced sex as the great, forbidden, taboo subject. The mixture of eroticism and death sought after from the 16th to the 18th centuries has reappeared in sadistic literature.

There is, however, a trend pulling in two opposing directions. Private associations as well as churches have cemeteries. The grave digger has become a funeral director or undertaker and manipulation of the dead is a profession. Embalming became known here in the mid-18th century and is now widespread in the United States, although it is almost nonexistent in Europe. Funeral directors advertise themselves as "doctors of grief," aiding mourners to return to normalcy. Death is once again becoming something to talk about: a current preoccupation concerns the desirability of a voluntary decision to die.

The perception of death is affected by the multiplicity of variables that affect the perception of any life event. Age and state of health are relevant, since death is perceived differently if the person is young and well, old and well, young and ill, or old and ill. The body part involved in the terminal illness influences the perception, since different body parts are valued to various degrees. Ethnic, socioeconomic, religious, or philosophical backgrounds, as well as life goals, also affect perceptions of death. In addition perceptions are different if the person is himself facing death, as opposed to facing the death of a loved one or even of an acquaintance.

Psychoanalytic Views

Perhaps the emotion most frequently associated with dying and death is fear. According to psychoanalytic theory, the unconscious cannot conceive of death because there is no direct experience with it. Hence, anxiety or fear about death can be theorized to be no more than a form of separation or castration anxiety (Greenberg 1965). Fear usually exists in relation to something known. No man knows death, so that death anxiety is directly related to feelings of anxiety caused by hurt or desertion (Feder 1965).

Since for the most part man wants to live as long as possible, various mechanisms of adjustment are used to cope with the feelings associated with the idea of death. Denial is a major mechanism for reducing fear of death, but it is difficult to maintain in the face of the sickness or death of contemporaries or personal declining capacities. Rationalization, suppression, regression, and withdrawal may provide a retreat from the source of anxiety, although the threat is not excluded from conscious awareness. Other coping mechanisms that may be utilized to master and resolve these overwhelming feelings (Choron 1964; Jeffers and Verwoerdt 1969) are intellectualization (suppressing feelings while superficially discussing the topic of death); counterphobic measures (such as avoiding fears and ideas of death by dressing or behaving in an inappropriately youthful manner); hyperactivity (frenetic pursuit of a phase of life which promises a sense of past achievement, an opportunity for continued usefulness, or an antidote to despair); life review, reminiscence, and recall of major events and relationships; sublimation (expressing feelings in creative efforts or by helping others); or the conscious acceptance of death (finding meaning and fulfillment in life and viewing death as peace, sleep, and release from suffering).

Societal Views

In stable, well-regulated, tradition-bound societies, customs exist that diminish the fear of death by giving a sense of control or mastery over the manner of dying. The dying person is better able to maintain a sense of self-esteem and purpose, and death is in more powerful hands than those of the doctor. In changing societies which are scientifically oriented, traditional values that served to provide a sense of personal control over events, including the manner of dying, may be lost. Help is sought from others. But when the provision of help is contingent upon the patient's residing in a setting most convenient to the provider, control is lost. Also, scientific medicine and institutions aim at preserving hope that illness and death will somehow be conquered, with the corollary that life has worth only when death is beaten. When it is perceived that death is not beaten this time, the interest of the therapist shifts to subjects more likely to survive, and the self-esteem of the dying individual is injured.

The American view of death has undergone radical change in the last few generations. The Cartesian perception of man as a biological being, subject to fate (including the fate of death), is now less dominant. Twentieth-century man has made himself the center of his own universe. He recognizes dying and death as part of living and sees himself as playing a conscious or unconscious role in his own fate and in his death (Jeffers and Verwoerdt 1969). Death has become secularized. Yet the modern American is not much different in one way from primitive man: he, too, fears death and tries various expedients to drive it away (Kübler-Ross 1973). The current attitude toward death appears to be one of ambivalence, combining awe and attraction; the love of life is combined with self-destructive habits. Contributing to the ambivalence is an urgent need to discuss death, a topic which many people do not know *how* to discuss, especially with an aged or dying person. Talk about death usually results in embarrassment, evasion, or pretense. In a study of attitudes about death, one-third of a sample of 30,000 subjects could not recall from their childhood a single discussion of death; one-third recalled uncomfortable discussions; and only one-third recalled open and easy discussion of death (Schneidman 1971).

Direct experience with death is also less likely during the last few generations In the past, dying occurred in the home; most adolescents had witnessed a death. Today most dying is done ascetically in hospitals, largely out of sight, and under the control of the institution. The physician has replaced the priest as the presiding officer, and the funeral industry rather than the family directs the mourning (Schneidman 1971). Since health-care providers have been reared in the current milieu, their behavior is influenced by the changing social attitudes.

Philosophic and Religious Influences

Religious beliefs strongly influence ideas about dying and death, especially if tenets of the religion are closely observed. However, many officially practicing adherents do not report the same beliefs about death as the religion proclaims officially. In one study, only 24 percent of those who belonged to one of the major American religions (Catholic, Protestant, or Jewish) stated that religion was significant in their attitudes toward death. One-third of the sample found introspection and meditation to be significant in their attitude formation; another third found existentialism to be the most significant guiding philosophy; and 15 percent of all subjects aged 20 to 24 years reported that hallucinogenic or narcotic drugs considerably influenced their beliefs about death. The threat of nuclear warfare had influenced more than half of the respondents in their thinking about death, and reading as well as presentations of the mass media were perceived as least influential. A distinguishing tenet of Christianity is belief in eternal life, yet only 42 percent of the Protestants and 55 percent of the Catholics expressed such as their belief — although 68 percent of the subjects desired that their images survive after them in some way, such as through children or philanthropic, literary, or artistic works (Schneidman 1971).

To the devout Christian, the suffering that accompanies terminal illness may signify God's way of singling out his soul for special honor, or to guide him in strengthening his faith. Yet other Christians, equally devout, may question suffering and death. Beliefs about sin, punishment, and the importance of faith may create fear of being eternally banned from the joys of heaven. For the strict Christian fundamentalist who believes that satanic forces surround him, that Jesus will soon bodily return to earth to proclaim his Kingdom, and that the end of the world is near, death is officially awaited as a step toward entering the Kingdom of God. Christian beliefs vary with region, race, and ethnic background. Even for believers, death is the ultimate and most comprehensive personal loss, the giving up of everything.

There are a growing number of people who do not profess traditional religious convictions; existentialism is probably the most influential of the secular philosophies influencing beliefs about death. Existentialism emphasizes becoming rather than just existing, along with the worth of the individual and his responsibility for shaping the self through the use of personal freedom. In order to be a free individual instead of one of a crowd, the individual must accept solitude, anxiety, grief, and his own death as a part of life. Special value is placed on facing adversity and suffering, because these choices result in personal growth. The specifically human task is to pass from existence, passively received, to being, which evolves through commitment to and acceptance of one's full share of life. For the existentialist, a death is a part of life; facing death provides a sense of freedom, a growth opportunity, to be and become. The existentialist chooses to be rather than to have, and will be open to suffering and death, just as he is open to love and life. To such a believer, lack of commitment means refusal to use the freedom to make a choice, to become involved with life, and in fact to live a life of meaningless conformity. For the uncommitted, death brings despair, for he is dying and he has not yet lived. Material wealth, social prestige, knowledge, and accomplishments used as shields from the realities of existence — joy, sorrow, love, dread, death — bring no real security. The dying person *has* nothing, he tenuously *is*. What he has been, and is, can sustain him. If his life has been inauthentic, death comes too soon, and he realizes too late that he remains responsible for shaping his own being until the very minute of death (Marcel 1949; Vaillot 1966).

The existentialist (Assell 1969) may subscribe to any one of the religions, or to no religion at all. Whether he is an atheist or a Christian will also influence how he views life and death. To the atheistic existentialist, man is nothing until he is born and has defined himself through his living. Life is seen as final and ultimate, hence death is final and removes all meaning from life. Death is a tragedy, an unjust affront, an emptiness and a loneliness. The mourning process which gives a mode of expression when a loved one dies also gives a mode to contemplate and mourn vicariously the death of the self. The Christian existentialist views being and living as two separate entities; man *is* before he can *live.* His being is in jeopardy from the moment life begins, but because he believes God exists he is convinced that through faith, social responsibility, and living to the fullest in this life he can be saved for another life. Death is not annihilation, but completion of life and a sign of hope of the future eternal life to be enjoyed. While the hope is real, equally real is the fear of the unknown, opening him to the realities of life and death. Whether the beliefs about death arise from a religious or a secular cognition, their intensity may be attenuated by the imminence of death, and fear of death occurs in believers and unbelievers alike.

The Influence of Age

In youth, death seems far away; by the middle years it has become more personal through the deaths of parents, friends, and siblings. The elderly may be likely to consider death daily, as exemplified in one study of 54 institutionalized and bedridden women, aged 65 to 85 years: 80 percent anticipated and hoped for death within five years (Davis 1972). Death takes on a different meaning at different life stages. The child, the adolescent, the adult, the aged—each perceives death differently, owing to differing abilities to conceptualize, differing expectations of self, and differing life experiences (Feifel 1959).

CHILDHOOD

Nagy (1959) identifies three stages in the child's concept of death: death is reversible, death is personified, and death is final and inevitable. The child under five years of age perceives death as separation, a temporary departure, like sleep, reversible; he conceives of the dead as being very still, less alive, unable to move. Death is disturbing to him because it separates people from each other and because life in the grave seems dull and unpleasant. The preschooler connects funerals, cemeteries, and absence. He thinks dead people still to be capable of growth, that they breathe, eat, feel, and that they know what is happening on earth. Because of his fantasy he tends to experience fear and guilt and make unlikely associations in the presence of death.

The child aged five to nine accepts death as final and unlifelike. He personifies death and conceives of an angel, a clown, a ghost, or a bogeyman who carries off people, especially bad people. He thinks death can be avoided by running fast, locking the door, hiding, or being very good. Death is feared, particularly if the child is threatened by his parents with punishment or if he experiences traumatic events (Nagy 1959).

The fatally ill child aged six to ten years appears to be aware of the seriousness of his illness, even though he may not be capable of talking about this awareness in adult terms. The child with a fatal illness shows preoccupation with threats to bodily integrity and functioning; he knows of his approaching death even when adults attempt to hide this from him (Spinetta 1973; Waechter 1971)

After the age of nine or ten, children begin to engage in conceptual thinking and can understand death in a more abstract sense (Nagy 1959). Death is realized as inevitable, final, and happening according to certain laws; the child begins to perceive that it will one day happen to him. Death is understood as the ending of life, like the withering of flowers or the falling of leaves, and as resulting from internal processes. It is associated with being in a coffin and being buried and slowly eaten by bugs or slowly rotting (unless information about cremation has been available). Children may express ideas about an afterlife.

However, as Dunton (1970) points out, not all children fit precisely into these descriptions, and some adults may continue to perceive death at a childlike level. The child's ideas and anxiety about separation and death and his ability to handle loss are influenced by many factors: parental reactions, situations of sibling rivalry, violence, loss, illness or death in the family, the behavior and teaching of significant adults, and his ability to conceptualize and assimilate the experience. By the time the child has reached preadolescence and learned to care for another as much as he cares for himself, he is capable of grief in the adult sense.

A study of midwestern children aged 5 to 18 years attending church schools and health clinics revealed somewhat different findings from Nagy's study (McIntire et al. 1972). By age 13 to 16, 20 percent of the subjects still thought that they would be cognizant when dead; 60 percent envisioned spiritual continuation; 20 percent saw death as total cessation. Those with frequent thoughts of suicide often denied death as final. Increasing age and religious training apparently resulted in a view of the significance of life beyond simple existence.

Evans (1971) reports that the death of parents during prepubertal years may cause great trauma in children who may perceive this event as deliberate abandonment caused by angry childish wishes for their death. Children fear personal death as retribution, or perceive it as contagious, and therefore avoid the body of the dead parent, or avoid a friend whose parent has just died. If death is perceived as sleep, sleep may be feared to the point of insomnia. Surviving parents or other family members are blamed for the parent's death, and this feeling is compounded when the surviving adults are so absorbed in their own grief that little attention is given to the children. Urgent wishing is somehow expected to bring about the return of the dead parent.

ADOLESCENCE

The adolescent is concerned about his future and because he is capable of conceptual and logical thinking he can understand death intellectually. However, his dependency–independency conflicts with parents and his efforts to establish his individuality result in a low emotional tolerance for death. He is not likely to think of death, at least not as something that will happen to him. Death happens to old people. If a young friend or his parents die, he feels acute loss; such a death means lack of fulfillment. He may inwardly grieve intensely, yet outwardly continue as usual. He may vigorously pursue studies or other activities, or withdraw and drop all of his previous interests. Mastery of feelings sometimes comes through such activities, or through a detailed accounting of the parent's death to a peer or interested adult, or through displacement of grief feelings upon a pet. The adolescent may fantasize the dead parent as perfect, or feel responsible for the parent's death, much as a child would (Evans 1971; Kastenbaum 1972).

MATURITY

In one of the earliest of the current discussions of dying (Feifel 1959), adult perceptions of death are identified. For the adult, fear of death is often more related to the process of dying than to the fact of death — to the mutilation and threat to body-image, pain, isolation, loss of control, fear of the unknown, and permanent collapse. Occasionally, death is seen as an adventure, as a way to punish others, to force others to give more affection than they were willing to give in the past. Premonitions, sometimes accurate, may occur about the coming death. Among adults in one survey (Schneidman 1971), death meant eternal loss of consciousness, the end of experiencing, the end of physical, mental, or spiritual existence. The older the subject, the less likely he was to be convinced that life after death existed, although he hoped for it very much. Respondents under 20 years of age were more likely to believe in heaven and hell. The greatest fear of death was expressed by subjects aged 25 to 29 years. Children under 12 were also very fearful of death, at least in the perceptions of their mothers. Two-thirds of the sample wished to die in old age; half of those who wanted to die at a younger age expressed feelings of depression. At any age, depression is related to preoccupation with death. Often the depressed person, unsuccessful at establishing supportive interpersonal relationships, will turn his thoughts to a dead person or commit suicide to reestablish a relationship with a significant person who is dead (Greenberg 1965).

Maturity demands integration of the idea of personal death, and recognition that dying and death are not separate, distinct states of being but phases of living and life. It demands recognition of limits: the perception of death as a necessary condition of life. The capacity to grasp the concept of a future and inevitable death may play a part in the determination of present behavior (Choron 1964; Feifel 1959, 1965; Jeffers and Verwoerdt 1969).

OLD AGE

The older person must either make some kind of adjustment to the approach of death or build up defenses which shield him from the awareness that he, too, must die. Death seems more frightening to people in general than to older persons, and fear of death is more common in older persons who do not report religious preferences, who score lower on intelligence-quotient (IQ) tests, who have experienced rejection in the past, or who are depressed. Generally, the elderly report they fear death less than they fear prolonged illness, dependence, incapacitation, or pain — all of which bring threats of rejection, isolation, and loss of social role, self-determination, and dignity. Some elderly persons look forward to death as a reunion with loved ones, or welcome it because they have already become socially dead in their own and others' eyes (Jeffers and Verwoerdt 1969). The progression through old age that precedes even a painless death may include much suffering. Society's attitude toward the aged and the dying may distress individuals whose functional capacities are declining with age; too, the treatment of younger persons who are dying is frequently not very different from the treatment of aging persons. To age, to decline, and to die are apparently synonymous.

Individual variations in adaptive behavior are greater among the elderly than in other age groups because of their longevity and breadth of life experience. Certain coping techniques may be adaptive for one person and maladaptive for another. Determinants of adjustment include: (1) previous patterns of coping with change and crisis; (2) chronological age and probable distance from death; (3) physical and psychological health and energy levels; (4) religious, socio-economic, and occupational experiences; (5) personal and family attitudes toward, and experiences with, death; (6) emotional commitments to significant others; (7) opportunities to talk about death with an attentive listener; and (8) community attitudes toward the aged and the dying (Jeffers and Verwoerdt 1969).

The Influence of Health

PERSONS IN HEALTH

No doubt all healthy persons who have formed close relationships think of the eventual death of parents, siblings, spouses, children, other relatives, and friends. Probably most contemplate death at some time, briefly, intermittently, or even frequently. Some may try to imagine what it would be like to be terminally ill. The well person may be able to speak calmly about personal death, although his reactions when actually faced with death may differ considerably from his earlier calm considerations. In one sample of 95 healthy subjects, intellectualization was the main mechanism used in thinking about death, and comfort while dying was sought from religion. When asked how they would spend their remaining lives if they had only six months to live, the majority wanted to create or accomplish something useful. Their death was not imminent; their answers were other-directed rather than self-serving (Feifel 1967). To most people in good health, even those who hold most tenaciously to religious beliefs in an afterlife, death is an enemy, representing a wall, a personal disaster, dependency, pain, and loss of consciousness. For some, the manner of dying rather than the actual death is perceived as most important. Death may be challenged by suicides or by the person who expresses omnipotence through involvement in an ideological movement: one triumphs over death by giving up his life when and how he chooses, and meaning is given to the death by the meaningfulness of the cause (Feifel 1965; Jeffers and Verwoerdt 1969). Age and sex are related to willingness to sacrifice; people under 20 years of age are more likely to report willingness to sacrifice their lives for an idea or a moral principle than older adults, and men more likely than women.

The healthy adult also tries to transcend and conquer death through belief in personal or social–historical immortality. He may believe that after death he goes to another world where his body and soul will live on forever. Or he may consider that while he is personally mortal, humanity is not, although in the age of possible nuclear holocaust that belief must be harder to maintain (Choron 1964; Feifel 1965).

PERSONS WITH CHRONIC ILLNESS

Advanced medical technology has given another chance for life to many people who were at one point critically ill or near death. Uncertainty about life and death is particularly felt by patients with cancer or heart disease who have received treatment and gained remission or recovery, but are not actually cured of the disease. Davis (1966) calls these people "patients in limbo." They live with the death sentence of cancer or a failed heart for an unpredictable number of years, assimilating the prognosis into their way of life. Life is prolonged, but it is different from life before the occurrence of the disease.

Certain behaviors are typical of persons who face sure death from a disease, but at an extended future date. They talk with ease and knowledge about the disease and its course, relating events sequentially as if they can be better integrated when they fit into a pattern. Time is structured around the disease: short hospitalizations, visits to the doctor, and reviews of subtle changes in symptoms. These patients are experienced interpreters of symptoms in relation to favorable or unfavorable progress. They tend to live from day to day, often with feelings of mild depression and loss of control, holding on to time and bidding for more of it, always considering the probability of a new drug or treatment. A gradual social withdrawal occurs, particularly for those persons with a diagnosis of cancer, for former friends frequently express fear of catching the disease or fail to offer needed support. Friends expect the patient to look deathlike, to be in constant pain, or to be unable to perform ordinary tasks or enjoy ordinary pleasures. These patients, therefore, are likely to conceal evidence of the disease from others in order to avoid their withdrawal or rejection. In spite of efforts to fight the disease and its effects, some incapacity results that necessitates role changes and altered social relationships both in the home with the family and at work. Eventually, work must be relinquished (Choron 1964; Davis 1966; Dovenmuehle 1965).

Patients with chronic diseases pick up the concern expressed by the medical team about the effectiveness of present treatment procedures, but they are not likely to receive much support from the team (especially from the foremost member, the doctor) in dealing with concerns about the future. The doctor tries to maintain the patient's optimism while encouraging him to avoid anxiety-tinged topics such as the illness, his eventual death, and his feelings of hopelessness and depression. The doctor simultaneously ignores his own and the patient's feelings. When the patient has no opportunity to express and handle his feelings, he is denied a chance fully to understand the problems, to integrate the concept of his vulnerability into his self-concept, and to work through the meaning of his death. Help with this derivation of meaning is likely to come from religion or from a significant family member rather than be part of the medical therapeutic effort (Davis 1966; Dovenmuehle 1965).

PERSONS WITH CRITICAL ILLNESS

Although the dying person drifts into and out of consciousness, he continues to live until the moment he dies. He continues to think and to feel — about the present, the future, and the past. He enumerates those who visit and those who do not. Sometimes he is accepting of his fate; sometimes he refuses the prognosis and cries "unfair!" He grieves; he pretends; he feels fright and despair. He may also know love, satisfaction, and enjoyment of what is until he no longer thinks or knows. His main concern while he can report concerns is not with death but with loss of control, separation, and pain in life. The early need to control the distressing events associated with the terminal illness gives way to the knowledge that control is not possible. As devastating loss becomes clear, hopelessness, despair, and intense grief follow as it becomes necessary for the dying person to accept that this pain is a part of life, even if he does not wish it to be so (Sobel 1974).

Those who face imminent death in a natural catastrophe or accident may experience death differently than those who linger in pain. Thoughts and feelings of beauty, sentiment, review of past life may be experienced in rapid sequence; pleasant illusions may crowd out the horror of the reality until unconsciousness occurs. If the person is in considerable pain, he apparently does not experience fear and dies willingly (Choron 1964).

In one comparison of attitudes toward death between healthy subjects and terminally ill subjects aware of their approaching death, more denial and avoidance of death topics was expressed by the dying group. The ill persons showed a fluctuating variety of behaviors: avoidance, anxious hope, hostility, uneasy resignation, panic, and calm acceptance. Belief in religion and an afterlife was strong. They expressed a wish to preserve body integrity and wholeness, to die nonviolently, quietly, with dignity, and preferably suddenly in such a manner as not to know death was occurring. These same wishes were expressed by healthy adults (Schneidman 1971). Fears of rejection, separation, and of the unknown were common, and feelings of loss regarding family, loved ones, and gratifications of life were expressed. Yet some attitudinal differences existed within the sample. Younger patients and patients with young children were more angry about, and rejecting of, death than older patients; they felt they had more to lose. Persons who had known of their impending deaths for six months or longer expressed less fear than those who had just learned their prognosis. A comparison of 52 subjects who knew they had an illness from which they *could* die with 40 subjects who knew they *would* die revealed more denial, more suicidal thoughts, and greater desire to be at home with their families in the latter group. The disease diagnosis and the proximity of death apparently influences attitudes toward death: a comparison of 38 patients with a diagnosis of cancer with 38 patients with a diagnosis of heart disease showed the cancer patients to be more conscious of the proximity of death and more accepting of personal death (Feifel 1967). The literature indicates that the diagnosis of cancer has many meanings: a death warrant, abandonment, separation, aloneness, punishment, silence, helplessness, pain, and destruction.

When asked how they would like to spend their lives if they had only six more months to live, critically ill patients expressed desires to travel, to spend time with their families, or to continue as usual. All wanted to live as fully as possible, to make peace with themselves and their Creator, and to help others if possible. The investigators suggest that travel may represent to them an effort to arrest time's passage and blunt death's threat by taking in life in huge swallows. Being with families or continuing to act as usual may represent a desire to hold onto life, taking refuge in the security of familiar things (Feifel 1959, 1965, 1967).

A pervasive issue is whether or not to tell the patient he is dying. Often diagnosis and prognosis are seen as a single entity by the doctors. The medical profession, the patient, and the family can acknowledge the diagnosis and the possibility of death. The patient and family may either deny or accept the implications as expressed in the prognosis, whichever fits their needs at the time, and may manifest frequent changes in the denial or acceptance of the prognosis from time to time. In one study, 82 percent of the patients studied stated they wanted to be informed of a terminal diagnosis; they believed they had a right to know about their own lives and to experience fully their own deaths, to settle financial and family affairs, to prepare themselves emotionally and spiritually for the end, and to spend the remaining time as they wished. They felt that knowing the diagnosis and the prognosis would help them to be more cooperative with the treatment (Feifel 1965, 1967). Incidentally, these same reasons were given by healthy persons who also affirmed they would like to be told if the illness were fatal. However, no group studied wanted to be informed of a specific date of death (Schneidman 1971).

In another sample of 105 patients with advanced malignancies who attended a clinic for treatment, Feder (1965) found that nearly all knew of their actual diagnosis, although they had been given false diagnoses by the staff. There was never complete denial of the progressive illness, the wasting, and the dying of the body, and depression was present to various degrees. The greatest fears expressed by these patients were of progressive isolation, aloneness, and being unloved and helpless. Although any cancer is a threat to the body-image because of its progressive destruction, those with more obvious effects of the disease expressed less threat. Apparently when the cancer is in view, it can be better observed, more carefully followed, and the patient feels some mastery in the situation. Depression and threat to body-image was greater when patients had had surgery or received drugs with defeminizing or emasculating effects.

Awareness of impending death was found in a study (Choron 1964) of 30 patients ranging in age from 24 to 74 years who were hospitalized for a fatal illness. A relationship existed between awareness and actual temporal distance to death, as well as hopelessness and decreased expectation of the future, although none of the patients could know exactly how long they still had to live. However, there is some evidence that patients may be subjectively aware of the rate of decline in physical status; by monitoring internal changes, they may be able to estimate the rate of decline from the present to the terminal point.

When an individual dies, his family and friends suffer a loss roughly in proportion to the quantity and quality of their relationships with him. The individual, however, is losing relatives, friends, and all significant others. His anticipatory loss should be equal to the sum of the anticipatory losses of those significant to him. The greater the number of significant others and the closer his relationships with them, the greater the feeling of loss and grief he must experience. Response to this suffering depends primarily upon earlier patterns of behavior in response to stress and the personality resources which should increase his tolerance to stress, although loss of these resources also causes stress (Aldrich 1963). As an individual's illness continues, he becomes more self-concerned and less interested in others. The significance of others to him is gradually reduced, so the anticipated loss is gradually reduced. The retraction of ego boundaries may continue to the point at which the patient no longer needs to deny or be depressed; he can then become more accepting of death.

THE MEANING OF DEATH TO THE FAMILY

Grieving for a family member often begins with the diagnosis of the terminal illness, although for a time family members are likely to keep hoping that the diagnosis is wrong. Or family members may initially deny the diagnosis and its impact as vigorously as does the patient. As the illness progresses in severity, its effect becomes intensely felt by the family, and the feelings expressed by the patient are likely to be expressed by the family as well. When the contributions of one member fail because of illness, other family members must take on the extra burdens and responsibilities. Constant adjustments and readjustments must be made, often before the family is ready to make them. Medical bills are often staggering, and so is the emotional drain. Feelings of helplessness, and often of guilt, are intense as the family relates to and tries to care for the ill member. The healthy parent may be distressed by his childrens' reactions to the approaching death of the other parent, which they manifest by changing personality, displaying detrimental habits, or attempting to escape through unusual activities, withdrawal from family relationships, or poor academic progress (Burnside 1971).

Yet the family can be inspired by the courage, sense of humor, or dignity of the dying individual as he bears the indignities of his disease, and feel thankful for the strength he manifests. At a time when the dying member is deteriorating, the family needs support and help from others; the lack of acceptance of the prognosis and talk about a miraculous recovery from well-meaning friends can be distressing. Emotions are close to the surface, and it is hard to remain stoic or composed in the presence of the dying individual or other family members. Death is sensitizing in that kindness and cruelty from others are more intensely experienced. A song or a phrase reminding the family of happier times and of what is being lost can trigger a flood of feelings that are difficult to control (Burnside 1971).

However, social death may occur before physical death, and the family may finish their grief work before the patient dies. When this happens to the families of institutionalized patients, visits and involvement taper off; family members reinvest their energies in each other, to the detriment of the dying member. At this point, the nurse may become the most significant person for the dying patient (Glaser and Strauss 1964). Several conditions may prompt a premature farewell between the patient and his family: distress in the family caused by seeing the suffering of the dying member, because the family prefers to remember the dying person as he was in health; realization by the patient that the family is distressed so that he withdraws to spare them suffering; and rejection by the family because the patient's overt behavior or slowly approaching death makes them uncomfortable (The living death syndrome, Newsweek, 1972).

THE MEANING OF DEATH TO THE CAREGIVERS

Health-care workers deal daily with dying patients. Much of what has been presented concerning the influence of various factors on the meaning of death in

American society applies to any individual worker. By virtue of the educational process — somewhere between entry as a student into a health profession and the practice of that profession — subtle changes occur in attitudes concerning dying and reactions to death.

Exposure to death may occur for the first time as one is a student and the experience may be overwhelming, depending upon the kind of support given by supervisors. All too frequently students are taught what to do in the event of death, but are given no opportunity to express their feelings, or to think about and talk about the feelings generated by the death experience. Because of the trauma commonly associated with this experience, death becomes a dark symbol, a stigma, an obscenity to be avoided (Feifel 1965; Phillips 1972).

There is some evidence to suggest that among the motivations for entering the medical profession is the fear of death and the need to control it. Similar data are not reported for nurses, but one can speculate that it is possible to obtain dominion over death anxieties by having the power to extend care as well as the power to cure. Doctors spend less time than the average person thinking about death; even doctors who study dying and death may be swamped by anxieties about dying, having either an antipathy for or an overidentification with certain kinds of patients. Doctors may have a sense of triumph about outliving some patients and a sense of guilt about the inability to help others. Overintellectualization is common, with physicians refusing to address any but the least emotionally tinged dimensions of what is happening. It has been pointed out (Greene 1974) that doctors doing studies on death and dying are generally those who are least likely to be providing therapy to dying patients. Whether these findings can be generalized to nurses is not yet clearly established; they operate in the same clinical arena and are exposed to the same stresses, but they do not exercise the same control. The practicing physician frequently refuses to admit his patients into a study on personal reactions to death, saying that it is too traumatic for them. Indeed, many doctors do not even want their patients to be informed that they are terminally ill. However, most patients report they have no objections to answering questions and prefer plain, honest answers to questions about their illness — including the information that the illness is terminal — and welcome the opportunity to talk about the impending separation (Feifel 1965). The feelings and reactions of doctors and nurses are usually sensed by patients; nonverbal communications speak loudly. Patients may become anxious and frightened by the grave, serious demeanor, the unspoken words, the avoidance, the lack of specific information about test results. Anger is generated by the enforced dependent role and the lack of opportunity to be involved in the decision-making about treatment.

One study of personnel working at a cancer research center (Greenberg 1965) revealed some interesting coping behaviors. The doctors formed a closely knit group, excluding nursing and other personnel. Their feelings of anger and helplessness about cancer and its effects were frequently displaced by active participation in games; they were enthusiastic players of golf, squash, and handball. They would compare cancer to heart disease when talking with patients. They avoided questions about death from both patients and nurses. The nurses coped in several ways: withdrawing from the patients, seeking consolation from their own families, and changing jobs. They referred patients' questions about their progress to the doctors; as the doctors did not answer such questions, no doubt the patients learned to obtain information in less explicit ways.

However, there is little malice in personnel who treat patients as objects; it is merely an attempt to defend against their own anxieties about death. The behavior may be more subtle in the professional groups than in the nonprofessionals, who have been reported to manifest cheerful, joking, superficial charm; a monotonous verbal banter; an uncaring friendliness; and a cute youthfulness (Private correspondence, 1972), but it is surely equally distressing for patients.

When nurses have not resolved personal feelings about dying and death, various defense mechanisms are used, resulting in distancing behaviors that can add to the distress of dying patients. These behaviors include: (1) the use of technical language that denies understandable communication to the patient and the family; (2) the use of social language, such as comments about the weather or the flowers in the room, which inhibit the patient from talking about his illness or his feelings; (3) the use of the doctors' authority to make it possible to ignore or dodge the questions or comments of the patient; (4) the use of treatment equipment such as oxygen masks, hypodermic syringes, and medications to focus on technical, ritualized activities rather than on the patient's feelings; (5) the development of an impersonal attitude manifested by referring to the patient as a case, a disease, or a room number; and (6) the use of sedation to reduce the patient's level of activity and communication. Using these mechanisms, nurses may feel more secure or even capable of facing death. The patient, however, is not deceived; he senses the superficiality of the behavior and withdraws to deal with his problems as best he may, alone (Kneisel 1968; Phillips 1972).

It is evident (Sobel 1974) that, in spite of the difficulties, working with dying patients may deepen personal insights and maturity in the caregiver, instill acceptance of what is painful in life, lessen the desire to control all that is painful, and strengthen the courage needed to stay with the dying patient while coping with personal anxieties, guilt, and despair. The caregiver *can* learn to drop pretenses and be able to do nothing but give of the self when that is what needs to be done.

When patients die, nurses may feel loss and grieve, although the professional ideal is still one of calm and composure. The loss felt by nurses for patients may be of three types: (1) personal loss, occurring if the nurse was involved emotionally with the patient and really cared, if there was strong transference and countertransference in the relationship, or if the patient was a personal friend or of a similar age; (2) professional loss, occurring if the nurse gave care frequently to the patient, or fought hard to save his life; and (3) social loss, occurring if the patient had characteristics highly valued by society. Characteristics of social value include beauty, youth, correct skin color, education, certain occupations and social classes, accomplishments, and specific personality traits. Each patient embodies these characteristics to some degree. The total of valued social characteristics indicates the amount of loss to the nurse, the family, and to society at large. Because social values are reflected in personal value systems, nurses react to the social loss of the patients in spite of having been taught that all patients must be cared for with equal commitment and competence. Equality of care is required; equality of grieving is not. Society (hence nurses) grieves more intensely when the dying person is young than when he is old. Living a full life has a high value, so a dying child is perceived as being robbed of the chance to live. The dying young adult or middle-aged person is missed because of his dependents and because he still has many contributions to make. Patients with the characteristics noted above — with their attendant charisma — may receive more than routine care and be grieved more intensely by staff. There is no doubt that some deaths can be rationalized more easily by nurses, thereby reducing guilt and grief feelings. Examples of patients whose death is more readily accepted by staff are: suicides, because these individuals can be considered to get what they asked for and deserve; criminals who are considered to be threatening or merely useless; patients with intense pain, or those who are incurably ill and are considered to be released from suffering; patients with damaged brains or permanent defects and who can no longer lead normal or useful lives; and aged patients who are considered to have lived a full life (Glaser and Strauss 1964). It is harder to rationalize death caused by an accident or caused by an unanticipated medical or surgical complication, or to rationalize the death of a patient who has truly become a significant other by long residence on the nursing division; these deaths take on a different meaning than those previously described.

Theological and philosophical positions state that all men fear death, although the unconscious is described as unable to accept the reality of death of self. Contradictory or ambivalent views about the meaning of death are apparently held simultaneously. Death is perceived as the end of life, or the beginning of eternal life; as an avenue of escape from certain problems, or the beginning of uncertainty and dread, as a final separation from loved ones, or a lasting reunion; as an instinctual wish, or an instinctual terror; as the attainment by man of ultimate harmony with nature, or the defeat of man by nature (Knutson 1970).

However it is perceived, the common bond among all mankind is the reality of the event of death. The impact of that event will be felt more than once, in more than one role, and with different intensities. Death is the last developmental stage, a goal, a fulfillment. Dying has an onset long before the actual death. How one faces death in others and what meaning is ascribed to it are influenced by culture, philosophy, religion, age, state of health, and distance from and relationship to the dying individual. Those persons whose vocation is the care of the sick must deal with the meaning of death both as individuals who will die and as members of the health-care disciplines with the responsibility of caring for the sick until they die, and extending that care in support of grieved families.

References

Aldrich C: The dying patient's grief. JAMA 184 (5):329, 1963
Anon: The living death syndrome. Nursing '72 2(8):13, 1972
Anon: Notes of a dying professor. Nurs Outlook 20 (8):502, 1972

Aries P: Western Attitudes Toward Death. Baltimore, Johns Hopkins University Press, 1974

Assell R: An existential approach to death. Nurs Forum 7 (2):200, 1969

Benoliel JQ: Nursing care for the terminal patient: a psychosocial approach. In Schoenberg B, Carr A, Peretz D, Kutscher A (eds), Psychosocial Aspects of Terminal Care. New York, Columbia University Press, 1972

Burnside I: You will cope, of course. Am J Nurs 71 (12):2354, 1971

Choron J: Modern Man and Mortality. New York, Macmillan, 1964

Davis B: Until death ensues. Nurs Clin North Am 7 (2):303, 1972

Davis M: Patients in limbo. Am J Nurs 66 (4):764, 1966

DeBeauvoir S: A Very Easy Death, New York, Warner, 1973

Dovenmuehle R: Affective response to life-threatening cardiovascular disease. In Group for Advancement of Psychiatry (eds), Death and Dying: Attitudes of Patient and Doctor. New York, Mental Health Center Materials, 1965, vol. 5, Symposium 11

Dunton HD: The child's concept of death. In Schoenberg B, Carr A, Peretz D, and Kutscher A (eds), Loss and Grief. New York, Columbia University Press, 1970

Epstein C: Nursing the Dying Patient. Reston, Va, Reston Publishing, 1975

Evans F: Psychosocial Nursing: Theory and Practice in Hospital and Community Mental Health. New York, Macmillan, 1971

Feder S: Attitudes of patients with advanced malignancy. In Group for Advancement of Psychiatry (eds), Death and Dying: Attitudes of Patient and Doctor. New York, Mental Health Materials Center, 1965, vol. 5, Symposium 11

Feifel H (ed): The Meaning of Death. New York, McGraw-Hill, 1959

Feifel H: Attitudes of the critically ill toward death and dying. Geriatric Focus 6 (5):1, 1967

———: The function of attitudes toward death. In Group for the Advancement of Psychiatry (eds), Death and Dying: Attitudes of Patient and Doctor. New York, Mental Health Materials Center, 1965, vol. 5, Symposium 11

Glaser B, Strauss A: The social loss of dying patients. Am J Nurs 64 (6):119, 1964

———: Time for Dying. Chicago, Aldine, 1968

Greenberg I: Studies of attitudes toward death. In Group for Advancement of Psychiatry (eds), Death and Dying: Attitudes of Patient and Doctor. New York, Mental Health Materials Center, 1965, vol. 5, Symposium 11

Greene WA: The physician and his dying patient. In Troup S, Greene W (eds), The Patient, Death and the Family. New York, Scribners, 1974

Hinton J: Dying. Baltimore, Penguin, 1967

Jeffers F, Verwoerdt A: How the old face death. In Busse E, Pfeiffer E (eds), Behavior and Adaptation in Late Life. Boston, Little, Brown, 1969

Kastenbaum R: The kingdom where nobody dies. Saturday Review: Science 55 (52):33, 1972

Kneisl C: Thoughtful care of the dying. Am J Nurs 68 (3):550, 1968

Knutson A: Cultural beliefs on life and death. In Brim O, Freeman H, Levine S, Scotch N (eds), The Dying Patient. New York, Russell Sage, 1970

Kübler-Ross E: On Death and Dying. New York, Macmillan, 1973

Marcel G: The Philosophy of Excellence (translated by Manya Harai). New York, Philosophical Library, 1949

McIntire M, Angle C, Struempler, L: The concept of death in midwestern children and youth. Am J Dis Child 123:527, 1972

Nagy M: The child's view of death. In Feifel H (ed), The Meaning of Death. New York, McGraw-Hill, 1959

Phillips DF: The hospital and the dying patient. Hospitals 46 (4):68, 1972

Schneidman E: You and death. Psychol Today 5 (6):43, 1971

Sobel D: Death and dying. Am J Nurs 74 (1):98, 1974

Spinetta J: Anxiety in the dying child. Pediatrics 52 (12):841, 1973

Vaillot, Sister Madeleine: Existentialism: a philosophy of commitment. Am J Nurs 66 (3):500, 1966

Waechter E: Children's awareness of fatal illness. Am J Nurs 71 (6):1168, 1971

Chapter 2

Institutions: An Introduction to Organizational Structure

The affecting death scenes described by early novelists — the dying individual resting in the bosom of his family — took place in upper- and middle-class extended families, who had enough space to house the invalid and enough money to hire necessary helpers to come into the home and aid with the more unpleasant aspects of the sick room. The poor may very well have done their dying surrounded by whatever amenities were provided by the poorhouse.

Studies of patients with terminal illness suggest that almost without exception they wish to die at home, in familiar surroundings, in the presence of their families. This wish may not be shared by the families; Elder (1973) has pointed out that institutionalization of the critically ill family member relieves the family of unpleasant tasks and responsibilities and minimizes the extent to which death interrupts the structure of everyday life. Also, because sick adults express a wish to die without pain and in a way which is least inconvenient for their families, they acquiesce to the transfer of their care from the home to the institution.

Since it is necessary to incorporate the process of dying and the crisis of death into an institutional routine, it is unrealistic to believe that life in a regulated setting among strangers will be the same as life within the family group. It is equally unrealistic to assume that all personnel are alike, any more than all family members are alike. It is also inappropriate to blame the fact of institutionalization, or an entity called "the institution," for all of the sorrow surrounding dying. Separation, grief, fear, loss, and pain will be experienced by the individual no matter where he dies, and the evidence of the effect of either family or staff activities on these feelings is subjective at best. Everyone experiences the event of death alone. One can wonder if those persons who complain of the behavior of staff would complain as bitterly about the behavior of family and friends if the ill individual were being cared for at home. However, there is no doubt that even with the constraints imposed by organizational requirements, care of patients dying in an institution can and should be improved.

In most nursing units, basic physical nursing tasks are carried out by licensed practical nurses and nursing assistants. In effect, professional nurses become managers who accomplish their functions through other persons. Head nurses, and perhaps team leaders, have been considered first-level managers: in fact, unless she is doing private duty, any registered nurse must develop managerial skills in order to carry out her nursing functions. Whether or not this is an ideal situation, it exists, and nurses who must assume this role in spite of their preferences require information about the concepts of management. They are frequently forced into situations which violate primary canons of management; some knowledge of these canons can support refusal to meet impossible demands. This section, therefore, focuses on the history, development, and current status of those organization and management theories which have particular relevance to nursing.

The study of organization has a long history; the beginnings are lost in time, but certainly must have occurred when the family grew into the tribe, necessitating some division of tasks among chieftains, counselors, medicine men, priests, and war leaders. Equally certainly, the interaction among these people involved some system of health care. When the priest and the shaman stepped between man and his environment; when the chieftain began to promulgate rules of procedure, leading to rules of law; and when more than one family occupied the same hunting grounds, the study of organization arose. In more modern times, organization theory has been studied and utilized in a variety of disciplines. March (1965, p. x), in an effort to identify the "first generation of current work in the study of organizational behavior," selected volumes from six different fields: sociology, anthropology, management, economics, political science, and psychology, and goes on to point out that organization study is evolving into a semidiscipline (p. xiv). Since the publication of this statement, the technological and theoretical advances of computer science and modern systems theory have made organization theory a major part of scientific and clinical thinking.

ORGANIZATION THEORIES

An institution can be defined as both the "corporate body or establishment instituted and organized for public use" and "the building occupied by such a corporate body." It is also "an established order, principle, law, or usage" and, popularly, "a well established custom, object, or person" (Funk and Wagnalls 1949). In these various definitions, the word can be used to refer to hospitals, to health-care systems, to professions, and to the bureaucracy which has developed in and around all of them.

Whatever else institutions generally, and hospitals particularly, are or are not, they are organizations in which people — patients, families, and staff — are differentiated into the statuses and roles that affiliation with an organization prescribes. The goals and functions of health-care institutions require a rather stringent regulation of behavior, as the nature of their activities necessitates that behavior be predictable. It is not conceivable that adequate care can be given unless both givers and recipients know when and under what circumstances that behavior and that care is available. Such organization is necessary in order that institutional objectives can be met. This presupposes management activity based on the needs of the institution, but also on some form of organization theory. Certain fundamental concepts of organization — for instance, planning and decision-making, division of labor, span of control, authority and leadership — are as relevant to the organization of health care as to any other business, and must be understood by those members of the health-care system who work within and around the system in activities of patient care.

Organization theory, like nursing theory, is still evolving; however, theories of organization are commonly listed as classical, neoclassical, and modern (Scott 1961; Massie 1965).

Classical Organization Theory

The classical doctrine deals with the formal structuring of organization and the process of general management; it is built around the division of labor, scalar and functional processes, structure, and span of control. The division of labor is a major element in classical theory and in health care. The scalar and functional processes deal respectively with the chain of command, delegation of authority and responsibility, unity of command and obligation to report (scalar process), and the division into specialized and compatible units (functional process). Structure introduces logical and consistent relationships among the functions, and generally in classical theory is described in terms of *line* and *staff*. Span of control refers to the number of subordinates effectively supervised. This theory does not address personality, informal groups, intraorganizational conflict, or the decision-making process (Scott 1961).

Definitions of terms commonly utilized are as follows.

> *Organization:* refers to structure, to the process of allocating jobs so that common objectives can be achieved. Relates to the formal relationships between positions and jobs, with the behavior characteristics of individuals treated separately. (This somewhat limited meaning became expanded with the neoclassical movement.)

> *Authority:* the right and power to act, usually viewed in classical theory as flowing downward.

> *Specialization:* deals with the division of labor.

> *Coordination:* prearrangement of a number of separate efforts in such a manner as to produce a definite end.

> *Line:* major functions which form the essential framework of organization.

Staff: organizational component existing for the purpose of providing advice and service to line units (Massie 1965, p. 402).

Following are several assumptions underlining classical theory; they are listed here to facilitate understanding of this section.

1. The efficiency of an undertaking is measured solely in terms of productivity; it relates to a mechanical process and economic utilization or resources, without consideration of human factors.

2. Humans are assumed to act rationally, and move in a logical manner toward clearly articulated goals.

3. Members in a cooperative endeavor are unable to determine the relationships of their positions without detailed guidance from a supervisor.

4. Unless clear limits to jobs are defined and enforced, members will tend to be confused and trespass on the domain of others.

5. Humans prefer the security of definite task assignments, and do not value the freedom to determine their own approaches to problems. They prefer direction.

6. It is possible to predict and establish patterns of future activities and relationships.

7. Management involves primarily the formal and official activities of individuals.

8. Activities of the group should be viewed objectively and impersonally, without regard to personal regard and characteristics.

9. Workers are motivated only by economic needs; incentives should be financial.

10. As people do not like to work, they must be closely supervised, and their accountability emphasized.

11. Coordination is not achieved unless it is planned and directed from the top.

12. Authority has its source at the top and is delegated downward.

13. Easy-to-master, simple tasks lead to higher productivity.

14. Managerial functions in varied types of activities have universal characteristics and can be performed in a given manner, regardless of the environment or the qualities of the personnel (Massie, 1965, p. 405).

Although the above set of assumptions are probably not vocalized, or even consciously ascribed to by hospital and nursing administrators, observation of the decisions and activities on a nursing unit suggests they are commonly held. Although other writers have renamed and added to their number, the five elements of administration in the framework developed by Henri Fayol continue to exemplify classical theory. These are considered to be the duties or functions of management, and include planning, organization, command, coordination, and control (Massie 1965). Planning, developed from the objectives of the organization, involves prediction of future events and arranging to meet them. Organizing involves the division of tasks and their grouping into a hierarchy. Planning and organization are preparation for operations; the functions of command and coordination exist to carry out the operation. Command involves the execution of plans; coordination is the correlation of all activities. Control is concerned with performance according to rules and instructions.

In current management thinking, coordination as a basic function is omitted because it is perceived as a result of the proper performance of other functions; nurses who perceive themselves as coordinators may wish to reevaluate their functions. The control function is receiving increased attention by classical management theorists and by professional standards and review boards. Management theorists suggest that, in any system of control, a predetermined goal, a means of measurement of current activity, a means of comparing current activity with a criterion, and a means of correcting the current activity to obtain the desired results are all required (Massie 1965, pp. 389–390). In view of the multiplicity of goals in the health-care system, the unreliability and invalidity of the measurements of health status, the lack of empirically sound criteria of health-care activities, and the lack of any real sanctions leading to change in professional behaviors, control as it is understood by management theorists is too rigorous for application to the health-care system. However, the concept of the control function is necessary to the development and implementation of standards of care.

The early developers of organization theories were operating executives and consultants, and the work of the analysts and academics followed the work of the practitioners. The classical framework was developed as a useful guide for practice, and before 1940 there was little effort to incorporate human interaction into the structure. There was some awareness that man was a key factor in management and should not be treated as a machine (Massie 1965), but human beings and human processes were not incorporated into the conceptual frameworks outside of the teaching of Mary Parker Follett. Massie (1965, p. 394) presents in summary Follett's four principles of organization: (1) coordination by direct contact with responsible parties; (2) coordination in early stages; (3) coordination as the reciprocal relating of all the factors in the situation; and (4) coordination as a continuing process.

The first two principles focus on the cross relationships between department heads; control is considered best maintained by increase of horizontal communications, with direct attention by low-level managers to matters involving their expertise. The third principle of coordination as the reciprocal relating of all the factors is concerned with the fact that it is not realistic to demand that department heads should subordinate the good of their departments to the good of the institution as a whole. The departmental point of view is necessary, but must be reconciled with other points of view through reciprocal contacts. It is not necessary to "de-departmentalize" thinking, but rather to "interdepartmentalize." The fourth principle of continuing process deals with the fact that the organization does not stand still while problems are resolved; rather the resolution generates new problems.

The Follett emphasis is on the dynamics of the management situation, in contrast to the structural emphasis of her colleagues. She indicated that it is not possible to learn from experiences unless experiences are observed, recorded, and related to the total situation. She perceived that authority belongs to the job and stays with the job and therefore cannot be delegated. Both authority and responsibility are dictated by the situation, and the subordinate gets his authority from the functions for which he is responsible. Authority is pluralistic and does not flow from the top, and management is perceived as a social process described by four terms: evoking, interacting, integrating, and emerging. *Evoking* is concerned with the duty of a supervisor to facilitate optimum performance from each individual, to draw him out to his fullest responsibilities. This involves educating subordinates to work with rather than to follow a leader. *Interaction* refers to the mutual impact of the situation on the individual and the individual on the situation, in which both are changed. *Integration* of divergent points of view is advised as the strategy for handling conflict which is perceived to be omnipresent. Managers may deal with conflict by domination, compromise, or integration. Recommended as most desirable, integration requires that differences are openly admitted, and conflicting desires are reevaluated so that resolution of conflict can occur. *Emerging* is oriented to the continually changing situation, and the evolving or emerging developments thereof (Massie 1965, p. 394).

Follett's surprisingly modern management concepts provide principles to support the activities nurses commonly carry out without knowing the principles. Horizontal communication between head nurses and nursing division supervisors, and other chiefs of departments (e.g., pharmacy, x-ray, and laboratories) is common procedure in the effort to protect department gains without jeopardizing institutional goals. The principle of continuing process is perhaps less fully understood, as nurses operating in administrative structures are likely to express frustration when the solution of one problem is followed not by a sigh of relief and a return to "normal" practice but by the prompt appearance of another problem related to the first solution. Her perception that authority flows from the job is included in the rhetoric of nursing, but it is not in the rhetoric of either hospital administrators or physicians. They are more likely to think that authority is invested in status, and do not understand nurses who resort to strike rather than continue to operate in situations in which physicians make nursing decisions. The principle that orders should be depersonalized — such that one person does not give orders to another but both agree to take orders from the situation — is violated on all hospital fronts. Orders are always the prerogative of the physician, and perhaps of the nursing supervisor. Follett's attention was chiefly in the areas of psychology and sociology, and she was not concerned about addressing the needs of a clinical situation; however, her thinking is relevant to nursing, and indeed her concepts of coordination articulate well with principles of nursing.

Follett aside, basic principles in current classical theories are summarized by Massie (1965, pp. 396–401) as follows.

SCALAR PRINCIPLE

This principle incorporates the notion of hierarchy and states that authority and responsibility should flow in a clear, unbroken line from the highest executive to the lowest operative. Obviously this principle in its pure form does not address problems that develop when other kinds of relationships are considered. The authority of the physician over the nurse, of the nurse over the patient, or of the patient over either professional, cannot be considered in terms of the scalar principle.

UNITY OF COMMAND

In its pure form, this principle states that no member of an organization should receive orders from more than one superior. This is not a realistic or comprehensive perception of organizations as they are likely to exist. The classical theorists ignored the informal influences operating in any organization, and concentrated on the formal line-authority relationships. This principle is basic to classic management theory, and when it is in conflict with other principles it is expected to take precedence. Because a principle which does not work in practice is not helpful to an operating manager, it is usually qualified to state that no member of an organization should report to more than one superior on any single function. Although this permits specialization, it does not provide guidelines for subordinates' behavior when there are conflicting instructions between functional superiors. A further qualification would state that there should always be a designated single position from which the subordinate is expected to obey orders under all circumstances. In an organization devoted to patient care, this position is likely to be inhabited by the physician rather than by the nursing supervisor.

EXCEPTION PRINCIPLE

The exception principle states that decisions that recur frequently should be reduced to routine and delegated to subordinates, with only important or nonrecurring issues referred to supervisors. This principle is important to the process of delegating authority, and of all the classic concepts probably comes closest to being valid across many situations. However, the routinizing of procedures may result in the routinization of people in the hospital setting.

SPAN OF CONTROL

This principle prescribes that the number of subordinates reporting to a supervisor be limited. Graicunas, who developed the concept of span of control (Massie 1965, p. 398), developed a mathematical formula to explain the potential increase in the complexity of relationships, identifying three types: direct single relationships, cross-relationships, and direct group relationships. Utilization of the formula to describe the potential relationships of a head nurse responsible for a division staffed by 30 nursing personnel, a situation which is not unlikely, indicated that the number of possible relationships for this nurse (excluding relationships with patients and doctors, and computing only possible nursing staff interactions) was 16,106,128,220.* However, use of the formula involves several assumptions: all of the various relationships of the subordinates must receive the attention of the supervisor; the relationship between supervisor A and subordinate B is different in the presence of subordinate C; focus is on the number of relationships weighted equally, without consideration of frequency or duration of any relationship. The number of subjects to which any manager can attend is limited, and a distinction is made (Massie 1965, p. 398) between attention to physical and mental activity, with the former demanding fewer changes in attention by the supervisor. Other limits are established by time and by the amount of available energy. Obviously any supervisor establishes priorities that rule out a major portion of the possible relations with subordinates; even so, the possibilities are astounding, and, in the case of the head nurse, they are confounded by the possible number of nurse–patient relationships, nurse–doctor relationships, nurse–patient–subordinate relationships, nurse–patient–doctor relationships, etc., in an astronomical progression. The head nurse managing a nursing division is in danger of being overwhelmed by interactions.

ORGANIZATIONAL SPECIALIZATION

The concept in this principle is the division of work into units with specialized activities. Classical theory assumes that it is possible to determine in advance all of the important tasks and processes necessary for the accomplishment of the objectives of the organization.

Four bases for departmentalization are identified (Massie 1965, p. 400): the purpose to be served, the process to be used, the clientele to be served, and the place where the activities will take place. Advantages of classification by purpose include focus of energy in the orientation of the group to the achievement of a common goal. The difficulty in avoiding overlap and the tendency toward overcentralization constitute disadvantages. Classification by process encourages the use of technical skills and labor-saving devices, and stimulates professional standards; however, the overemphasis on how things will be done may be at the expense of what is to be done, and segmented approaches to common goals may develop. Classification on the basis of clientele to be served brings together all

---

*If the number of subordinates reporting to a superior is n, then the number of direct relationships is n. The second type (cross-relationships) involves interactions between two subordinates and is given by $n(n-1)$. The third type involves interactions between the superior and various subsets of subordinates and is given by $n\left(\dfrac{2^n}{2} - 1\right)$ (Massie 1965, p. 398). In the case of the head nurse supervising a 24-hour staff of 30 nursing personnel, the arithmetic is as follows:

$$n = 30 = \text{possible single direct relationships}$$
$$n(n-1) = (30)(29) = 870 \text{ possible cross-relationships}$$
$$n\left(\frac{2^n}{2} - 1\right) = 30\left(\frac{1,073,741,823}{2} - 1\right) = 16,106,127,320$$
$$= \text{possible direct group relationships}$$

The sum of the three sets of possibilities is 16, 106, 128, 220.

activities relating to a given type of customer, reducing the number of depart-ments that must be visited by the client. However, such classification minimizes the advantage of specialization by functions and requires greater duplication of facilities. Departmentalization by place is the easiest to visualize and to apply. It is necessary only to establish territories on a geographical basis and define all activities within this physical area. While this improves the adaptability of any organization to local needs, it also increases the difficulty of maintaining uni-form policies and increases the cost of supervision.

PROFIT-CENTER CONCEPT

This principle has more relevance for hospitals than is immediately evident; it dictates that various parts of a large organization should be departmentalized into integrated self-contained units, each with its own facilities and staff sup-port, operating on a competitive basis in an effort to maximize profit. The closing of expensive obstetrical units, or their modification into gynecological units; the bookkeeping that shows laboratories making a profit when emergency rooms do not; or the separation of out-patient departments from in-patient de-partments, so that each operates with its own staff, are all procedures that draw upon the profit-center concept disguised as a cost/benefit analysis that may dic-tate certain kinds of decentralization activities in large hospitals.

Neoclassical Theory

The neoclassical doctrine is identified with the human relations movement, and adds to management as primarily a normal hierarchy the idea of management as primarily a social process. This approach incorporates the postulates of the clas-sical school as they are modified by persons operating either independently or within the context of the informal organization. Management prerogatives are qualified by consultation and participation of subordinates in decision-making. The concentration on command and on the delegation of authority is qualified by emphasis on horizontal and informal communications. The emphasis on di-rection from a single individual is changed to emphasis on decision-making by a group of executives. The traditional organization theories dehumanized the working individual by assuming that one person was the same as another, and minor differences would cancel out; they leaned heavily on the assumption that men rationally pursued their own self interests. A single standard of values (pro-ductivity) was pervasive. The neoclassical approach either ignores the classical concepts or uses them as points of departure, treating them as having little value in present situations (Massie 1965, p. 407). A more pernicious practice, however, is to give lip service to new concepts of management but operate the institution on the basis of the classical assumptions.

The neoclassical approach is of particular interest for nursing, as two aspects which have been studied in this framework are (1) the delegation of authority and responsibility and (2) gaps in the overlapping of functional jurisdictions. The difficulties caused by insufficient delegation of authority combined with over-assignment of responsibility and accountability are certainly familiar components of nursing status and discussions of role.

Perhaps the major contribution of the neoclassical view to nursing is to be found in the work on informal organization, as the characteristics of informal organizations are basic to the understanding of the health-care system. These are briefly described by Scott (1961) as having their own leaders and acting as agents of social control within the formal organization. The distribution of relationships is not necessarily predictable from distribution in the formal group, and informal organizations have status and communication systems not necessarily derived from the formal system (e.g., the grapevine). The interaction between the formal and informal organizations is an important study of the neoclassical school.

Massie (1965, p. 414) identifies three common neoclassical approaches to management: (1) the management process and human behavior approach, (2) the comparative approach, and (3) the challenge-and-response approach. Management process and human behavior theorists continued to build on classical foundations but treated the human factor as a variable instead of a given. The comparative approach has many variations, but it is based on empirical study of management activities in two or more firms in an effort to develop guidelines for predicting what will work well in comparable situations. The objective is to build parts of a theory that could be useful at the present time and might later be developed into universally valid propositions. Those who espouse the challenge-and-response approach do not attempt to build a framework of knowledge, but stress that management is a practice that should employ all the ideas developed by science and the arts to increase achievements in business. A major contribution to this school of thought is Drucker's concept of management by objectives (Massie 1965, p. 417). The job of management is divided into three parts: managing business as a whole, managing managers, and managing workers and work. The first involves setting specific objectives for performance, the second the establishment of a system by which managers may monitor themselves and develop future managers, and the third involves the management of workers by providing challenges and motivation to work. This approach differs from the others in that it focuses on actual performance rather than on normative theories, and does not offer much encouragement for the development of general theory.

In spite of the attention given by the neoclassicists to the human components of organizations, Scott (1961) suggests that neoclassicism suffers from incompleteness and lack of integration; he supports the development of modern organization theory, distinguished by a conceptual-analytical base and reliance on empirical research data and on its integrating nature.

Modern Organization Theory

Modern organization theory is associated with general systems theory in that both study the movements of individuals in aggregates into and out of the system; the interaction of individuals with the environment and with each other;

and system growth and stability. However, general systems theory is concerned with every level of system,* whereas modern organization theory focuses primarily on human organization (Scott 1961).

Modern organization theorists accept as a premise that the only meaningful way to study organization is to study it as a system. System analysis treats organization as a system of mutually dependent variables.

The basic components of the human system are the individual and whatever history and personality he brings to the organization; the formal structure, that is, the interrelated tasks making up the system; the informal organization, status and role patterns; and the physical setting in which the work is performed.

The processes by which interaction among these parts is achieved is addressed by role theory. Three other linking activities that appear to be universal factors in human organizations are communication, balance, and decision-making. Communication involves information exchange between the parts of the system, the receipt of messages from outside the system, and the storage and retrieval of information. Balance refers to mechanisms developed to maintain system equilibrium. However, because human organizations are open systems, and thereby vulnerable to stimulus from their environments, they must also develop methods for achieving innovation and regulated change; balancing mechanisms must be such that change can occur. The goals of a human system are met by the decision-making activities of the individuals comprising the system and impinging on it. The decision process is basic to the survival of the organization (Scott 1961).

In summary, the classical theories of organization are concerned with principles common to all organization. The neoclassical view adds to concern with the anatomy of the formal organization the analysis of human behavior, but in doing so tends to lose the concept of the social system itself. Modern organization theories study organization as a whole, including structures and function, as these are affected by human behavior.

DECISION-MAKING

Theories of organizational decision-making assume that organizations and individuals are purposive, and act to accomplish or maintain goals, values, objectives, or ends. Economic theories are likely to assume that the organization is guided by a single decision-maker with a single goal. Other theories (e.g., theories

---

*Kenneth Boulding has developed the following hierarchy of classifications of systems: (1) static structures, the level of frameworks, of the anatomy; (2) simple dynamic systems, the level of clockworks, of predetermined necessary motions; (3) cybernetic systems, the level of the thermostat with self-regulation; (4) open systems, the level of self-maintenance, including living organisms; (5) genetic-societal systems, the level of cell society, characterized by a division of labor among cells; (6) animal systems, the level of mobility with evidence of goal-directed behavior; (7) human systems, the level of symbol interpretation and idea communication; (8) social systems, the level of human organization; and (9) transcendental systems, the level of ultimates and absolutes, unknowable in essence (Boulding 1956, pp. 200–202).

of bureaucracy) allow for the aspect of individual behavior but assume that goals are set by a single individual, or a small controlling group. The theory of bureaucracy assumes the existence of an organizational structure that neutralizes behavioral differences among individuals. A third group of theories assumes that the organization is composed of multiple decision-makers, each with separate goals, demanding conflict resolution; this group is exemplified by approaches describing the organization as a game, or as a political coalition (Feldman and Kanter 1965). Probably the descriptive model which best fits the hospital is one of multiple decision-makers with multiple goal structures, a coalition of groups with conflicting goals. The problem addressed by this model is the nature of the process by which the members of the institution resolve their differences. The tripartite structure of Board of Trustees, hospital administrator, and medical staff is one in which the formal lines of authority are at any time subject to medical override.

Feldman and Kanter (1965, p. 642) state that

> the most important problem standing in the way of the understanding of organization decision making is incorporation of available empirical information into theories adequate to the task. There are two major stumbling blocks to the development of such theories: (a) their formulation involves sifting evidence of a heterogeneous and sometimes casual nature; (b) the derivation of the predictions of such theories involves formidable computational difficulties.

There is a striking resemblance between the problems of organizational theorists and the problems of nursing theorists which generates the assumption that nurses will benefit from some understanding of the elements of a decision-making problem. The elements include goals, alternative courses of action, outcomes for each alternative, and choice procedures.

Goals: Thompson (1965) suggests that in dealing with goals it is useful to think in terms of maximizing and minimizing certain identified factors, in order to identify effective attainment of the goal. This may be simple enough when only one goal is to be considered; however, in an organization individuals and departments are not likely to espouse the same goals — regardless of the stated goals of the organization. In a health-care institution there may be a stated meta goal called "healthy and satisfied patient" or the frequently stated medical-center trio of "Service, Education, Research." But the nursing-department goals differ from the goals of the other departments; even if they did not, departmental tactics to reach the goals will certainly differ. The meta goal may be shared, and all departments may agree that the path to reaching the goal includes increased budget and increased numbers of staff. They may even agree on how the responsibilities for meeting the goal are assigned to different departments (although none of this agreement is likely in a hospital setting), but there is still the problem of limited resources. There may be agreement between departments that increased staffing is required to meet the patient care goal, but if all departments need staff, the department of nursing is not likely to consider that the greater need is in the department of pharmacy. Straitened means provoke interdepartment and even intershift skirmishes for scarce resources. These difficulties are present even in the situation in which there is agreement concerning institution goals. In the face of multiple goals, all demanding a large part of the economic and human portions of the resource pool, the difficulties are compounded. The goals of the researcher are not the goals of the therapist in the clinical setting, although the meta goals of research and service may both be espoused by the institution. At a different level, the patient-care goals developed together by the nurse and patient may never be met if they are in conflict with medical goals. When there are conflicts, the goals of the most powerful individuals, departments, or systems will override other goals — even if the goals of the powerful are less appropriate. A frank realization by nurses that in the institution other goals will take precedence over nursing goals is an important factor in deciding among alternative courses of action; however, the depressing effects of such realization must be subdued.

Alternative courses of action: There are different ways to attain any goal, and the course chosen is best based on some measure of the probable effectiveness of each course. Such measures cannot be developed without consideration of the relationships between alternative courses and probable outcomes. There is some question as to whether in health-care institutions decisions are really made by selecting alternative actions on the basis of their consequences for a set of goals. It is quite likely that decisions may be made on the basis of expediency, fatigue, attitudes, organizational constraints, and other rational and nonrational considerations. Although the nursing goal may be to meet a patient need, thus articulating with an organizational goal of satisfied patients with satisfied needs, the decision (course of action to attain the two goals) of a nurse to stay or not to stay with a dying patient may be made because the nurse is tired, busy, or frightened of the impending death. The tendency of decision models to explain the rational processes and ignore the nonrational realities inhibits their usefulness; as will be discussed later, Games theory overcomes this disadvantage, and may prove useful in nursing because it incorporates nonrational components into the decision-making process.

The decision problem is to select some path to move the system (the individual, the organization) from one state to another more desirable state. The problem may be complicated by the existence of more than one initial state, and more than one final state. Criterion for the choice of paths is the achievement of the most preferred final state, leading to the attainment of the goal(s). The best course can be identified only if all alternative courses and the consequences for the goals of each final state are known. In most decision situations, the possible alternatives are not obvious, and it is difficult to estimate their consequences (Feldman and Kanter 1965).

Outcomes: The relationship between alternative courses of action and outcomes may be a relationship of perfect knowledge, partial knowledge, or complete ignorance (Thompson 1965). The first and third relationships do not need to be considered in nursing as they seldom exist in reality, and when they do exist matters are clear. If you have complete knowledge of the relations between paths and outcomes, the preferred outcome dictates the choice of path, and in a state of complete ignorance, any choice is as good as any other choice. The usual relationship is one of partial knowledge, which must be used to establish choice procedures.

Choice procedures: Chance and the existence of other decision-makers add to the number of possible outcomes of alternative courses chosen by an individual to attain his goals. Multiple outcomes for given alternatives have led to the classification of decision problems into those dealing with certainty, risk, uncertainty, and competition. In decision-making under certainty, there is a "measure of effectiveness, a set of alternatives, and a model which relates each alternative to the measure of effectiveness. Only one outcome is possible for each alternative" (Thompson 1965, p. 138). The decision-maker ranks the alternative choices in the order of their effectiveness and chooses the most effective. In the health field, any decision which can be made under certainty is likely to address either problems that are trivial or problems with an already-determined resolution.

Decisions under risk and uncertainty involve interaction between the choice of an alternative and the existence of some variable(s) not under the control of the decision-maker, which affects outcomes (referred to as "states of nature"). In this case, for each alternative choice, there are as many outcomes as there are states of nature. The distinction between risk and uncertainty can be made in terms of knowledge of the probable distribution of states. In the case of decision under risk, the probability distribution of the states is known; in cases of decision under uncertainty, the possible distribution is known, but not the probabilities of occurrence of each state (Thompson 1965).

The consequences of the various alternatives depend on the action of "nature" (chance, predetermined states) and on the activities of other decision makers. The individual must consider in *his* choice of alternatives, the alternatives open to *other* decision-makers, and the likelihood of any of these being chosen; the nature of the resultant final state; and his own preference in the ordering of these states (Feldman and Kanter 1965). In a situation of individual decisions under competition, or group decisions, the existence of multiple goals may dictate the expressions of the outcomes in utility terms. Alternatives may be ranked differently by different individuals, and group decision can only occur if individual rankings can be combined (Thompson 1965). However, situations in which decision-makers are of equal power are not common in health-care organizations, and the choice of alternative actions may be geared to the preferred outcomes of the most powerful member of the group rather than to the preferred outcomes agreed upon by less powerful members. There is no need to labor here the ability of physicians to dictate procedures and policies which meet medical goals at the expense of the goals of the other members of the health-care system.

Decisions are also affected by the actions of the organization, the physical and mental characteristics and the previous experience of its members, and by the social, political, and economic environments (Feldman and Kanter 1965).

In institutions, decisions are made in an already-established framework of rules, regulations, procedures, and system traditions in both the formal and informal organizations. They are made in the absence of adequate information and in the presence of multiple mutually exclusive goals. Goal displacement occurs and rules are internalized to the extent that the purpose of the rule is ignored and the primary emphasis is on the rule itself. Rules and procedures impose constraints on staff and patient behaviors, and while treatment and other decisions are not entirely determined by organization rules, they are certainly affected. The number of alternative courses of action is reduced by the limited capacity of the system to carry out an exhaustive search for alternatives; in the face of economic, legal, and administrative reasons for keeping things as they are, the search for alternatives may take place only in the neighborhood of present activities. Most alternatives considered may be only slight variations on present choices, as these are likely to be obvious and relevant. The principle stimulus to a comprehensive search for alternative courses of action is to be found in dissatisfaction with available alternatives (Feldman and Kanter 1965). However, such dissatisfaction must occur in persons with the power to implement alternative courses of action. It is a question whether the dissatisfaction of nurses and patients presently has any real impact on health-system goals, courses of action, or outcomes. As more nurses understand the theoretical bases of various organization activities, and become comfortable with, and expert in, the manipulation of activities to attain nursing goals, they may develop the power necessary to advance toward their goals. Movement away from the commitment to a "health-team" approach is probably requisite to the development of any real power in the system, because the team concept of colleagues working together is obviously not espoused by any group but nursing. The reality is more in keeping with the foreman–laborer model; the physician is in charge, and dictates the activities of the rest of the group. He makes those decisions he chooses to make, and reserves the right to monitor and change decisions made by others. As patients are more likely than not to perceive this as how things should be, the decision-making powers of nurses are triply constrained: by medical directives, institutional procedures, and patients' perceptions.

In the preceding section decision-making has been discussed in terms of goals, alternative courses of action, outcomes of alternatives, and choice procedures. Nurses may be more familiar with decision-making presented as problem-solving, in which one identifies the problem, lists possible alternative solutions, evaluates the alternatives, selects the one most suited to the solution, and evaluates the outcome (Plachy 1973).

Because problems *are* problems only in the light of the existence of certain goals, and outcomes can only be evaluated in terms of the same goals, the more comprehensive discussion is useful in making explicit exactly what goes into the decision procedure. "The Nursing Process" (Assessment, Planning, Intervention, Evaluation) as it is usually described is a form of *clinical* decision-making which nursing students are taught to consider their domain. What may be lacking in the teaching is the perception of the impact on nursing decisions of other decision-makers with other than nursing goals.

Pellegrino (1972, p. 301) suggests that everyone who works in a hospital may be involved in clinical decision-making, although he uses the term primarily in reference to "the processes whereby the most prudent and beneficial actions are chosen to meet the medical needs of the patient when he seeks aid from the hospital." He includes not only decisions "made at the bedside" by physicians, nurses, and others, but also "those policies and decisions made at a distance, i.e., by the institution as such and by the community, which alter the context of clinical decisions and impinge necessarily upon the relationship of patient and physician. . . ." He examines the necessity to move away from the concept of a private physician–patient relationship. The institutionalization of the decision setting and the intrusion of other previously silent groups into the clinical decision arena now make it impossible for physicians to operate apart from procedures and goals which they did not establish. The team concept of care itself challenges the privacy if not the power of the physician decision. When this is combined with institutional regulations and latterly with the demand for accountability (at least to peers) for medical decisions, it is obvious that the historical physician–patient relationship is no longer viable. However, the physician remains the central and powerful figure in clinical decisions, and the team concept may receive only lip service, without implementation.

In addressing the problem of delivery of health care, Pellegrino defines a team as a group of persons cooperating for the attainment of a defined goal. He suggests (1972, p. 308) the identification of three kinds of teams with differing goals, differentiated by closeness to the patient: patient-care teams, medical-care teams, and health-care teams. The patient-care team is composed of members of any group of care givers jointly providing needed services in a program of patient management that brings them into personal contact with patients. The medical-care team provides needed services, but members are not brought directly or personally into contact with patients. Included here, for example, are hospital administrators and operating-room supervisors. The health-care team includes all those who provide or plan some service that will improve general or community health. Pellegrino does not provide examples of members of this team, but it is apparent from the definition that it will include legislators and insurance representatives, since the improvement of community health will depend on financing by these groups. It is obvious that nursing is necessarily represented on all of these teams. However, patients are identified as the concern of the teams rather than as team members.

Who captains any of the teams at any time is determined by the patients' needs, as the captain must possess the "skill and knowledge most consonant with dominant features of the clinical condition exhibited by the patient" (Pellegrino 1972, p. 310). In the acute or emergency clinical situation, physicians captain the teams, although they are not likely to have the skills in coordination and the knowledge of community needs required to captain the medical-care and health-care teams as they are defined by Pellegrino. However, physicians' technical skills are always so relevant, and they have for so long dominated decisions related to health, that they are not likely to accept the idea of shifting captaincy, or of shared authority.

In any case, even on the patient-care team, the decision as to what constitutes the "dominant features of the clinical condition" must be made. The dominant features of the clinical condition of dying patients do not respond to curative procedures, and there is some evidence in the nursing literature that the care of dying patients is properly under the auspices of nursing rather than medicine. However, medical control of palliative strategies suggests that physicians are in fact, if not in name, captains of the team — regardless of the dominant clinical features — simply because they retain the power to monitor the activities of all members of the team, although refusing to coordinate those activities. Physicians may depend upon others to undertake major responsibilities for patients' care, but presently they are in charge when they choose to be. There is no doubt, however, that shared responsibility for patient care is basic to the care of patients in institutions, and the dynamics of the group are usurping the benevolent despotism of the physician–patient relationship. Shared responsibility demands shared authority and shared accountability.

However tempting the concept of "team" may be, nurses should examine the authority structure with care. In the past, their concept of themselves as team members and coordinators has inhibited them in the development of power bases from which to practice.

HOSPITALS

History

MacEachern (1951) provides a brief and interesting overview of the history of the development of the hospital. As suggested in Chapter 1, the first known hospitals were the outgrowth of religion, rather than of medicine. The great East Indian convert to Buddhism, King Asoka, built hospital temples throughout his lands. The attendants in these early institutions were ordered to give gentle care to the sick, to furnish them with fresh fruits and vegetables, to prepare medicines, to give massages, and to keep their own persons clean. They were required to be adept at surgery, to take daily baths, to keep their hair and nails short, wear white clothes, and to promise to respect the confidence of the patient.

Early Greek and Roman temples of the gods were also used as hospitals. If the patient was cured, his cure was laid to miracles and divine intervention. If he died, he was lacking in piety, and unworthy to live. This idea of disease as an entity controlled by the gods remained a popular one, in spite of the fact that it put the burden of cure on the patient.

In later Greek temples some medicine was practiced, but the emphasis was on occupational and physical therapy. There were large gymnasia and amphitheatres for amusement. The temples were built to admit sunshine, sea air, and pleasant vistas, and they included libraries and rooms for visitors. They were religious institutions supported by gifts and controlled by the priests.

After Hippocrates, with his emphasis on facts rather than faith, the temples came more and more to resemble the present-day concept of hospital. Teaching was carried out, and diet and moderation in living habits were stressed. Ambulant sick were treated in out-patient clinics, and there was some practice of both medicine and surgery. Administration, however, remained in the hands of the priests.

In Western Europe, hospitals began as houses of hospitality for pilgrims and for the indigent (see Chapter 1). Care of the poor, and of the sick poor, was an integral part of the Christian religious policy. Hospitals, even those built and endowed by rulers or other persons of wealth, were controlled by the clergy. Doctors were members of the priestly orders, subject to the control of their superiors and a part of the hospital they served. During the Crusades many hospitals were built, staffed, and administered by military-religious orders such as the Knights Templar and the Hospitalers of Saint John of Jerusalem. Throughout the Middle Ages, the majority of hospitals remained religious institutions. There were usually too few beds and too many attendants. As beds were at a premium, there frequently were as many as five patients in one bed, with no effort to segregate by sex or by disease. There were "plenty of woolen bed coverings which were needed, as patients were usually kept unclothed except for linen turbans. The patient's garments were kept in a locker room where they were cleaned, mended, and returned to him immediately prior to his departure" (MacEachern 1951, p. 9) — assuming, of course, that he survived his treatment and his environment, and was *able* to depart.

Education at this time was confined almost entirely to monks and clerics; they were the physicians. Thus the Church edict of 1163, forbidding clergy to perform operations which necessitated the shedding of blood, lost to medicine its best practitioners and ushered in the dark age of the uneducated barber-surgeon. Hospitals, with their close ties to the church, became houses of death.

A non-Christian light in the darkness was the Al Mansur hospital, built in Cairo in 1276. It had separate wards for the more serious diseases, diet kitchens, and out-patient clinics. The hospital provided both music and story-telling for sleepless patients, and operated separate convalescent homes. Each patient was given a small sum of money when he was released.

Civil hospitals were built in Europe during the Renaissance, and the practice of allowing apprentices to walk the wards for clinical teaching under experienced surgeons was begun. The duties of the medical staff were explicit. There was a doctor of physic "upon whom rests the duty of visiting all poor patients in the building, females as well as males" (MacEachern 1951, p. 10). The doctor of surgery had a duty "to apply ointment to all the poor people in the hospital who have wounds of any kind; a barber who is competent to do for the women as well as the men all the other things that a good surgeon usually does" (1951, p. 10).

In the 18th century, hospitals were built by parishes or counties for the relief of the sick poor. A free medical dispensary, established by the Royal College of Physicians in England at the beginning of the 18th century, was brought to an untimely end by controversies and law suits; however, the idea was picked up by other societies, charitable rather than medical, and the clinic came into existence. The Westminister Charitable Society built an infirmary by voluntary subscription in 1719, where the medical services were gratuitous; the hospital was neither civil nor religious, but charitable in origin.

Cortez built the first hospital on the American continent in 1524; the first hospital in the United States of America was built for sick soldiers on Manhattan Island in 1663. Most large cities built pesthouses and alms houses, and their scope was expanded to include the care of the sick. Conditions were unbelievably bad in these institutions, and "hospitals resembled the worst type of prisons where those who were so unfortunate as to be ill were at the mercy of attendants who were both heartless and ignorant" (MacEachern 1951, p. 17). Four persons may be noted as influential in the establishment of modern hospitals: William Morton, with his work on anesthesia; Louis Pasteur and Joseph Lister, who developed concepts of antisepsis, asepsis, and sanitation; and Florence Nightingale, who created both modern nursing and the concept of hospital administration. As hospitals improved in the care they gave, they were more frequently utilized, and their functions changed. In the late 19th century, "hospital" was synonymous with "operation" in the lay mind. But the treatment and cure of communicable diseases required laboratories; this, in conjunction with the use of x-ray, with its expensive apparatus, contributed to the founding of community hospitals, with both medical and surgical functions, where physicians could share in the use of the expensive and unwieldly diagnostic and treatment equipment.

The development of adjunct services and the greater confidence of the public in hospitals led to the building of bigger hospitals with diagnosis, therapy, social services, out-patient clinics, research, and medical and nursing education becoming more and more a part of the hospital framework. Rosengren and Lefton (1969, p. 15) describe what hospitals have come to be. They are: (1) of massive economic importance in both the national and personal economy; (2) the locus of technological and ideological innovations; (3) places which manifest social change early; (4) concerned with fundamental values of modern society, i.e., the maintenance of life, support for the incapacitated, and guidance for the dying; (5) the most professionalized of modern formal organizations; (6) settings for the confrontation of concern for clients with the ethic of scientific manipulation of materials; and (7) organizations in which the collaboration — or, at the least, the acquiescence of the client — is mandatory to the delivery of service. Also, of course, they exemplify the control dilemma of modern complex organizations, which is to combine technological efficiency with humane service.

Structure and Economics

The responsibility assumed by the community to protect the health of its members is embodied in federal and state constitutions. The maintenance of hospitals and protection of health are not spelled out as obligations in the United States Constitution, but the general welfare clause is interpreted as providing the power to safeguard the public health. State constitutions generally give the states

> . . . what is called jurisdictionally "police power," permitting State governments to protect the health, welfare, safety, and morals of their citizens. The rational foundation of this power may be the need to protect individuals from the harmful acts of others or even from personal imprudence. Hence the State exercises its police power over the sale of drugs or the wages and hours of working people. It may require vaccination

> *against smallpox and quarantine of persons with diphtheria. Likewise it*
> *may regulate hospitals since these institutions may intimately affect the*
> *life and well being of the people. (Shain and Roemer 1961, pp. 401–402)*

Hospitals derive special privileges from the state, and the state imposes certain obligations on them. They are incorporated bodies, subject to a charter granted by the state, and with responsibilities of corporation defined by law. Because of their charitable and nonprofit character they are exempt from federal income taxes, local property taxes, many excise taxes, and sometimes from local sales taxes. They may receive tax-deductible gifts from donors; they may receive public money for construction purposes.

At a local level, boards of citizens may examine hospital operations; for instance, community councils may look into the way the hospital uses community-donated funds. The College of Surgeons approves hospitals meeting certain standards of organization and practice. The American Hospital Association has established limited standards for membership. The American Medical Association has a system of approval of hospitals for internships, residencies, and post-graduate education. Nursing-school programs are monitored by The National League for Nursing, which may withhold approval. Approval of such services as tumor clinics, blood banks, and schools are given by other professional societies. Internal controls are provided by various in-house committees: tissue committees, medical records committees, medical and nursing audit committees, utilization review committees, and the like. In 1952 an overall system of hospital accreditation was established by a joint commission that included representatives of the College of Surgeons, the American College of Physicians, the American Hospital Association, and the American Medical Association.* This group, known as the Joint Commission on Accreditation of Hospitals (JCAH), inspects hospitals throughout the nation. In order to receive accreditation, an institution must meet a list of minimum essential service and structural standards. Size is related to accreditation in that smaller hospitals are not likely to be able to meet the standards.

Previous to the Medicare–Medicaid legislation, accreditation by JCAH was more a matter of prestige than necessity; however, because Medicare certification requirements are considered to be met by JCAH accredited hospitals, the impetus to accreditation is greater.†

The interests of the public in the hospital are protected by a variety of governmental agencies and laws. The principal means of governmental supervision are the laws defining the power of the state to license hospitals and,

---

*The Canadian Medical Association was also part of the original Commission.
†JCAH accreditation is not the only way that Medicare certification requirements may be met. Marginal institutions *may* be certified if there are no other hospitals servicing an area, as may hospitals which are too small to receive JCAH approval. Regional needs and standards are considered. Medicare certification requirements are met by osteopathic hospitals if they are accredited by the American Osteopathic Association.

since July 1966, the economic clout provided by the Medicare and Medicaid programs.

The Federal Hospital Survey and Construction Act of 1946 contains a stipulation that every state receiving federal grants for hospital construction should have a law governing minimum standards of maintenance and operation. The legislatures pass laws which declare, generally, that every hospital must have a license granted by a particular state agency, usually the health department. The department may then issue regulations to carry out the broadly defined legislative intent. The older hospital regulations concentrated on protecting the safety of the patients; they were explicit about fire hazards, building maintenance, water supply, sewage disposal, and requirements for maternity departments. The newer regulations are concerned with broader aspects of hospital organization: the functions of the governing board and administrator, the medical-staff organization, medical records, laboratory and x-ray departments, nursing service, dietary management, and infection control.

The scope of hospital licensure regulations in most states is broad enough to determine that the hospital is properly built, organized, equipped, staffed, and maintained. In fact, most state regulatory agencies now have the authority to set standards for medical care. However, the problem is in the implementation; inadequate standards of quality and inadequate budgets almost dictate laxity in enforcement by state regulatory agencies. With few exceptions, states do not really assume responsibility for monitoring the quality of medical care, delegating such responsibility to the federal government or to the physicians (Worthington and Silver 1970). The problem is to implement these regulations. In an effort to be practical, while striving for an ideal organization, published licensure codes set out certain standards as mandatory. Others are only recommended, although recommended standards may, in time, become mandatory. Regulations cannot be stated generally. "A regulation with the force of law must be specific and clear enough to enable the person or organization being regulated to know what he must do to comply, and what he must not do to avoid violation of the law" (Shain and Roemer 1961, p. 406). This means that as knowledge increases and standards change, the regulations must also be changed; the time lag is likely to be substantial.

Another problem in hospital regulation is the frequent multiplicity of regulatory agencies in a state, and the inconsistencies in the rules issued by each of them. For example, in an early examination of agencies, Shain and Roemer (1961, p. 407) point out that

> In New York, for instance, general hospital regulations are issued by the State board of social welfare. Specific rules, however, on newborn nurseries, vital statistics, communicable diseases, laboratory and radiology departments, and the handling of cadavers are issued by the State health department for hospitals outside New York City; still other rules on these subjects for hospitals in New York City are issued by the city health department. Educational programs in hospitals are regulated by the State board of regents. State and local fire regulations, multiple dwelling laws, and zoning ordinances affect hospitals through still other jurisdictions.

Licensure of hospitals is done by the states. In addition, accreditation may be done by one of several voluntary accrediting bodies; certification is provided by the Department of Health, Education and Welfare (DHEW). The term accreditation is used to signify that a hospital has "met the standards of some recognized group whose sole or primary function is to promulgate and apply standards to hospitals" (Worthington and Silver 1970, p. 310). Hospitals are certified by DHEW to receive reimbursement for services provided to Medicare beneficiaries.

Some comment is relevant here concerning the quasiregulatory function of JCAH in the hospital setting. Although JCAH is a private agency, the law specifies that an institution meets the Medicare certification requirements if it is JCAH accredited (Long 1972, p. 37). Because JCAH hospital reviews are confidential and not subject to federal scrutiny, in effect there is federal delegation of authority over hospital standards to JCAH. Although state certification agencies *may* survey JCAH-accredited institutions, and may be provided on request with the JCAH survey report, these validation surveys are expected to include cooperative activity with JCAH. Certification is dominated by JCAH such that DHEW cannot set up its own standards for Medicare participation. As JCAH decisions are made by physicians and hospital administrators, it is only reasonable to assume that the standards and requirements will be implemented for the benefit of the medical profession and/or the institution rather than the patients — institutional review boards not withstanding.

"In sum, though functioning in a quasi-public status, by virtue of the substantial standard-setting functions delegated to it by Congress under Title XVIII, the Joint Commission has operated as a totally private body unaccountable to the public or to the government" (Worthington and Silver 1970, p. 325).

The supply and the location of hospital beds are not presently regulated by the state. The licensure laws specify only that a hospital to be constructed must meet certain standards. If these standards are met, the hospital must be licensed regardless of whether those kinds of additional beds are needed in that area. The formation of various municipal and regional health-planning councils has to date had little apparent effect on hospital boards' decisions to move into or remain in an area, although various insurance plans may affect the kinds of hospital beds made available.

In the United States today there are a little more than 7,000 hospitals, providing an estimated one- to one-and-one-half-million beds. More than two-and-one-half-million persons are employed in the service of more than 33 million in-patients per year, and over 200 million out-patients (Somers and Somers 1967; Fuchs 1974). There is a great variation in the size, location, function, and locus of control in the system of hospitals. A hospital with fewer than 200 beds is considered to be small; middle-range hospitals may have from 200 to 500 beds, while the large, university-affiliated, medical centers may number beds in the thousands. Hospitals are distributed in a somewhat arbitrary pattern throughout the country; the rationale of the distribution is not logical but political in nature. They may provide short-term or long-term care, and may be operated by federal, state, or municipal governments, religious bodies, or corporations composed of physicians and/or others. They may be, although they usually are not, profit-making institutions.

Community short-term hospitals account for more than half of the hospital beds and are responsible for 92 percent of all hospital admissions and 78 percent of hospital expenses. They are distinguished from all other hospitals by the short average length of patient stay: typically eight days (Fuchs 1974, p. 82).

The concept that society is in any way officially responsible for individual problems is a fairly recent one, and it was preceded by a long history of community indifference to the woes of the indigent. Wealthy persons paid for whatever medical and nursing skills were available; the sick poor were exposed to the mercies of religious or other charitable institutions. The development of private insurance programs changed this to some extent; the cost of medical catastrophe to any individual was spread among contributors to the program, and insured employed persons were removed from the ranks of the medically indigent. However, the elderly and other unemployed groups unable to afford the high costs of private medical insurance remained at risk of financial ruin as a result of illness.

Somers and Somers (1967) have reported the history of federally sponsored health insurance in this country, and discussed in interesting detail the political maneuvers surrounding the evolution of Public Law 89-97, the Social Security Amendments of 1965, which include Titles XVIII (Medicare) and XIX (Medicaid). This bundle of legislation has, to some extent, removed the concept of indigence from considerations of care, as patients now are likely to be equally indigent. The Medicare legislation is financed and administered through the Social Security Administration, with its Bureau of Health Insurance assuming responsibility for the administration and policy.

A hospital that can be approved for Medicare payments is one which

> . . . *(1) is primarily engaged in providing diagnostic, therapeutic, or rehabilitation services; (2) maintains clinical records; (3) has by-laws for the medical staff; (4) requires every patient to be under the care of a physician; (5) provides 24-hour nursing service under supervision of an RN or has a licensed practical nurse or RN on duty at all times; (6) has a utilization review plan in effect; (7) is licensed pursuant to state or local law; and (8) meets other requirements for health and safety, as found necessary by the Secretary of HEW, except that such requirements may not be higher than those prescribed by JCAH, unless such higher requirements result from state initiative. (Somers and Somers 1967, p. 84)**

Conditions of participation in the Medicare program are provided in various manuals for hospitals, extended-care facilities, home health service, and private laboratories. Each condition is made up of several standards; each standard may have several factors. The conditions are modeled on those established by the professional organizations. Because state agencies are responsible for certifying institutions in their states, there is some flexibility in the implementation of

---

*Compliance with the discrimination requirements of the Civil Rights Act of 1964 is also required.

the conditions of participation. In any case, it was federal intent to be inclusive rather than exclusive, to the extent that hospitals not meeting certification requirements may still be paid for the care of Medicare patients in localities where there are no other available institutions, or for emergency services.

Medicaid funding is delivered to the states in the form of federal grants to expand or consolidate programs for medical care for persons on public-assistance rolls or those who are otherwise unable to withstand major medical expenses (Stevens 1971). From Medicaid's inception, it was perceived that the plan would be ineffective because it served as both a health-service program and as an expansion of public assistance (Stevens and Stevens 1970, p. 420). The present concern with the integrity of the entire Social Security funding mechanism reflects the accuracy of these perceptions.

The debates about health-insurance legislation are frequently carried out in an atmosphere of passionate concern for the problems of persons needing care; however, the basic issue is always one of compensation for those who provide the care. Medicare and Medicaid are no exceptions to this rule; they merely added federal funds to the third-party reimbursement schemes already available in the health-care system (Somers and Somers 1967; Stevens 1971). Both programs have been under attack for "extravagance, fraud and waste" (Stevens 1971, p. 444), but the attacks are geared to promulgation of control techniques rather than to any real consideration of change in the provision of care. Medical practitioners may be chastised because their fees are large and the amount of time and compassion given to patients is small. However, suggested improvements are usually in terms of training auxiliary personnel to carry out many physicians' tasks — the concept of the physician extender. The allopathic medical model — which gives physicians trained mainly in drastic pharmacological or surgical curative techniques complete control over all health-system functions — is in itself seldom addressed. The problems are perceived to be present because there are too few such physicians and they have become somehow less compassionate. Whether other medical theories (for example, homeopathy, osteopathy, naturopathy, chiropractic) or other health disciplines (for example, nursing or pharmacology) *should* become viable and powerful components of the system is not generally considered a relevant question by insurers, who continue to support various physician-dominated health-care plans. The complex and extensive administrative set up between the federal government and the health providers in the Medicare legislation follows the usual model, with separate hospital and physician funding mechanisms (Appendix C).

Nonfederal hospitals may be classified into three categories based on locus of control: (1) state, county, or municipal hospitals, owned and operated by political subdivisions; (2) proprietary hospitals, money-making institutions owned and operated by corporate medical or lay groups; and (3) voluntary hospitals, with a somewhat ambiguous ownership. Capital for the voluntary hospitals is usually raised through community drives, and administered by a Board of Trustees composed of prominent community figures and/or religious groups. These hospitals are considered private — in that they are not government owned and are not accountable to any public instrumentality. However, they are quasipublic in character, with some public-institution privileges.

The traditional distinctions among the three kinds of institutions are becoming blurred, particularly as regards patient populations and sources of revenue. Government hospitals are tax-supported, and historically have cared for indigent patients; however, they are now caring for a fully insured clientele. Voluntary hospitals are receiving a large part of their funding from tax-supported programs (Medicare and Medicaid), and even proprietary institutions may be accepting low-income patients with full-pay insurance status (Somers and Somers 1967).

In spite of the influx of federal monies into these establishments, and the enrollment in 1966 of 19-million persons in the Medicare coverage (Somers and Somers 1967), consumer complaints about the quality and quantity of both medical and nursing care have never been more intense. Fuchs (1974, p. 4) has suggested this is in part due to a misunderstanding of the nature of the resources, which will always be scarce in relation to human wants. No matter how well run the system is it is never possible to give everything to everyone. Resources have alternative uses: schools may be perceived as more important than meals for the elderly. Certainly the exciting field of operative intervention in cardiac dysfunction drains health-care resources from use in techniques of prevention or care of chronically ill patients. The instrumental needs of the few take precedence over the expressive needs of the many. It is also clear that not everybody wants the same thing with the same intensity. Health is obviously not a primary goal for those otherwise intelligent citizens who habitually eat too much, drink too much, smoke too much, and drive too fast. Also, the desire of professionals to practice in the most fully equipped hospital in the country may not be in line with community needs.

Along with the constant gap between what is demanded and what it is feasible to supply is the question of the productivity of the system, the efficient use of available resources. Fuchs (1974, pp. 82–84) reports an emerging consensus among those studying hospital-based health care that there is a strong relationship between hospital size (measured by number of beds) and efficiency (measured by expenditure per patient day). Generally, there is an increasing efficiency associated with increasing size, up to the middle range of 200 to 500 beds, although this varies with the number of services and facilities offered. Very small and very large hospitals are not likely to be economical. As 40 percent of the hospital beds in this country are found in institutions with fewer than 200 beds, and 20 percent are in institutions with more than 500 beds, there is certainly loss of efficiency, which is compounded by the average occupancy rates. Hospital administrators suggest 85 percent of capacity (or slightly higher) as an optimum occupancy rate; the average rate in small hospitals is 70 percent of capacity; in medium-size and large hospitals it exceeds 80 percent of capacity. Small hospitals have a lower number of personnel per patient (2.7) as compared with medium-size (3.0) and large (3.4) hospitals, and a smaller average stay figure (small, 7.2 days; medium, 8.1 days; large, 9.8 days). However, larger institutions are more likely to have sicker patients, as well as research and teaching responsibilities not shared by smaller institutions. When the smaller institutions limit services and facilities, they are less expensive to maintain.

Regardless of their stated goals or their size, hospitals today are very likely to be serving as health centers — providing emergency and ambulatory care and rehabilitation services in addition to the care of the acutely sick and injured within the institution (which is usually considered the task of the hospital). This expansion into a multifunction center is relevant to the care of dying patients because care in such a setting is expensive, and the patients will be in the position of paying for services they will never utilize. Also, the sick role — which requires the individual to try to recover — is precluded in the case of the terminal patient, who may be required to assume behavioral norms that are inappropriate.

Goals and Functions

The goal of the general hospital is to provide the requisites for the maintenance and restoration of health for individuals in the community. This duty involves four functions, the first of which is the care of the sick and injured. Although care of the sick is the main objective of the hospital, it cannot be licensed for this purpose; care of the sick is the responsibility of the medical and nursing staffs. Other hospital functions — such as the maintenance of scientific standards and the advancement of research in scientific medicine — may be provided for by the governing board, but must be implemented by the professionals attached to the institution. Two other functions of the hospital, the education of physicians, nurses, and allied personnel, and the prevention of disease and promotion of health in the community, are also dependent upon the health professions (Shain and Roemer 1961).

Further definition of goals would include those shared with any organization devoted to human service: organizational efficiency, excellence in members' practice, and continued viability.

The hospital is like other organizations.

> *An arrangement of interdependent parts each having a special function with respect to the whole . . . . The members assemble on schedule, each person engages in a limited number of activities, the range of interpersonal transactions is restricted and stable over time and the style of social interaction is patterned. Behavior has a reasonably high degree of predictability and people know rather well what to expect of one another. Moreover the activities of different individuals tend to combine in such a way as to result in organizational accomplishment (Cartwright 1965, p. 1).*

Mauksch (1975) suggests, however, that while the hospital is a place which must routinize the emergencies of clients, the different occupations tend to isolate themselves from one another.

Wilson (1963) points out that

> Hospitals are among the most complex organizations in modern society, characterized by extremely fine divisions of labor and an exquisite repertory of technical skill. The major hospital embraces multiple goals, chiefly patient care, teaching and research. It is at once a hotel, a treatment center, a laboratory, a university. Because the institution's work is so specialized, staffed by a variety of professional and technical personnel, there are very important problems of coordination and authority. Paramount in the social structure are relationships between patients and hospital staff and among staff members. The patient, both the client and the product of the organization, enters a therapeutic situation in which his style is largely passive. He encounters the physician, like himself a guest of the hospital, and the nurse, who is the full-time symbol of the organization's atmosphere. The physician is undergoing a shift from his older charismatic role toward a more nearly bureaucratic niche in the hospital. Staff relationships are distinguished by unclear patterns of authority and intense competition for spheres of competence and prestige. The physician is implicated as the professional least amenable to hierarchical control, and the leading figure in skill and status.

In spite of advances in scientific, research-oriented medicine, the increased numbers of nursing and other health specialists who require clinical educational facilities, and the growth of outreach community health, home care, and other out-patient functions, the main objective of the hospital is to render direct, individualized medical and nursing care to patients housed in the institution. Some planning of work is possible, but the requirements of patient care are such that it is difficult to mechanize, standardize, or preplan many of the system tasks. Emergencies are common, leading to management by crisis; work problems are variable, and there is little tolerance for ambiguity or error (Georgopoulous 1972). Deviation from standard procedures is not encouraged.

The focus on adherence to rules and regulations only confounds the problems inherent in the fact that the goal of the hospital is cure. Dying patients not only do not reach that goal but also demand that regulations and routines be changed to meet their needs (Mauksch 1975; Castles and Keith 1979). Hospitals are set up to fight death, not to let it occur, and care-givers who are trained to deal effectively with disease do not know how to cope with the anger and distress of persons whom no techniques will save. Acute-care institutions are organized to cure, to handle short-term or emergent patient activities with great skill. Those patients who are dying must either adapt to procedures designed to ensure living, or move to institutions considered less important by the professional community. Since positions in these institutions lack both excitement and prestige, abandonment by the more highly educated professionals is likely to occur. The repetitive tasks and the waiting—inseparable from the care of the dying—become the responsibility of the least powerful, least prestigious, and least well-educated members of the care system.

Professionals as Personnel

Although comprehensive medical care is now viewed as any citizen's right, and patient compliance cannot be assumed, doctors and nurses are also now considered to have their own private interests, which must be accommodated to the demands of the institution and the patients (Rosengren and Lefton 1969). Three categories of personnel are considered in their roles and functions within the hospital structure: hospital administrators, nurses, and physicians. The therapeutic activities and the needs for system support of nurses and physicians caring for terminal patients are treated in detail in Chapter 6. In this section the three major professional groups are examined as they function in the institution.

HOSPITAL ADMINISTRATORS

The Board of Directors constitutes the governing body of most hospitals. Directors are community representatives, although they cannot usually be said to represent all groups in the community: business and professional people predominate. In the case of a municipal hospital, the governing board of the community may also function as the governing board of the hospital. The Board of Directors employs a manager, the hospital administrator, to implement its policies.

The ancient historian Herodotus observed the Babylonians in his travels, and reports the following:

> They bring their sick to the market place, for they have no physicians; there those that pass by the sick person confer with him about his disease, to discover whether they have themselves been afflicted with the same disease as the sick person or have seen others so afflicted; thus the passersby confer with him and advise him to have recourse to the same treatment as that by which they escaped a similar disease, or as they have known to cure others. And they are not allowed to pass by a sick person in silence without first inquiring into the nature of his distemper. (Bochmeyer and Hartman 1943, p. 5)

Harrassed hospital administrators must manage institutions that are always too costly, for the benefit of patients in various stages of illness and who know what they want but not what they need. They manage through the efforts of various professional guilds and other unions who know exactly what they want and do not really care what it costs the hospital. They operate in a confused network of tradition and laxity and have responsibility for patient care without either the knowledge or authority to dictate what that care should be. They must occasionally perceive many advantages in the Babylonian market-place system of care.

The administrator is under surveillance by his own governing board, by insurance boards, by government agencies, by various professional associations, and by the general public. In a large hospital he manages with or in spite of the help of five different groups with varying amounts of power: the private physicians, the hospital-employed chiefs of staff, the nursing service adminis- trators, the funding agencies, and the patients who are the objects of the orga- nization. In this very loosely integrated system in which semiautonomous cooperators and competitors meet to use common facilities and provide services for each other, it is a question whether further integration into an hierarchial organization is desirable or possible. However, planning and consideration of policy must occur and organizational decisions must be made. Consent and agreement rather than logic or command is required in the presence of a medical group that does not usually care to concern itself with "organizational decision," but which can sabotage any decision by declaring a "medical emergency."

Administration by consent rather than command fits well with concepts of civil rights and democratic processes; however, efficient administration by consent demands administrative control of communication networks. The organization maximizes its assets to the degree to which it secures the full emotional and intellectual attachment of its members. To secure this attach- ment, the members must know what is going on and why. Obviously this concept of administration imposes heavy burdens on the administrator. Ad- ministration conceived as a problem in interpersonal relations may be appro- priate for the hospital, with its ambiguous authority structure, its 24-hour operation, low pay for all but the top levels of personnel, and traumatic working conditions for personnel at all levels. On the other hand, the characteristics of the work call for more command and less representation of a total group than is required in most work settings.

Wilson (1963) has suggested the hospital resembles a federal system: "a federation of departments, each department enjoying considerable autonomy and discretion in its management of work."

The administrator and the medical staff are the primary authority figures, although day-to-day decisions are likely to be made by nurses. The current trend toward more organization control of tasks and functions was perceived by Wilson more than ten years ago.

> There are two persistent reasons why the hospital can perhaps never approach the degree of formal controllability, of symmetrical power and task arrangements which distinguishes industry and government. One is the nature of the work flow, the temporal and ethical constraints imposed by intractable human material: the patient. The other is the nature of the medical profession, which resists bureaucratization and is the un- changing repository of certain fundamental decisions about the care of the ill. Despite these strictures, however, the hospital is now exhibiting many more of the faces of bureaucracy. Specifically it is becoming ra- tionalized and specialized to an unprecedented extent. Rationality is expressed in such features of the modern hospital as cost accounting and written personnel policies, quality control and job descriptions; a loose benevolence is yielding to calculated, planful, organization of services. Specialization already acute in medicine itself, is now seen in adminis- trative as well as technical guises. Task assignments and spheres of dis-

cretion are increasingly narrowed and legitimized in formal rather than accidental ways. Most hospital jobs are increasingly constricted as the assumed prerogatives of general helping roles are replaced by the deliberate mandates of announced organizational functions. (Wilson 1963, p. 74)

In spite of the "mandates of announced organizational functions," and even the development of the interdependent as opposed to the entrepreneurial professional model, the authority of hospital administrators is "severely limited when compared with the heads of almost any other type of organization; in fact it is not quite accurate to call them 'heads' nor can any other person in the hospital generally be identified in that capacity" (Somers and Somers 1967, p. 123).

PHYSICIANS

Members of a hospital medical staff could be expected to take issue with the last-noted quotation. The traditional authority of the physician, recognized by patients and nurses, as well as doctors, when combined with the rapid advancement in the technology of medicine, has resulted in a change in the power structure of hospitals. As Perrow expresses it:

Trustees dominate when the technology is fairly simple and few skills are required, doctors dominate when they provide most of a complex, high level technology, and the administration is in a position to dominate when critical tasks are performed by other specialists as well as the doctors and a high degree of coordination is required. Goals are thought to reflect this shift, moving from a humanistic concern with palliation, to a concern with technical proficiency and the remunerations derived from service to private patients to, finally a concern for the social as well as the physical aspects of medicine. (Perrow 1965, p. 965)

Although physicians in the hospital are becoming increasingly more bureaucratized, and hospital administration is becoming a profession (Perrow 1965), the medical decision still takes precedence over all other decisions.

In the past the physician has been the privileged guest rather than the employee of the institution, with his activities parallel to rather than an intrinsic part of the hospital activities. There are two sets of activities " . . . the general administrative and technical medical which are manned in overlapping fashion and which generate something close to two lines of authority" (Wilson 1963, p. 71). The private physician is not subject to control by the administration; even when medical staff are employed by the hospital, as is more and more the case, the employed physicians are subject to the medical authority of the chief of staff, rather than to the organizational authority of the administrators. Who monitors the chiefs of staff is an interesting question. It is doubtful if they report in any meaningful way to the head of the formal organization, the hospital administrator. While the hospital Board has ultimate legal responsibility and authority, it would be an intrepid trustee who gave orders to the chief of surgery in a large university hospital. The constraints on the chief's behavior come from cooperation and competition with his peers. However, in spite of the power of the medical professional, some changes in his role are occurring. If he wishes his patients to receive care within the institution, he must be willing to have his care scrutinized by others — members of various institutional review committees.

In a setting that is necessarily bureaucratic, physicians describe quality medical care as "customized, individualized care under the direction of a competent practitioner" (Scott 1972, p. 152). The needs of individual patients take precedence over an organization's need for routine and predictability in work arrangements that are required to care for an aggregate of patients. This concept of quality in medical care supports the continuation of autonomous practice within an organization and provides a rationale both for medical independence of hospital rules and regulations as well as medical input at all levels of decision-making.

There are many reasons for the continuing dominance of hospitals by physicians. Their array of curative techniques is sophisticated; they may no longer be the benign comforters of tradition, but they postpone death and make people well. They control access to hospital beds, so that hospital administrators as well as patients must await their decision to institutionalize the patient. They control access to drugs, so that pharmacists cannot function without their prescriptions and patients cannot indulge to any great extent in self-medication for cure or relief of pain. They control access to patients, so that nurses cannot be paid to give nursing care without the authorization of physicians. They are wealthy — in contrast both to patients and to any other member of a health team — and in this country their social standing is high. This very real dominance complicates both the lines of authority and the social efficiency of the system. Physicians can demand and receive personnel and equipment resources essential for what they perceive to be optimal care for any of their patients; medical staff may make the same demands in the name of all patients (Pellegrino 1972). Clinical decision-making is considered the prerogative of the physician, but the managerial and economic complications of any decision are not his responsibility.

Evaluation of medical performance by the organization is difficult because an audit of professional behavior can only be carried out by other members of the profession. If an effort is made to exercise control through some nonmedical hierarchy, there is resistance from the physicians; if evaluation is turned over to professional peers, the organization loses control. In any case, administrators cannot ever say or even know exactly what the professional contribution should be. This is resolved to some extent (Hall 1972, p. 223) by allowing the professionals to control themselves (e.g., through institutional review boards) with some member accountable for the work of the unit collectively.

NURSES

Nurses are employed by the institution to care for patients residing in the institutions. They ascribe to professionalism, indicating that they can identify and utilize a body of knowledge specific to nursing in the care of patients. They identify only one dependent function: implementation of physician directives regarding the medical treatment of patients. Realistically, their status as personnel, with responsibility to the institution, is much more clearly defined than their status as professionals who control their own practice. The position of the nurse in the institution is dominant in that nursing is the only group caring for patients 24 hours a day, 7 days a week; further, nurses are the largest group in the health-care system. However, there is some confusion as to their position. There is considerable ambiguity concerning nursing responsibility and nursing authority. Nurses themselves indicate they are responsible to their patients and to their profession. However, they are paid by the institution and are responsible for carrying out those functions for which they are paid. Because their professional organization may serve (at the state or local level) as a bargaining agent between institution and nurses, the ambiguity is confounded. They are responsible for the care they give, but that care may be inhibited or stopped by a physician or a hospital administrator.

Multiple subordination is obvious, and it generates difficult working relations. Nurses report to their nursing supervisor, but also to physicians. Clearly they control their own practice only when that practice is accepted by physicians as appropriate, and by hospital administrators as something they are willing to fund. Generally, when compared with personnel policies in other institutions, hospital wages are low and conditions of employment are unfavorable. Pension plans are lacking, working schedules are awkward, and there is little room for upward mobility (Somers and Somers 1967). The overwhelming predominance of women in nursing is seen as a special characteristic of hospital employment contributing to complacency in administration. Somers and Somers (1967, p. 125) suggest that employers—in an effort to solve problems without addressing structure, guildism, or tradition—think answers are to be found in more money and more people rather than in more productivity. The increased militancy in women is reflected in an increased militancy in nursing. Hospital authorities are now required to deal with collective bargaining, and even strikes, by nurses. It is interesting to note that when nurses do strike, the issues are usually productivity and control of nursing practice, rather than wage and pension increases.

The personnel status of licensed practical nurses and nursing assistants is clear: they are hired by the institution to carry out certain division and/or patient-care activities. The personnel status of registered nurses is perhaps less clear because their tasks and functions are expected to be respondent to patient and physician needs. They are, however, employees of the organization, rather than visitors and entrepreneurs. As they do not bring in patients or prescribe drugs, and because they do not have the technological armamentarium of the physicians, their power vis-à-vis the organization resides in their numbers and in patients' need for their constant presence. They are ubiquitous, and when they become less so (as, for instance, when they strike), their absence is felt. However, their current status is such that the rules for employees take precedence over the rules for professionals. While this is not entirely appropriate, when professional goals are accomplished in an institution, some attention must still be given to the responsibility of the professional to incorporate duties to the institution into the activities of patient-care management.

POWER BASES

There is general agreement among social scientists that power is concerned with relations between two or more persons in which the behavior of one is affected by the behavior of the other (Hall 1972, p. 204). The essence of the concept is that one person has power over another if the other is influenced to do what he otherwise would not do; that is, power is relational, and cannot be exercised in isolation. Weber (Hall 1972, p. 206) differentiates power from authority in terms of force as opposed to judgment; power implies force or coercion, and authority involves suspension of judgment. Directives of authority are followed because of the belief that they should be, and compliance is voluntary because there is a common value system among organizational members. This differentiation is not particularly useful in examining the role of nurses in the hospital system, as there are neither common values nor common goals among organization members. Also, of course, there are many kinds of coercion. Nurses are subject to economic coercion by administrators; physicians coerce both by law (medical orders are legally directive to nurses) and by tradition. Within the structure of nursing it is appropriate to consider authority and leadership; when nursing is understood to be an element in the health-care system, in interaction with other elements, it is necessary to talk of power.

In the typology developed by French and Raven (1968) power is interpersonal, based on the relationship between the power-holder and the power-recipient. They identify (1) reward power, in which meaningful reward for the recipient is involved; (2) punishment power, in which punishment can be meted out to the recipient by the holder; (3) legitimate power, in which the recipient perceives that he has the obligation to follow directions the holder has a right to give; (4) referent power, given by a recipient because he identifies with the power holder and tries to be like him; and (5) expert power, held when special knowledge claimed by the holder is necessary to the recipient. All of the power bases described above are utilized in the hospital setting.

Because the amount of power in a system is not a fixed amount for all time, it may be possible to expand the amount of nursing power within the system without subtracting from that held by others (e.g., physicians, administrators, patients). However, at least some of the authority desired by nursing is at present explicitly held only by physicians: e.g., information control and clinical decision-making. Sharing of this authority with nursing is not likely to be encouraged by any of the three other groups, although they are not particularly in agreement with each other either. The demands of physicians for the resources of the hospital for individual patients must now be adjusted somewhat to the perceptions of hospital administrators, who allocate resources to meet the needs of aggregates of patients. However, the power of physicians to alter hospital policy, goals, or commitments by addressing any decision as a *clinical* decision is evident, as they determine what is "good" for patients, and the good of patients is the organization goal.

Administrators may consider the implementation of policies set by professional staff to be their domain, but the reward-and-punishment power bases from which they operate affect only the lower echelons, and their legitimate power is not well recognized by those who operate from referent and expert power bases.

Nurses may imagine that they can derive power from assuming the role of patient advocate, thus further legitimizing their attempts to develop professional autonomy. There is, however, some question as to whether patients perceive nurses as advocates. They may indeed mediate between the patient and the system, but the tendency to align with the most powerful persons (thereby providing a referent power base to these persons) leads patients to refer to "my" doctor but "the" nurses; they tend to believe that when they want something that is denied or given grudgingly by the nursing staff, complaint to their physicians will procure what they wish. This is not unrealistic. The patient pays the physician to protect him as an individual; he does not pay the institution or the staff for this. His well-being and his comfort he perceives to be dependent on his physician. The myth of Dr. Welby is comforting and difficult to relinquish.

Whatever the bases of power, power relationships do not always follow hierarchical organizational lines. Those departments or systems that are most critical to the viability of the organization are likely to be those with the most power, regardless of their placement in an organization chart. Dornbusch and Scott (1975) identify two kinds of professional organization: (1) autonomous, in which participants enjoy autonomy from administrative control; and (2) heteronomous, in which professionals are subordinates to the administrative framework, although not so much so as in patently bureaucratic organizations. It is obvious that for physicians the hospital is an autonomous professional organization; for nurses it is heteronomous.

However, lower-echelon participants may also exercise power over the system. Their power is based on their technical expertise, difficulty in replacement, personal relations with power figures outside of the work setting, a physical location or position in which they have control of access to information, the formation of coalitions and meticulous knowledge of the organizational rules under which they operate (Hall 1972, p. 229). All of these sources of power are open to individual nurses, but they do not advance the expert power base of nursing as a whole.

No power arrangement is optimal for all organizations, and power frameworks in any organization change through time. Hall suggests (1972, p. 235) that the nature of the personnel, the tasks of the organization, and the conditions of technology and environment determine which power arrangements are optimal for a given institution. Shifts in allocations of power may or may not be accompanied by conflict. The kinds of shifts that would result in nursing autonomy almost certainly would generate conflict, as the power bases of nursing (legitimate power and expert power) can expand only at the expense of both hospital-administrator and physician groups. If nurses with power continued to espouse the concept of caring for the holistic person that is now advanced by nurses without power, patients would gain by the expansion. Hall (1972, p. 325) states that conflict is vital to organizations: they do not remain viable when conflict is not present. This conflict may also be vital to the profession of nursing, which cannot remain viable without power.

Authority

Authority can be distinguished from power in that power is the ability of a system member to distribute valued sanctions to other members, and authority is the normative regulation of this relation (Dornbusch and Scott 1975, p. x).

The Weberian typology of authority is still widely used in organization analysis. Weber identified legal authority, which is based on belief in the right of those in authority to exercise power over subordinates; charismatic authority, based on personal characteristics; and traditional authority, based on a belief in established order. Peabody (Hall 1972, p. 215) distinguishes four forms of authority: (1) the authority of position (power is based in rewards and punishment); (2) the authority of legitimacy (power based in the obligation to follow the directions given by someone with the right to give them); (3) the authority of competence (power based on content expertise); and (4) the authority of person (power based in identification with power holder). Disruption occurs if employee characteristics (e.g., number of professionals and degree of professionalism) demand one class of authority structure and the organization operates under another class. Hospitals — in which large numbers of personnel in varying stages of professionalism, guildism, and unionism must work together in the same setting — exemplify institutions with multiple overlapping authority structures that are frequently in conflict.

The concept of authority requires the concept of *acceptance;* there is no authority without willingness to accept another's decision. Simon (1957) has suggested four motivating factors in the acceptance of authority: rewards and sanctions; legitimacy; social approval; and confidence in competence. Rewards and sanctions are present when the person exercising authority can dictate consequences of acceptance or refusal; for instance, hiring, firing, demotion, or promotion. Perception of the legitimate right to give orders and the obligation to accept them is a strong motivator in a hospital setting. The undoubted right of the physician to give medical orders to personnel is a strong support to the authority structure. Whether an order is "medical" merely because it is given by a physician is a possible source of conflict. Authority is accepted when rejection would generate disapproval by a reference group, and it is obvious that one difficulty in the development of power bases in nursing is the difficulty in identifying a nursing reference group. Presently there is evidence to suggest that in the institutional setting the approval of physicians is more important to nurses than the approval of patients, and both are more important than the approval of nursing peers. Acceptance of the authority of confidence is motivated by perception of technical competence. In the hospital setting, the "legitimate" order-givers belong to that group with the best developed technical competence, providing strong motivating factors for the acceptance of physician authority by all personnel in all situations. Whether authority is categorized on the basis of the motivational bases for the acceptance of authority or on the power bases of those exercising authority, it is obvious that in itself authority is value-free. It is the consequences of the exercise of authority which become value-laden. Simon (1957) suggests that authority can be regarded as coercive when it is primarily based in sanctions and used to promote the interests of the holder at the expense of the interests of the recipient. It is manipulation when it is based on disparity between the parties in techniques of persuasion or negotiation, and used to promote the interests of the stronger against the weaker. However, authority perceived as legitimate is not likely to be experienced as either coercion or manipulation by either party.

Authority is utilized to control the behavior of subordinates rather than the supervisors; employees, however, have options of minimal performance, literal performance, and nonperformance to help resist the exercise of authority perceived as illegitimate (Simon 1957). Nurse employees unfortunately lack this range of behaviors, as their performance is in response to patient needs. Nonacceptance by nurses of the exercise of authority they perceive to be illegitimate is compounded by perceptions of the need to protect patients from the consequences of nursing struggles to establish power bases in their effort to avoid acceptance of illegitimate authority.

If active participation in decision-making by those who will be affected by the proposed changes is a necessary component to acceptance of changes, nurses employed in institutions may find themselves unable to institute expanded power bases for their practice. Presently it is difficult to identify a source of nursing authority in the institution setting. Nurse-administrators have the authority of sanction and legitimacy only as these are provided by organization rules and procedures. Their authority is over nurses; but this is not specifically a *nursing* authority, as is evidenced by the trend toward employing directors of nursing and nursing division managers who are not nurses. The lack of an easily identifiable technology of nursing weakens the claim to the authority of competence, and while charismatic nurses who can exercise the authority of person exist, they are not likely to be found in an institutional setting.

Authority is a function of the formal organization, with its status and norms; the right and the obligation to exercise authority is attached to certain statuses. Bierstadt (1954) suggests that authority may only exist when it is not questioned; when questions start to be asked, authority is undermined. He believes the rationale for authority is to be found in the factors that induced individuals to associate. Associations are formed to meet needs, and sick individuals who need care accept the authority of care-givers in order to meet the needs generated by ill health. However, care-givers in institutions do not all occupy the same status or meet (or even identify) the same patient needs. The power variable is a basic component of the relationship among nurses, patients, and physicians — most particularly when patients are institutionalized. In this situation, in which both conflicting and parallel interests are present, nurses and patients — as the weakest members of the triad — will depend on persuasion rather than the exercise of authority to move toward their goals. Indeed, the nurse who is system-wise and persuasive may be able to accomplish more nursing goals with her patients than the nurse who has merely nursing competencies to offer.

Leadership

Most investigators (e.g., Hall 1972; Bierstadt 1954) differentiate in some way between authority and leadership, although Simon (1957) argues that authority depends on the acceptance by a subordinate of a supervisor decision and is therefore strongly related to leadership. Within an organization, the distinction is usually made between the formal right to direct others' performance given by some contractual agreement and the ability to influence others to act in a desired fashion. Authority is found only in the formal organization, while leadership may occur in either formal or informal organizations. Bierstadt (1954) contrasts authority (which *requires* competence on the part of a subordinate as a right and obligation derived from the organization) with leadership (which depends upon the personal qualities of an individual that enable him to influence others). He considers the exercise of leadership to contain three dimensions: the leader (including competence, attitudes, intellect, needs); the followers (including competence, expectations, attitudes, needs); and the situation (including societal or group values, and formal or informal organization and communication channels). Leaders cannot require obedience, and the leader-follower relation is always personal. The authority relationship is one of superordination and subordination; the leadership relationship is one of dominance and submission. Authority is a function of power, while leadership is a species of influence (Bierstadt 1954).

Hall (1972, p. 244), however, perceives leadership as the exercise of a particular kind of power: referent power. Leadership implies change of preference in followers to agree with leader preference, while power implies only that preferences are held in abeyance.

Two contrasting approaches to the role of leader are identified: authoritarian (task or instrumental) and supportive (socioemotional) approaches. The two forms are likely to conflict, and the organizational demands will determine which is successful. Etzioni (1965) suggests that it is not possible for first-line supervisors operating as task leaders to improve their socioemotive leadership qualities because they will then come in conflict with already-present socioemotive leaders in the informal organization. Head nurses — who are certainly first-line supervisors and task leaders — are also required to provide socioemotive leadership by virtue of the fact that they are nurses. In effect, if the Etzioni views are accurate, the two kinds of leadership are virtually exclusive. This certainly has implications for nurses, who are required by the nature of nursing to excel at both simultaneously.

Leadership traits are apparently not standard across all conditions (Hall 1972, p. 247), and by whom, and in what manner leadership is expressed will depend on the situation. Different situations will demand different forms of leadership, so that individuals with particular skills and behaviors will be called for; leadership depends on congruence between the situation, and the characteristics of the person who is appointed, elected, or assumes the leadership role (1972, p. 248).

Although authoritarian leadership is currently not fashionable, it is not clear that socioemotive leadership results in higher levels of production — although it is likely to generate positive attitudes in subordinates. Filley and House (1969) suggest that supportive leaders are best (1) when decisions are not routine, but need not be made rapidly; (2) when required information is not standardized or centralized; and (3) when subordinates believe in the legitimacy of their decision-making and are comfortable working without close supervision.

There is some difficulty in applying these theoretical and empirical notions to nurses working in the hospital setting. Etzioni (1965) has suggested that in socializing and other expressive organizations, socioemotive leadership is appropriate; it is less so in coercive and segregating organizations, because of the predominance of instrumental power sources. A hospital has socializing, expressive, coercive, and segregating components, and both instrumental and socioemotive leaders. It is tempting to assign the label of "instrumental leaders" to the physicians, operating with their advanced technology developed to meet task goals, and the label of "socioemotive leaders" to the nurses, whose major function in any situation may be supportive. However, this assignment of role does not articulate well with the perceptions of the patients, who are likely to want physicians to operate in a supportive role and who are not willing to accept support from anyone else. Further, this concept is not a realistic perception in that presently head nurses and supervisors are explicitly assigned to an instrumental role by the institution — although they are also expected to behave in a supportive way to personnel, physicians, and patients.

In a predominately female discipline it is perhaps necessary to differentiate very clearly amongst socioemotive leadership behavior, supportive nursing behavior, and the seductive and persuasive behaviors manifested by persons of least power in situations in which they wish to meet their own goals.

Golembiewski (1961) identifies three leadership styles: leader-centered (autocratic or authoritarian), group-centered (democratic), and individual-centered (each group member operates at his own initiative). He does not identify any "best" style, agreeing with other writers that styles and even leaders must change to meet situations. His description of the four conditions to take into account when choosing a leadership style (and therefore a leader from a group of potential leaders) is useful to nursing. The conditions are: (1) personality (not all persons function well under the same style); (2) task characteristics (tasks of different complexity and the need for coordination may require different styles for completion); (3) task roles (supervisor, subordinate, mixed); and (4) characteristics of the group (group norms and goals).

There is evidence that while a group-centered style may be appropriate when tasks are complex and require interpersonal cooperation, the leader-centered style may be useful at other times. Situations are not uncommon in nursing in which tasks are complex and require cooperation, but at the same time require the immediate making and implementation of decisions. When institution regulations are added there is some question as to which leadership style is most appropriate. Also, in its task roles, nursing, more than other groups in the hospital system, is likely to function in mixed roles.

It is clear from the preceding discussion that leadership is not easily reduced to a set of guidelines that are always appropriate. Gross (1961) suggests it is best not to speak of a leader at all, but rather to identify leader behaviors. He believes that such behaviors may be concentrated in one person or spread out over many. His dimensions of leader behavior include: goal definition, goal clarification, means clarification, task assignment and coordination, motivation, and integration. Gross contends that some of these dimensions may be incompatible, and that one person is not likely to be able to do them all. The problem is not to find a leader, but to decide which dimension is called for by the current goals and tasks. However, it is possible that a leader who is called in for one dimension may be extremely reluctant to move out of the leader role when another dimension is called for. The emergence of generals on the political scene when an active war is followed by an uneasy peace and generals can no longer make unilateral decisions is a matter of record. While the impact of persons endeavoring to enact a leadership role regardless of the demands of the situation may be diluted on a national scene, it is bound to make itself felt at the organization level.

Kline and Martin (1958) have pointed out that in situations that demand management it is not easy to retain freedom. The authoritarian leadership styles get the institutional tasks accomplished in most cases, although in hospitals patients and personnel may be uneasy with such controls. The dilemma found in the cultural stress on individual freedom and the institution's stress on authority, direction, and control, is compounded for nurses. The profession stresses the freedom to nurse and the necessity to use the nursing body of knowledge; the institution stresses the dependent function of implementing physician directives and the task of regulating visitors and patients. Progress in nursing, meeting nursing goals, and giving high-quality care to patients depend on the utilization and expansion of nursing knowledge. Institutions, however, foster the least expensive use of some part of nursing knowledge (that which is most visibly reflected in patient outcomes and physician satisfaction) and inhibit creativity and innovation, which are likely to be expensive and probably threatening to system stability.

Kline and Martin (1958) suggest that the freedom-control dilemma may be resolved if the concept of delegating *authority* to act gives way to delegating *freedom* to act. A person with the delegated authority to act may indeed have the power to do so, but the implication is that she acts in an approved manner. The person with the freedom to act has clearly defined boundaries, but within those boundaries she can accomplish the task in her own way. The real test of freedom in this instance is whether the supervisor will support a subordinate in carrying out a task in a manner different from her own. For this to work, the supervisor must maintain and assure noninterference for the subordinate, and the structure must be such that the freedoms of different individuals do not clash. The delegation of freedom to act requires at least five conditions: (1) an appropriate attitude on the part of the superior; (2) the development of a comprehensive system of rules; (3) maintenance of adequate systems of communication and information; (4) comprehensive followup activities; and (5) an atmosphere sympathetic to the exercise of freedom.

The first condition — the supervisor's supportive attitude toward subordinate freedom — may be difficult to achieve in a health-care institution. Because the supervisor does not lose responsibility for outcomes, she may not be willing to lose control over the means of achieving them. The supervisor must be able to see herself in the role of teacher rather than as an authority and action taker, and this may not be considered realistic in the patient-care situation. The system of rules is twofold: rules aimed toward structuring the situation, and rules addressed directly to the behavior of personnel. The former are situational rules, and they influence behavior indirectly. Behavioral rules demand certain fairly specific actions, and state what should be done in the event of stated occurrences. Behavioral rules may be rules of duty ("must" or "shall" statements, in which disobedience incurs penalty) and rules of reason, stated in "should" or "ought" form. The implication is that any rational person would act as is set forth in the rule, and there is no penalty for disobedience because the responsibility for action is with the individual rather than a higher authority. For subordinates to have freedom to act, the use of situational rules — with a strong mix of behavioral rules of reason — is probably the most appropriate structure. Behavior according to rules of reason demands knowledge to predict the consequences of behavior; the right information at the correct time is crucial to the general exercise of freedom to act. Follow-up becomes the responsibility of the subordinate to whom freedom to act is granted, and should be in terms of whether or not goals are met. The final condition — the atmosphere of freedom which must permeate the institution — is not a condition likely to be found in a hospital because patients are a basic part of the hospital system, and they, along with physicians, would have to be educated into comfort with the explicit delegation of freedom to act to both nurses and patients.

Nonetheless, nurses working in institutions must develop and maintain legitimate power bases from which they can make and implement nursing decisions. In a paper that addresses the development of a framework for professional collective bargaining, Cleland (1978) has proposed an adaptation of the Baldridge (1971) political model of university governance as an appropriate scheme for nursing administrators in hospital settings. The following material draws heavily on the Cleland paper; her suggested schema for shared governance is presented here as a means to the development of nursing authority to make nursing decisions in the health agency.

As Cleland points out, the professional nurse is licensed by the state, giving her a legal base for expert power that is independent of any institution. Professional licensure also makes her accountable for her activities and the activities of those under her direction. In this period of health-system development and civil-rights legislation, health-care providers — although they retain authority over technical aspects of care — are no longer able to make unilateral policy decisions. A format for shared decision-making is required. In reference to university decision-making, Baldridge (1971, p. 12) advances the political model of governance, the essence of which is that it voluntarily and formally recognizes that divergent interest groups — having different values and bringing pressures to bear upon the goals and practices of the institutions — must come to some consensus. Cleland has adapted the assumptions and framework of the model to hospital governance. She compares the two institutions and notes that health agencies and universities have in common the organization of large numbers of highly trained and specialized professionals; their product is human service; and work units are difficult to define. The public has a valid concern for quality and cost of services in both institutions, but at the same time cannot ascertain effectiveness independent of professional input.

Cleland's model (Fig. 1) utilizes a pattern of nursing committees and councils; it stresses the necessity for clarity as to which positions and committees are advisory and which have decision-making authority. The following material is quoted from Cleland's paper (pp. 39–43).

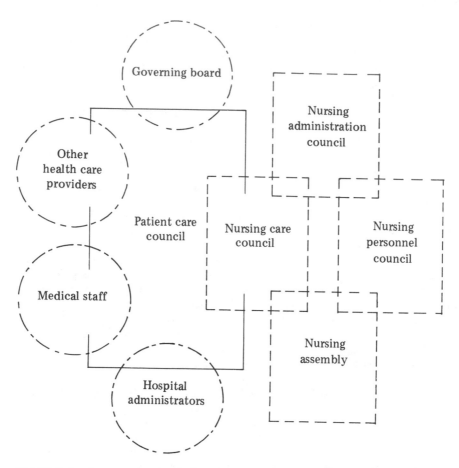

FIGURE 1. Suggested schema for shared governance. *(From Cleland: J Nurs Admin 5:39, 1978)*

The Nursing Assembly would consist of not only general duty nurses, but also head nurses and even supervisors if it can be shown that the majority of their day-to-day decisions derive from patient care data or information. The Nursing Administration Council would consist of those nurses whose day-to-day decisions derive from information originating in the nursing office. From these two groups, members would be elected to serve on either the Nursing Personnel Council or the Nursing Care Council.

The Nursing Personnel Council would be responsible for developing and maintaining a system of evaluation of all nursing personnel. Merit increases in salary and staff terminations could be tied to these evaluations. In addition, this council would make recommendations in the areas of salary schedules, modification of fringe benefits, and the approval of educa-

tion leaves and travel requests. Another important responsibility of the Personnel Council would be to appoint small search committees who, after internal and external survey, would recommend two or three persons for vacancies in head nurse or supervisory positions. The director of nursing should make the final appointments.

The Nursing Care Council would be responsible for developing the policies relating to standards of practice. Changes in nursing procedures, practices, and staffing ratios would be developed by this group. This council would be responsible for approving both the goals of nursing service and the standards used in the institution for evaluating the quality of nursing care.

One or two members from the Nursing Care Council would be elected to serve on the institution's Patient Care Council, which would have representation from every professional group in the institution directly involved with care. In addition, there would be representation from hospital administration and, most importantly, consumers from the institution's governing board.

Until board members become involved in the issues of patient care, not much will happen in most hospitals. The board cannot meet its responsibility to the public by merely studying the ledger sheets and adding new and exotic treatment facilities in competition with those of other institutions! The Patient Care Council must in some manner have direct communication to the board separate from that of hospital administration and the medical staff.

The Patient Care Council should provide the board with its own recommendations for priorities in the development of new programs of care or the curtailment of services no longer needed. Among other responsibilities the Patient Care Council should provide the mechanism and procedures for hearing cases involving patients' rights. The Committee which approves research protocols should be a sub-committee of the Patient Care Council rather than of the medical staff.

Cleland suggests that such modification of bureaucracy will make the hospital a more attractive work setting for professional nurses, and involve staff in control over conditions of work. Nurse leaders can be identified, but perhaps the primary benefit of shared governance will be an increase in the real power of nursing administration, in that recommendations dealing with nursing care and patient needs are more likely to be acceptable when they are made by the appropriately constituted Councils. Cleland perceives the development of such a system of shared governance occurring slowly because of the education that must accompany the changes; however, professionally autonomous employees in nursing will assist in meeting organization goals.

However, because it involves the development of power in the nursing system at the expense of the medical and administrative systems, there is some question as to whether Cleland's rational pattern of organization will ever be realized in the hospital setting. Hospital administrators currently coping with one autonomous professional group are not likely to welcome the advent of another such group, however well motivated, and Board members do not yet understand that nursing is separate from medicine. However, the Nursing Assembly and Councils can be developed within the nursing system, which would provide a union and a sense of community to nurses that may well give them the strength to move the development of an interdisciplinary patient-care council.

Communication

Kline and Martin (1965) suggest that while institutions are supposed to be organized for the most effective use of knowledge and skills, it is probable that the chief characteristic of the command hierarchy is not knowledge but ignorance. It is possible to know only a fraction of what is going on, and perceptions of "facts" may be erroneous. Kline and Martin state that at any given time vastly more is not known than is known either by one person in a command chain or by all the organization; further, organization into a hierarchy of authority for the purpose of increasing efficiency may merely institutionalize ignorance.

In spite of this depressingly realistic assessment, there is no doubt that the exercise of power is related to control of the amount and accuracy of relevant information, and therefore to the control of information networks.

In his discussion of the characteristics of communication flow in organizations, Guetzkow (1965) examines the combination of organization components involved; whether the process is simultaneous or serial; and whether the form is transitory or storable. In the hospital setting, communication is likely to be from one to several (doctor to nurse, patient, family; head nurse to several team leaders; team leader to team); this occurs because numbers of personnel are likely to be utilizing the same information, particularly in the patient-care situation. The timing may be either simultaneous or serial (when different members of the organization get the same message at different times); for instance, the physician tells several nurses about a terminal prognosis but does not provide the patient or the family with the same information. Serial provision of relevant information has implications for the functioning of individuals in relation to each other, and problems in coordination arise at the system level because of time lag within information flow. Correction of messages may be delayed, and may only be possible through informal channels. In the hospital, the original message may be given from one to many, but the correction of the message may be given only to one, who is responsible for sending it on. Oral messages compete with written messages for attention, but they do not provide a permanent record unless they are on tape. However, written information may not be permanent either; it may be filed incorrectly or not at all, and may not reflect the actual information in any case. Patients' records, particularly the nursing portions, are notoriously incomplete and incorrect in terms of situations that are discussed orally at shift-change reports. Whatever the format of information delivery, there is a relationship between organization size and effectiveness: the larger the organization, the less effective the communication flow.

Whether relevant information is provided through vertical or lateral communication nets is important to nursing. When communication is through contacts between status circuits (lateral) rather than along administrative lines (vertical), nursing may not receive the message simply because nurses are not part of status circuits. If the hospital administrator, two members of the Board of Trustees, and the Chief of Surgery get together for dinner and cards, and talk, incidentally, about how to spend a fifty-thousand-dollar gift which one of the Board members has just been told about, the decision is not likely to be to spend the money for nursing.

Communication channels in organizations are not single; they consist of a number of networks varying from well-structured nets carrying task-related messages to *ad hoc* nets developed in response to organization emergencies. Guetzkow (1965, pp. 543–548) discusses communication channels in organizations in terms of authority, information exchanges, task expertise, friendship, and status.

AUTHORITY

Channels of interaction in the authority net are defined in terms of the legitimacy that one individual or group has vis-à-vis another with respect to issuing directives. The dominant feature of such nets is directionality: orders flow vertically from a few individuals at the top. The authority network in nursing is not so clearly defined, as orders flow to nurses from the top and also from all sides.

INFORMATION EXCHANGES

Messages on this net are usually concerned with knowledge about the state of affairs with respect to the internal operations of the organization and its external environment. However, this net can be used by those in authority to supply information to lower-echelon members. Also, whether a message is regarded as a command or as information may be a matter of interpretation, and authority may regard itself as handing down directives that subordinates perceive as information and advice. The lateral communications are probably essential to proper functioning of the vertical system. When regularized vertical channels do not function adequately, new specialized channels may be developed. Difficulties are encountered when formally prescribed means of communication are at variance with the informal operating actualities in an information system.

TASK EXPERTISE

This net handles communications involved in bringing technical knowledge to task performances. The dominant feature of this network is segmentation, as islands of expertise are constructed throughout the organization. As technical bases for organizational activities become increasingly salient (as they are in hospitals), problem-solving communication seems to develop channels of its own. Organization members with special technical expertise consistently evade official prescriptions in order to accomplish their own goals. Authoritative channels are avoided by the experts when they bring their own knowledge to bear upon their specialized tasks. There is overlap in the communication structures involved in transmission of messages concerned with authority, information, and expertise because all three are involved in task specialization.

FRIENDSHIP

This is perhaps the most segmented of all the nets, existing as localized linkages among clusters of individuals who find each other's company rewarding. Messages devoted to authority, information, and expertise also carry overtones of feeling of one individual for another; this double usage illustrates the manner in which nets devoted to different kinds of messages share the same communication channel.

STATUS

These nets are even less well defined than friendship nets, but appear all pervasive. They are used by all members of the organization in interactions with each other. When contact between individuals of differing status takes place, communication from superior to subordinate takes place more easily than communication from subordinate to superior. Those who serve effectively in liaison roles must be well linked into two or more networks.

Information exchange is a major component in organization, and exchange occurs within the units of a system (departments, groups, and individuals) and between a system and its external environment. Hall (1972, p. 271) says:

> Communication is most important, therefore, in organizations and organizational segments that must deal with uncertainty, are complex, and have a technology that does not permit easy routinization. . . . The more an organization is people and idea-oriented, the more important communication becomes.

It is clear from this quotation that information exchange is paramount in the patient-care setting.

The process of communication is relational in that it always involves a sender and a receiver, and message content is affected by the social impact of one on the other. The content of a message will be perceived differently by two receivers, one of whom is afraid of the sender.

In order to be best implemented, information should be provided to all system members to whom it is relevant, in an affectively appropriate manner. As Hall points out (1972, p. 272) this means that "neither too much nor too little information is in the system, and that it is clear from the outset who can utilize what is available." He describes social and organizational factors impinging on the perception and use of information.

Social factors common to all perceptual situations are basic conditions in the communication process in organizations. These elements include response to cues of which one is unaware, the influence of emotional factors, the use of irrelevant cues, unequal weighting of information, and decisions made on the basis of inadequate information. Personal needs, values, and interests are part of the process, as is perception of the other in the information relation. The phenomenon of stereotyping also affects communication (Hall 1972): the exercise of authority based on expertise is more difficult for a group that has been perceived in the past as powerless and dependent on physicians' direction for task completion. Social factors affecting information exchange are compounded by organizational factors. "Vertical and horizontal considerations greatly affect the communication process" (Hall 1972, p. 275).

In vertical communication, information flow is both downward and upward. Kinds of downward flow include (1) job instruction (a subordinate is told what to do); (2) rationale for the task, including its relationship with the rest of the system; (3) information regarding organization procedures; (4) feedback to the individual regarding his performance; and (5) ideology, the socialization into acceptance of system goals (Katz and Kahn 1966, pp. 239–242). In this information system, the superior decides who gets what information and when, a crucial role in the organization.

Katz and Kahn (1966) reduce the form of upward communication to what an individual reports about his own performance, what he reports about others' performance, comment about policy and procedure, and comment about what tasks need to be accomplished and how this can be done. Information flowing upward is influenced by considerations of rank and power. It is condensed and summarized by middle managers before it reaches the top, providing a source of middle-managerial influence in both directions.

Vertical communication is carried out through formal organization channels; horizontal communication among peers is necessary for the coordination of effort to accomplish system goals. Horizontal communication may be task oriented or affective in nature, and may take place among peers in the same unit or across units. The implementation of directives handed down through vertical channels is impossible without horizontal information exchange, as is exemplified by the logistics of the patient-admission process. Coordination between units that may be in conflict as to both means and goals requires a horizontal information flow. Chiefs may issue orders, but the implementing Indians must have their own coordinating discussions, providing or withholding information to each other as either action is appropriate to meet their own goals along with the organization's goals.

Aside from the structure of information flow, and the effect of structure on message content, the intent of a message can also be changed within the message itself. Guetzkow (1965, pp. 550–561) identifies two major types of message transformation: omission and distortion. Omission can occur as information is passed through the system when any recipient is unable to grasp all the content and relays only that portion he understands, or when communication overload occurs and there is more information in the system than it can accommodate. Omission may also be deliberate; parts of a message may be deleted in order to keep various segments of the organization in ignorance.

Messages are distorted — that is, meanings are altered — because individuals are selective, either consciously or unconsciously, about what they perceive. Altered meanings are recommunicated, compounding the problem. This occurs in all communication systems, but it is particularly crucial for organizations because they depend upon accurate communication as a basis for rational decision-making (Hall 1972).

Accuracy may be maintained, or restored, by repetition; redundancy is achieved either by repeating the messages, by varying their form, or by using more than one channel. However, repetition itself may also interfere with accuracy, as it will add to the system load. If the repetition itself is not entirely accurate, the recipient will not know which of several messages is correct.

Verification by means of testing the understanding of earlier messages requires feedback from recipient to sender, which may not be feasible in an institution such as a hospital, where much information is based in specialty expertise and deals with emergent situations.

There is no distortion-proof information system as, along with the errors in understanding dictated by the human organization components of the system, intentional distortion may be a source of power. The individual who controls information relevant to the operation of the system is in a position to control the behavior of other members of the system.

The intent of this brief overview of organization theories and components is to point out that hospitals *are* organizations and thus subject to the same functions and dysfunctions as other organizations. While it might seem gratuitous to make such a statement, the tendency of patients and physicians to blame nurses for organization dysfunctions — and the tendency of nurses to assume responsibity and guilt for events and consequences they cannot control — makes it necessary to gain clearer insight into how an organization actually works.

References

Baldridge J: Models of university governance: bureaucratic, collegial and political. Stanford, Ca., Stanford Center for Research and Development in Teaching, Research and Development, Memorandum No. 77, 1971

Bierstadt R: The problem of authority. In Berger M, Abel T, Page C (eds), Freedom and Control in Modern Society. New York, Van Nostrand, 1954

Bochmeyer A, Hartman G (eds): The Hospital in Modern Society. New York, Commonwealth Fund, 1943, p. 5

Boulding KE: General systems theory — the skeleton of a science. Management Sci 2 (3):197, 1956

Cartwright D: Influence, leadership, control. In March JG (ed), Handbook of Organizations. Chicago, Rand McNally, 1965

Castles M, Keith P: Patient concerns, emotional resources and perceptions of nurse and patient roles. Omega 10, 1979

Cleland V: A framework for professional collective bargaining. J Nurs Admin 5:39, 1978

Dornbusch SM, Scott WR: Evaluation and the Exercise of Authority. San Francisco, Jossey-Bass, 1975

Elder R: Dying in the USA. Int J Nurs Stud 10:171, 1973

Etzioni A: Dual leadership in complex organizations. Am Sociol Rev 30 (5):688, 1965

Feldman J, Kanter HE: Organizational decision making. In March J (ed), Handbook of Organizations. Chicago, Rand McNally, 1965

Filley AC, House RJ: Managerial Processes and Organizational Behavior. Glenville, Ill.: Scott, Foresman, 1969, p. 399

French JRP, Raven B: The bases of social power. In Cartwright D, Zander A (eds), Group Dynamics, 3rd edition. New York, Harper and Row, 1968, pp. 259-269

Fuchs VR: Who Shall Live: Health, Economics and Social Choice. New York, Basic, 1974

Georgopoulous BS (ed): Organization Research on Health Institutions. Ann Arbor, Institute for Social Research, University of Michigan, 1972

Golembiewski RT: Three styles of leadership and their uses. Personnel 38 (4):34, 1961

Gross E: Dimensions of leadership. Personnel J 40 (5):213, 1961

Guetzkow H: Communications in organizations. In March J (ed), Handbook of Organizations. Chicago, Rand McNally, 1965

Hall RH: Organizations: Structure and Process. Englewood Cliffs, N.J., Prentice-Hall, 1972

Katz D, Kahn RL: The Social Psychology of Organizations. New York, Wiley, 1966

Kline BE, Martin NH: Freedom, authority and decentralization. Harvard Bus Rev 36 (3):69, 1958

Long RB: Social security and welfare reform: Summary of the principal provisions of H.R. 1 as determined by the Committee on Finance. Committee print: 92nd Congress, 2nd Session. Washington, D.C., U.S. Government Printing Office, 1972

MacEachern M: Hospital Organization and Management. Chicago, Physicians Record, 1951

March JG: Introduction. In March J (ed), Handbook of Organizations. Chicago, Rand McNally, 1965

Massie JL: Management theory. In March J (ed), Handbook of Organizations. Chicago, Rand McNally, 1965

Mauksch H: The organizational context of dying. In Kübler-Ross E (ed), Death: The Final Stages of Growth. Englewood Cliffs, N.J., Prentice-Hall, 1975

Peabody RL: Perception of organizational authority: a comparative analysis. Admin Sci Quart 6 (4):463, 1962

Pellegrino ED: The changing matrix of clinical decision-making in the hospital. In Georgopoulous B (ed), Organization Research on Health Institutions Ann Arbor, University of Michigan, 1972, pp. 301–328

Perrow C: Hospitals: technology, structure and goals. In March J (ed), Handbook of Organizations. Chicago, Rand McNally, 1965, pp. 910–971

Plachy R: Delegation and decision-making. Mod Hosp 120 (2):73, 1973

Rosengren WR, Lefton M: Hospitals and Patients. New York, Atherton, 1969

Scott WG: Organization theory: An overview and an appraisal. Acad Management J 4 (1):7, 1961

Scott WR: Professionals in hospitals: technology and the organization of work. In Georgopoulous B (ed), Organization Research on Health Institutions. Ann Arbor, Institute for Social Research, University of Michigan, 1972

Shain M, Roemer M: Hospitals and the public interests. Public Health Rep 76 (5):401, 1961

Simon HA: Authority. In Arensberg CM et al. (eds), Research in Industrial Human Relations. New York, Harper, 1957

Somers HM, Somers AR: Medicare and the Hospitals: Issues and Prospects. Washington, D.C., Brookings Institution, 1967

Stevens R: American Medicine and the Public Interest. New Haven and London: Yale University Press, 1971

Stevens R, Stevens R: Medicaid: Anatomy of a dilemma. Law and Contemporary Problems 35 (2):348, 1970

Thompson HE: Management decisions in perspective. In Schlender W, Scott W, Filley A (eds), Management in Perspective. Boston, Houghton Mifflin, 1965

Wilson RN: The social structure of a general hospital. Ann Am Acad Polit Soc Sci (March 1963)

Worthington W, Silver LH: Regulation of quality of care in hospitals: the need for change. Law and Contemporary Problems, 35 (2):305, 1970

Chapter 3

Institutionalized Dying Patients

Before we present and discuss interview material concerning institutionalized patients who are dying, and nurses who are caring for them, it is prudent to introduce the reader to an overview of philosophical and clinical definitions of death as well as information about patients' rights.

DEFINITION OF DEATH

Philosophical Perspectives

In his proposed definition of "natural death," Callahan (1977) describes it as the point when life work is accomplished, moral obligations are discharged, others will not despair, and the process of dying is not unbearably painful. He suggests that it is not reasonable to invest social money in expensive life-extending therapies; however, supportive care of the elderly should be financed, the goal of which is not to extend lives but to make them as comfortable and free of pain as possible. The concern in this instance is not with distinguishing life from death, but rather with recognizing when it is appropriate to refrain from trying to extend life.

Fulton (1972) points out that death is primarily an experience of the aged, a group of persons who are no longer central to the lives of their families. The modern technology that cures childhood diseases and repairs accident-induced injuries in young adults also allows the prolongation of biological function in the elderly or in persons suffering from degenerative disease (past the time when they manifest self-awareness or self-control).

74

Morison (1971) has addressed the concept of death in terms of process rather than event. As in other movements of human organisms from one stage (e.g., childhood) to another (e.g., adolescence), there is no one moment to be identified as the moment of transition. The process of growth and decay is continuous. Therefore "death" occurs at different times in the various sub-systems of the organism, making it difficult to attach the label "dead" to the entire organism at any one time. He suggests that "the 'life' of a complex vertebrate like man is not a clearly defined entity with sharp discontinuation at both ends . . . life is certainly not an all-or-none phenomenon" (1971). Because physiological function can continue indefinitely in the absence of human interaction, Morison suggests the necessity to "make judgments about the intactness and value of the complex interactions themselves" (1971). Clearly, in this philosophical view, the definition of death is more than cessation of respiration and circulation. In response to Morison, Kaas (1971) points out that "we should not take our bearings from the small number of unusual cases in which there is doubt. In most cases there is no doubt. There is no real need to blur the distinction between a man alive or a man dead or to undermine the concept of death as an event." Kaas believes that the question of whether death has occurred is a question of medical-scientific fact which can be answered by physicians. Veatch (1975) blames analytical confusion for disputes centered around whether death has occurred and proposes a formal definition: "Death is the irreversible loss of that which is essentially significant to the nature of man." (His contentions concerning *what* is essentially significant will be presented in the section on neocortical death.)

Philosophical perspectives of death generate useful discussion related to the development of legal definitions and of public policy — whether or not such policy is expressed in statutes. Currently, legal definitions of death vary (see Appendix C for a discussion of statutes in several states), and are tied to clinical rather than philosophical notions. In effect, the definition of death is directly related to which physiological functions can be measured, and how well. As finer measurement became possible, philosophical problems became more evident. When the event of death was tied to respiration (as indeed it still is) but respiration could only be measured grossly with a mirror at the lips, a *last* gasping breath could be identified as the end of mortal life, with no conflict between the clinician and the philosopher. The presence or absence of a soul might be a point of conflict, but it was a conflict separated from the argument as to whether an individual was alive or dead. In an institutional setting, death was clinical death and was determined by a physician to be present when respiration and heart beat could no longer be seen, felt, or heard. Death is still clinical death in the institution, but as measurement techniques and technological control of biological events improved, clinical certainty decreased, and it became necessary to involve philosophers in medical discussions and decisions.

Williams (1973, pp. 147-149) has suggested four stages of death as follows:

1. *Impending death which begins when maintenance of life seems rela-tively hopeless; this may last for weeks, months, or years. The person*

may feel relatively comfortable, and continue working. The diagnosis is known by the family; medical therapy is directed to relief of symptoms. In the stage of impending death, the person and the family can make psychological, financial and other plans for eventual death.

2. *Imminent death is present when death is expected soon, within a few days, and seems certain. Preparations for death are made by the patient, family, and others, and suffering is relieved as much as possible.*

3. *Cardiorespiratory failure, which may last for hours, occurs when the person is unconscious, when the heart stops, and successful resuscitation may or may not be possible. This stage may have a sudden or a prolonged onset. Great anxiety and horrible sensation may or may not be associated with this stage, although actual pain and suffering may be no more in this stage than in the other two.*

4. *The Hereafter, which lasts infinitely, and which is a mystery.*

Presently, the institution will probably be involved only in the second and third of these stages, although if the Hospice movement remains viable, the first stage may also be of concern in the future. For most patients, the third stage could be prolonged indefinitely, with the use of cardiopulmonary devices and intravenous infusions. The question arises as to why such prolongation is *ever* desirable. Aside from the philosophical or legal impact on physician decisions to initiate, continue, or discontinue the devices, and aside from a very real fear of movement into the fourth stage, there is at least one utilitarian reason for the use of the support machinery with selected persons. Barnes' (1974) positive evaluation of organ donation and transplantation describes that reason. He states that many persons have benefited by means of different organ transplantations provided by organ donations from deceased individuals. The organs that can be transplanted include the kidneys, skin, liver, heart, and cornea of the eye; kidney and cornea donations are most needed because these transplantations are done most frequently.

Organs can be accepted only from healthy individuals. Permission to harvest an organ must be easily available for emergency workers or physicians at the site of an accident or medical emergency; therefore, Barnes suggests that a special permission card designating organs to be donated should be carried in the wallet. He believes that organ donation can be comforting to the survivors of the deceased, as organ transplant helps another person return to living and health, and further points out that virtually no religion in the United States restricts organ donation to help another person regain health.

Only healthy organs are worth the effort to transplant. In order to provide the best chance for the recipient, they should be perfused with circulating blood for as long as possible. How much treatment, then, should be imposed on the donor, to keep an organ in good shape for a recipient? And, of course, when is the donor deceased? On which criteria do physicians base the pronouncement "deceased," regardless of whether organs are harvested?

Clinical Definitions

HEART-LUNG DEATH

In the majority of cases, and particularly in those instances in which respirators and electroencephalogram equipment are not immediately available, the definition of death is in terms of cessation of respiratory and cardiac activity. Even if dying — and death — occur in an institutional setting, the measurement of "brain death" is not likely to be carried out outside intensive-care units. In hundreds of nursing homes, extended-care facilities, and small community hospitals, patients move from the status of "living" to the status of "dead" without causing staff difficulty in deciding to which category the patient should be assigned.

Traditional criteria related to a heart-lung definition of death include cessation of vital functions, of respiration, of circulation, and the impossibility of resuscitation. These criteria are not dictated by law, although court decisions have been based on them, but are a conventional, historical basis for certifying death. However, with the development of techniques that will allow organ systems to function in the absence of conscious awareness in an individual, the issue of when or whether such an individual is dead has arisen (High 1972). A beating heart and respiration may no longer indicate that life is present.

CEREBRAL DEATH

Discussion of the state known as cerebral death has been part of the medical literature for many years. The improvement in resuscitative and supportive machinery (leading to continued biological function in comatose patients) and the growing popularity and success of transplant operations made it desirable to modify the traditional definition of death. Criteria have been developed for a definition of death based on altered states indicative of cessation of whole brain function. The Ad Hoc Committee of the Harvard Medical School to Examine the Definition of Brain Death suggested irreversible coma as a new criterion for death, and noted the characteristics of irreversible coma. They considered these to be the characteristics of "a *permanently* nonfunctioning brain" (Ad Hoc Committee 1968), although in the report of the collaborative study sponsored by the National Institute of Neurological Diseases and Stroke, an explicit distinction is drawn between cerebral death and irreversible coma. This distinction states that "Cerebral death implies total destruction of the brain so that both volitional and reflex evidences of responsivity are absent. Irreversible coma refers to a vegetating state in which all functions attributed to the cerebrum are lost, but certain vital functions . . . may be retained" (Collaborative Study 1977). The distinction has practical importance, as a number of states allow cerebral death but not irreversible coma as a means of certifying death.

The report of the Harvard group (Ad Hoc Committee 1968), states that a patient with a permanently nonfunctioning brain appears to be in deep coma. The condition is "satisfactorily diagnosed" by the first three points given below, with the fourth (electroencephalogram) giving confirmatory support. The criteria are:

1. *Unreceptivity and unresponsivity to externally applied stimuli.*
2. *No spontaneous muscular movements or spontaneous respiration.*
3. *No reflexes. Pupils fixed and dilated, no ocular movement or blinking, no postural activity, swallowing, yawning or vocalization, absent corneal and pharyngeal reflexes. The stretch of tendon reflexes not elicited.*
4. *Flat electroencephalogram.*

Criteria are not valid in the presence of hypothermia or central nervous depressants, and measurements should be repeated in 24 hours (Ad Hoc Committee 1968).

There have been some modifications in this set of criteria in the last several years (for instance, the time of the repeated measure), but basically they remain the standard. The 1977 report of the Collaborative Study group, which assessed the validity and reliability of the criteria of cerebral death, made the distinction between this and irreversible coma described above. The study identified three criteria of cerebral death to be validated. These are:

1. *Cerebral unresponsivity (deep coma): in which the patient does not respond purposively to external stimuli, obeys no commands, and does not vocalize.*
2. *Apnea: absence of spontaneous respiration for at least 15 minutes (patient makes no effort to override the respirator in that time).*
3. *Electrocerebral silence (ECS): presence of a flat EEG.*

The investigators addressed the validity and reliability of the above criteria for indicating cerebral death, as well as the prerequisites that must be met before the criteria are applied — that is, the *absence* of four conditions: sedative drug intoxication, hypothermia, cardiovascular shock, and a remedial primary disorder. On the basis of the study findings, they recommend for clinical trial the following criteria.

Prerequisite
All appropriate diagnostic and therapeutic procedures have been performed.

Criteria (to be present for 30 minutes at least six hours after the onset of coma and apnea).
Coma with cerebral unresponsivity
Apnea
Dilated pupils
Absent cephalic reflexes
Electrocerebral silence

Confirmatory Test
Absence of cerebral blood flow (Collaborative Study 1977).

The confirmatory test is suggested when an early diagnosis of cerebral death is desired. The investigators indicate that the above criteria identified subjects in the study who died within a week with evidence of a dead brain. They state that:

> *[despite] difficulties in the determination of drug intoxications, the fallacies in clinical and laboratory tests, and the inevitable observer errors . . . the chance of even temporary survival if the proposed clinical and EEG criteria are met for 30 minutes is small (Collaborative Study 1977).*

Comfort with the assessments of the indicators of cerebral death described above rests in the assumption that when brain cells die (as indicated by the criteria) the person is dead, and in consequence the behavior of the living may change to reflect this event. Assessment of the criteria is a medical function; the rationale for accepting the criteria as indicators of death is a function of values and beliefs about what constitutes humanness, and what medically identifiable loss indicates loss of the person. Veatch (*see below*) advances a conceptual clarification of the concept of death, and explores the question as to what is of critical importance in the functioning of the brain.

NEOCORTICAL DEATH

Veatch (1975) identifies four factors any one of which may be "so essentially significant to the nature of man that its loss is called death and appropriately initiates death behavior." These factors are the capacity to integrate bodily function, the capacity for rationality, the capacity to experience, and the capacity for social interaction. After presenting a persuasive argument, he combines the third and fourth factors and settles on the capacity for experience of social interaction — adding that there must be an embodiment of the capacity. The element essential to human life becomes "embodied capacity for experience and social interaction." Acceptance of this description of what is essential suggests that it is the neocortical function that must be measured, as empirical evidence suggests that the locus of the capacity to experience social interaction is to be found in the neocortex. The neocortical function is reliably measured by the electroencephalogram (Silverman et al. 1970); thus the EEG is moved from its status as a confirmatory criterion to status as the primary criterion. The findings and recommendations of the Collaborative Study move the EEG to a position of equal importance with the data of the clinical assessment. Veatch (1975) suggests that the legal structures should allow the patient or his agent to "choose among the plausible death concepts: those related to body fluid flow (heart and lung oriented), to integrating capacity (whole brain oriented), or experiential and social interaction capacity (neocortically oriented)."

Whatever comes of the debates among philosophers, theologians, and lawyers concerning the concept of death, or where it is located, or how it might best be measured, two facts are of salient value in nursing terminal patients in an institutional setting. (1) For the great majority of dying patients, nursing and medical clinicians are in very little doubt as to whether the event of death has occurred. (2) In any event, death has occurred if it is so certified by the physician.

This is not to suggest that nursing input into the philosophical discussions is not worthwhile, but merely that in the usual practice of nursing the traditional criteria are reliable (and utilized). At the abstract level of cognition and discussion that should precede the pronouncement of public policy, the concept and locus of death in humans requires precise definition (the measurement criteria probably remain a technical issue). However, at a concrete or clinical level, for most patients suffering from a terminal disease clinicians can and do recognize the change from the process of dying to the event of death.

PATIENTS' RIGHTS

The premise that institutionalization does not deprive a patient of his civil rights is fairly recent, and is related to the premise that characteristics of race, religion, gender, age, or physical condition should not inhibit rights. The rights of patients have not been advanced with quite the momentum of other rights, and Annas (1975) suggests this may owe to the impact of illness, a hospital stay that is too short to develop an in-patient organization, and the tendency not to think of hospitalization after the fact. Those persons who must spend more time in institutions usually belong to categories of persons — aged, terminally ill, physically handicapped, mentally retarded — who have little power in the community. Fear of retaliation must also be considered; the hospitalized person is literally at the mercy of the staff.

Annas points out that there is no single absolute definition of what is meant by "right." He suggests a continuum at one end of which is all of those rights that are recognized as *legal* rights; these include the rights of citizenship, and exist because they are created by the Constitution, legislative action, or prior court determination. In the middle of the continuum he places rights that would probably be recognized as legal rights by a court of law; i.e., there is a reasonable expectation that if the court is presented with the issue, it will recognize the right. Annas calls these *probable* legal rights. At the far end of the continuum are "statements of what the law ought to be, based on a political or philosophical conception of the nature and needs of man" (Annas 1975, p. 6). He terms these *human* rights.

Patients' rights are considered by the JCAH in the preamble of their Standards, which states that patient rights include equitable and humane treatment at all times and circumstances; privacy; confidentiality; participation in clinical training programs only on a voluntary basis; knowledge of the identity of the physician; information as to the nature of and purpose of any technical procedures performed and by whom such procedures will be carried out; communication with those responsible for care, and adequate information from them concerning the nature and extent of the medical problem, the planned course of treatment, and the prognosis. The patient also has a right to adequate instruction in self-care to cope during the time he is outside the hospital (Annas 1975).

The American Hospital Association (AHA 1973) promulgated a patients' bill of rights as a national policy statement in 1973; this, or a similar statement, has been adopted by many hospitals (Annas 1975). The AHA Patients' Bill of Rights is given below.*

> *The American Hospital Association presents a Patient's Bill of Rights with the expectation that observance of these rights will contribute to more effective patient care and greater satisfaction for the patient, his physician, and the hospital organization. Further, the Association presents these rights in the expectation that they will be supported by the hospital on behalf of its patients, as an integral part of the healing process. It is recognized that a personal relationship between the physician and the patient is essential for the provision of proper medical care.*
>
> *The traditional physician–patient relationship takes on a new dimension when care is rendered within an organizational structure. Legal precedent has established that the institution itself also has a responsibility to the patient. It is in recognition of these factors that these rights are affirmed.*
>
> *1. The patient has the right to considerate and respectful care.*
> *2. The patient has the right to obtain from his physician complete current information concerning his diagnosis, treatment, and prognosis in terms the patient can be reasonably expected to understand. When it is not medically advisable to give such information to the patient, the information should be made available to an appropriate person in his behalf. He has the right to know by name, the physician responsible for coordinating his care.*
> *3. The patient has the right to receive from his physician information necessary to give informed consent prior to the start of any procedure and/or treatment. Except in emergencies, such information for informed consent, should include but not necessarily be limited to the specific procedure and/or treatment, the medically significant risks involved, and the probable duration of incapacitation. Where medically significant alternatives for care or treatment exist or when the patient requests information concerning medical alternatives, the patient has the right to such information. The patient also has the right to know the name of the person responsible for the procedures and/or treatment.*
> *4. The patient has the right to refuse treatment to the extent permitted by law, and to be informed of the medical consequences of his action.*
> *5. The patient has the right to every consideration of his privacy con-*

---

*Adopted in 1973 by the American Hospital Association. Reprinted by permission of the American Hospital Association.

cerning his own medical care program. Case discussion, consultation, examination, and treatment are confidential and should be conducted discreetly. Those not directly involved in his care must have the permission of the patient to be present.

6. *The patient has the right to expect that all communications and records pertaining to his care should be treated as confidential.*

7. *The patient has the right to expect that within its capacity a hospital must make reasonable response to the request of a patient for services. The hospital must provide evaluation, service, and/or referral as indicated by the urgency of the case. When medically permissible a patient may be transferred to another facility only after he has received complete information and explanation concerning the needs for and alternatives to such a transfer. The institution to which the patient is to be transferred must first have accepted the patient for transfer.*

8. *The patient has the right to obtain information as to any relationship of his hospital to other health care and educational institutions insofar as his care is concerned. The patient has the right to obtain information as to the existence of any professional relationships among individuals, by name, who are treating him.*

9. *The patient has the right to be advised if the hospital proposes to engage in or perform human experimentation affecting his care or treatment. The patient has the right to refuse to participate in such research projects.*

10. *The patient has the right to expect reasonable continuity of care. He has the right to know in advance what appointment times and physicians are available and where. The patient has the right to expect that the hospital will provide a mechanism whereby he is informed by his physician or a delegate of the physician of the patient's continuing health care requirements following discharge.*

11. *The patient has the right to examine and receive an explanation of his bill regardless of source of payment.*

12. *The patient has the right to know what hospital rules and regulations apply to his conduct as a patient.*

No catalogue of rights can guarantee for the patient the kind of treatment he has a right to expect. A hospital has many functions to perform, including the prevention and treatment of disease, the education of both health professionals and patients, and the conduct of clinical research. All these activities must be conducted with an overriding concern for the patient, and, above all, the recognition of his dignity as a human being. Success in achieving this recognition assures success in the defense of the rights of the patient.

The thrust of this Bill of Rights is obviously toward relationships between the physician and the patient, and there is some question as to authority of an institution to address that relationship. Even if that authority is granted, the items themselves, as Annas has pointed out (1975, p. 28), address merely matters of courtesy, or of informed consent. The legal standing of the statement is ambiguous, but Annas states that it has been used in court at least as evidence of custom (1975, p. 29). Thus, to achieve more precision and comprehensiveness than the AHA Statement, the following Model Patient's Bill of Rights was developed (Annas 1975, pp. 233-235).

As you enter this health care facility, it is our duty to remind you that your health care is a cooperative effort between you as a patient and the doctors and hospital staff. During your stay you will have a patient's rights advocate available. The duty of the advocate is to assist you in all the decisions you must make and in all situations in which your health and welfare are at stake. The advocate's first responsibility is to help you understand who each of the people are who will be working with you and to help you understand what your rights as a patient are. Your advocate can be reached at any time of the day by dialing _____. The following is a list of your rights as a patient. Your advocate's duty is to see to it that you are afforded these rights. You should call your advocate whenever you have any questions or concerns about any of these rights.

1. *The patient has a legal right to informed participation in all decisions involving his health care program.*
2. *We recognize the right of all potential patients to know what research and experimental protocols are being used in our facility and what alternatives are available in the community.*
3. *The patient has a legal right to privacy respecting the source of payment for treatment and care. This right includes access to the highest degree of care without regard to the source of payment for that treatment and care.*
4. *We recognize the right of a potential patient to complete and accurate information concerning medical care and procedures.*
5. *The patient has a legal right to prompt attention especially in an emergency situation.*
6. *The patient has a legal right to a clear, concise explanation of all proposed procedures in laymen's terms, including the possibilities of any risk of mortality or serious side effects, problems related to recuperation, and probability of success, and will not be subjected to any procedure without his voluntary, competent, and understanding consent. The specifics of such consent shall be set out in a written consent form, signed by the patient.*
7. *The patient has a legal right to a clear, complete, and accurate evaluation of his condition and prognosis without treatment before he is asked to consent to any test or procedure.*
8. *We recognize the right of the patient to know the identity and professional status of all those providing service. All personnel have been instructed to introduce themselves, state their status, and explain*

their role in the health care of the patient. Part of this right is the right of the patient to know the physician responsible for his care.

9. *We recognize the right of any patient who does not speak English to have access to an interpreter.*

10. *The patient has a legal right to all the information contained in his medical record while in the health-care facility and to examine the record upon request.*

11. *We recognize the right of a patient to discuss his condition with a consultant specialist at his own request and his own expense.*

12. *The patient has a legal right not to have any test or procedure, designed for educational purposes rather than his direct personal benefit, performed on him.*

13. *The patient has a legal right to refuse any particular drug, test, procedure, or treatment.*

14. *The patient has a legal right to both personal and informational privacy with respect to: the hospital staff, other doctors, residents, interns and medical students, researchers, nurses, other hospital personnel, and other patients.*

15. *We recognize the patient's right of access to people outside the health care facility by means of visitors and the telephone. Parents may stay with their children and relatives with terminally ill patients 24 hours a day.*

16. *The patient has a legal right to leave the health care facility regardless of physical condition or financial status, although he may be requested to sign a release stating that he is leaving against the medical judgment of his doctor or the hospital.*

17. *No patient may be transferred to another facility unless he has received a complete explanation of the desirability and need for the transfer, the other facility has accepted the patient for transfer, and the patient has agreed to transfer. If the patient does not agree to transfer, the patient has the right to a consultant's opinion on the desirability of transfer.*

18. *A patient has a right to be notified of discharge at least one day before it is accomplished, to demand a consultation by an expert on the desirability of discharge, and to have a person of the patient's choice so notified.*

19. *The patient has a right, regardless of source of payment, to examine and receive an itemized and detailed explanation of his total bill for services rendered in the facility.*

20. *The patient has a right to competent counseling from the facility to help him obtain financial assistance from public or private sources to meet the expense of services received in the institution.*

21. *The patient has a right to timely prior notice of the termination of his eligibility for reimbursement for the expense of his care by any third-party payer.*

22. *At the termination of his stay at the health care facility we recognize the right of a patient to a complete copy of the information contained in his medical record.*

> 23. We recognize the right of all patients to have 24 hour a day access to
> a patient's rights advocate who may act on behalf of the patient to
> assert or protect the rights set out in this document.

Item 23 implies the existence of a patient advocate, and Annas sees this
as a status and role separate from the line authority of both medical and institutional administration. The goals of a patient-rights advocate program include
protection of patients, particularly those with the least power; to make available
to those who wish it the opportunity to participate with the doctor in a personal
health-care program; to restore to proper perspective technological and pharma-
ceutical advances, and to confront the exaggerated expectations of the consumer;
and to reflect in the physician–patient relationship the reality of the health-
sickness continuum, reasserting the humanness and naturalness of death. The
advocate has the powers that belong to the patient, and assists the patient in
exercising his rights. He must have access to medical records and the ability to
call in a consultant; participate in hospital committees responsible for monitoring care; be able to exercise patient rights through the Executive Committee, or
other agencies that deal with patient complaints; and be granted support services
for all patients who request them. The advocate must be available to all patients
who request his help. Because this position is one in which the primary responsibility is to the patient, and the function is to assist the patient in asserting or
protecting his interests, support and supervision should come from outside the
health-care facility (Annas 1974). Payment mechanisms are not considered in
any detail, but are likely to cause difficulty in implementing such a program.

Sullivan, writing in the *New England Law Review* suggests that as a mechanism for enforcing the preferences of a terminal patient, a proctor could be
provided by law — at the request of the ill or dying individual.

> The proctor will act as the court regulated agent of the dying person. . . .
> among other things he can deal with the family and inform them in no
> uncertain terms what the dying person expects from them. He can relate
> to the physicians . . . and tell them what the dying person demands. He
> can act as authoritative intermediary between physician and patient . . .
> make the wishes of the dying person known unequivocally to the hospital
> staff or nursing home staff (Sullivan 1973).

The proctor's further duties would include assisting the patient to exercise
his rights in support of his preferences, even to the point of "legal standing in
the estate to enforce his late charge's funeral orders" (Sullivan 1973).

The established need for such positions in the health-care system is an
index of the many faults in that system. If patients were treated as equals by
caregivers, there would be no need for a specified advocate; the patient would
be supported by all those caring for him, who are, after all, being paid to help
him to regain whatever health is possible or to die with as much comfort and
dignity as dying allows. Nurses have in the past proclaimed themselves as patient
advocates and have tried to serve in that role as part of their *nursing* function.
However, physicians, patients, and hospital administrators have not perceived
them as advocates; the fact that they are paid by the institution and do not

serve on the more powerful hospital committees makes them weak advocates even if they are recognized as such.

The prevalent attitude toward the dying patient is reflected in the denial of the patient's right to privacy, to consent to treatment, to choose the place and time of his death, and to determine the disposition of his body after death; he is frequently denied his basic right of knowing his diagnosis and prognosis. Annas (1974) has described how each denied right adversely affects the patient by adding to his anxiety — preventing him from planning for care of his family and material assets and denying him close communication with his family and his friends. Annas maintains that the dying patient must be offered the human rights of the living.

The Right to Information

DIAGNOSIS AND PROGNOSIS

Perhaps the major difference in the treatment of terminal and nonterminal patients is the professional reluctance to discuss diagnosis and prognosis with the former group. Not only do physicians withhold such information from patients, they require that other health workers do so. Even when disclosure of the diagnosis is made to the patient, it is frequently in technical terms that do not really inform; the prognosis is seldom recorded in the patient record, although presumably it will affect the therapy.

Glaser and Strauss (1965) identify and discuss four information contexts in the staff-patient interaction: these are closed awareness, suspicion awareness, mutual pretense, and open awareness. These contexts are defined in terms of the amount of information concerning *whether* and *when* a patient is going to die that is held by physicians, nurses, patients, and families.

The physician is the only person who has the authority to define the patient's condition and to provide patients or families with the information. Nurses make use of physiological cues in the patient and behavioral cues from the physician, and also have access to the patient's record; they may therefore know both diagnosis and prognosis before they are officially informed, and this knowledge can and should affect their nursing activities. It may, indeed, affect their behavior in such a way that patients may infer a good part of the information that is being withheld. However, the provision of information to the patient about his condition is the prerogative of the physician, and if he chooses not to inform, and the internal and external cues to the patient are such that *they* do not inform, the patient may not recognize his impending death, and interactions will take place in a situation of closed awareness. This may or may not be protective for patients; physicians are likely to assume that it is, although there is some evidence that most people wish accurate information about the process of their dying. In a situation of closed awareness, great care must be taken by staff working with the patient not to disclose by mistake. Because honest interaction is basic to any nursing functions that are other than superficial, nursing may meet only physical needs.

Physicians are not malicious; they defend withholding a terminal prognosis from their patients on the basis of protecting them from despair and loss of hope. The evidence that patients need this kind of protection is individual and anecdotal in nature; it does not appear that the closed context is in any way more therapeutic than an open context. Also, physicians who defend closed awareness on the basis of protecting their patients from the information at the same time point out that patients know anyhow. In any case, the perception that dying adults are not able to cope with the explicit information has in it an element of contempt: they are perceived as weak, with a childish need for reassurance when very little reassurance is really appropriate.

Closed awareness in a conscious, competent adult is not likely to last; the process of dying is such that some degeneration of the body is likely to occur. This, together with the perception of unusual treatment by staff and family, is generally enough to move to a context of suspicious awareness: in this context, staff knows that the patient is dying, but the patient merely suspects it. His efforts to become informed without asking directly, in the presence of the directive not to inform, is likely to be painful for both staff and patient.

Mutual-pretense awareness is the state in which both patient and staff are aware of the prognosis, but both pretend that the patient will recover. A game of make-believe is set in motion, which can continue only when great care is taken by all parties to the pretense. Professional rationales for taking part in the pretense are stated in terms of what is best for patients; nurses and doctors take part in the pretense if they believe that the patient should not be forced into an awareness he does not wish to sustain. The mutual-pretense context provides a certain amount of privacy to the patient; he need not discuss the difficult and emotion-laden topic of death if he chooses to ignore the likely future. Although this inhibits closer relationships with staff, he may be more comfortable in the less personal interaction.

Open awareness is present when both staff and patient know the patient is dying and acknowledge it in their actions. Whether these actions are acceptable to each party is another question; patients who know their fate may behave in hostile, angry ways that staff does not perceive as appropriate, and staff responses may provide less reassurance than patients would like to have.

The context of awareness in which staff and patients interact has implications for nursing. There are some nursing behaviors that cannot take place in a closed or merely suspicious context. Because interaction with patients is the basis of nursing practice, nursing intervention is inhibited when one party to the interaction lacks relevant information about the conditions of the interaction.

What rights do terminal patients have to explicit statement of diagnosis and prognosis, and from whom can they expect to attain the information? Physicians traditionally control dissemination of information concerning medical diagnosis and prognosis. If families, physicians, and nurses are in a benevolent conspiracy to deny information to the dying adult, what are his other sources? His fellow patients, although they might be sources of information concerning other topics, are not likely to inform concerning a terminal prognosis, although they may have overheard conversations of family or staff. Records may be a source of information, but the medical record is the property of the hospital. Annas states (1975, p. 116) that in 41 states the only legal right the patient has to see his hospital record is by instituting a lawsuit and having the records subpoenaed for evidence. Hospitals generally will make medical records available to the doctor of the patient's choice, but they are less willing to make records available to the patient. Nine states give the patient or his attorney the right to inspect hospital records: however, in three of these, access is limited to the attorney. Common hospital policy requires the consent of the physician for the patient to have access to his own record, although this is in violation of law. There is some trend to change this ridiculous situation, and courts are beginning to decide that the information on a patient's medical record should be available to him without his having to go to court (Annas 1975, p. 118). At present, however, the only legal right the patient has is to demand to see his record and have it explained, before consenting to treatment; a competent patient may refuse to allow a procedure to be performed at any time, and can make willingness to submit to treatment dependent on full information about the reason for and the probable consequences of treatment. It is important to note that nurses who tell the patient his rights, or inform him of his documented medical diagnosis or prognosis, are liable to censure by nursing, medical, and administrative colleagues.

It is also important to note that the prognosis is never entirely certain, and dying patients appreciate knowing that. Stewart Alsop, himself a leukemia victim, made poignant reference to this.

> My own view is that a patient should be told the truth and nothing but the truth — but not the whole truth. I find scribbled in my notebook: "a man who must die will die more easily if he is left a little spark of hope that he may not die after all. My rule would be: Never tell a victim of terminal cancer the whole truth — tell him that he may die, even that he will probably die, but do not tell him that he will die." (Alsop 1973)

INFORMED CONSENT

Informed consent is defined by Annas (1975, p. 58) as consisting of

> . . . two separate elements: (1) information and (2) consent. . . . the doctor must first disclose a certain amount of information to the patient concerning the proposed treatment, its risks and alternatives, and thereafter must obtain the consent of the patient before going ahead with the treatment. . . . in general terms . . . the information conveyed must include all the material facts of the treatment proposed, including risks of death or serious bodily harm, the probability of success, the alternatives to the treatment (including nontreatment), and their risks and probabilities of success. . . . the patient's consent must be competent, understanding and voluntary. Specifically, the patient must be legally capable of giving consent . . . must comprehend the information disclosed, and must not be coerced into consenting.

The purpose of informed consent is to protect the patient's right of self-determination; the intent is to give the patient enough information so that he can decide how and if he is to be treated. Obviously, in the case of a dying patient, such information must include a specific prognosis as well as the diagnosis. The desire to protect the patient from anxiety-producing information is not an adequate legal reason for not informing. Because a physician is also constrained from abandoning his patient, it would seem that he cannot refuse an informative interaction with a patient who demands more details than that physician really cares to give. The presumption is that all patients are capable of dealing with complete disclosure, and the trend is

> . . . for the courts to view the doctor–patient relationship as a partnership in decision-making rather than as a medical monopoly. Under this view the doctor is obligated to disclose not what other doctors customarily disclose to their patients in similar circumstances, but what the individual patient needs to know to intelligently make up his own mind concerning the proposed treatment. (Annas 1975, p. 64)

Consent must be given out of understanding of relevant facts. In view of the fact that the second function of informed consent is encouraging rational decision-making, Annas believes these facts include risks, success probabilities, and alternatives. He points out that the doctor and the patient are not in an equal bargaining position; the position of strength of the physician requires him to take care. Annas upholds the presumption that the physician "always inform the patient of all material information, but that the manner in which the information is conveyed (time, place, language used, etc.) be permitted to vary depending on the patient's circumstances" (1975, p. 68). If the patient indicates he does not wish to know information the physician considers relevant, Annas advises putting the patient's request to remain in ignorance in the written record.

The blanket consent form that most patients are asked to sign on admission is considered legally inadequate, although it might serve as proof of consent to routine hospital procedures if specific forms are signed for nonroutine activities (Annas 1975, p. 70). However, legal consent can be given without signed forms, as the reason for writing the consent is merely to maintain a permanent record of the agreement. Consent may be implied by voluntary submission to treatment if the situation is such that the patient understood what was going on and was aware that action would be interpreted as consent. Annas (1975, p. 73) cites the example of the woman who was given a smallpox vaccination, after standing in the vaccination line, observing what was happening, and holding up her arm for the injection. Her actions were construed by a court as consent to be vaccinated.

If it is impossible to obtain consent and the life or health of the patient is in immediate danger, treatment may be rendered without consent.

The patient always has the right, within practical limits, to change his mind and withdraw consent to treatment, even if he has signed a written form. If the treatment cannot be aborted (for instance, if a drug has already been injected), or if the patient becomes unable to change his mind (for instance, following the administration of an anesthetic), the right is necessarily curtailed.

Obviously, the right to informed consent implies a right to know both the diagnosis and the prognosis. The habit of withholding this information from terminal patients is notorious, although both theoretical and empirical data suggest that as a general rule dying patients want to know and should be told the truth about their condition and the limits on treatment objectives. The power of caregivers to constrain patients into biddable and nonthreatening behavior is frightening. Patients who demand information are likely to be labeled uncooperative; nurses who try to support patients who demand their rights are likely to be removed from the system. Even when "rights" have some legal recognition, a sick and dying patient, accompanied by a distraught family, or without any family at all, is not likely to try to exercise them. Real and well-publicized support for the initiation of open interaction among staff and patients is required before either patients or nurses can feel comfortable in the exercise of the patients' right to information.

The Right to Refuse Treatment

For terminal patients, the right to refuse treatment may, by some clinicians, be equated with a right to die. There is much in the literature on this particular right, and even on "the right to die" in some specific manner — e.g. "with dignity" is a common statement. Herter (1969) makes the points common to this attitude. He states that many wish for death to come quickly, without warning or deliberation. The fear of lingering death associated with chronic diseases and the fear of prolonged suffering are universal, and anxiety about being an emotional or financial burden to the family is common. However, death frequently follows a variable period of illness with physical suffering or mental anguish, and often with tenacious clinging to life. Death seldom comes peacefully and without resistance; dying is a series of slow, painful steps, characterized by preoccupation with symptoms or rigors of treatment with little or no opportunity for quiet contemplation. Preoccupation with physical comfort may preclude serious examination by the patient of his approaching death. Physicians are often frenetically following various routines and experiments as they vigorously resist death, more so than does the patient. As discussed above, physicians seldom give patients credit for being able to accept approaching death; yet most people can accept the truth. A stated prognosis can be realistic without conferring complete hopelessness and can be accomplished without being dishonest. The truth comes as relief to many, as they can then bring forth their reserves of courage and understanding, and begin to cope as they are able.

Alsop (1973) has reported his own experience as follows:

> when death is due to occur at some time in the fairly near but indefinite future — in a few months, or a year or two years, or maybe even later, it is possible to forget about death for many hours at a time.

Indeed, death can be postponed, and patients continue to live; however, the patient, the family, and society may be faced with intolerable financial and emotional burdens when life is prolonged when the disease is irreversible. The dying patient may prefer fewer life-prolonging treatments. On the other hand, he might prefer more. Theoretically, the decision is his.

Any competent adult has the legal right to refuse medical treatment, and to refuse to stay in the treatment setting regardless of the opinion of medical staff that treatment is necessary to life. These refusals may not be construed in such a way that the patient is labeled incompetent merely because he refuses to be treated. If a patient refuses a specific treatment, the hospital is responsible to see that no member of the staff imposes it; it is also obliged to continue the best medical care possible within the limitations imposed by the refusal of a specific treatment (Annas 1975); that is, refusal by the patient to carry out one treatment does not absolve medical and nursing staff from all other necessary treatments. Although the above is considered to be a general rule, the application by practitioners and by courts in individual situations has varied. The institution of possibly inappropriate heroic life-saving measures in intensive-care settings is too well documented to need discussion here. In fact, treatment may be and frequently is imposed against the wishes of the individual being treated.

A right that must be exercised against the position of a power elite is not very real. Dying patients informed only of a general diagnosis, but not at all sure of the prognosis, may be subject to professional whim in the way of treatment. A "new" therapy may be tried; the patient may submit because he believes it will help him, or because he believes he will receive better care if he does as he is told. Analgesics and narcotics may be withheld, or given in small dosage, because staff is afraid of addiction or of suicidal tendencies in patients. In the interviews reported later, it will be seen that patients submit to the practices mentioned above because they believe that the doctor always knows best, and because they *are* afraid of addiction.

The current outcry against the depersonalizing treatment of institutionalized individuals is mainly addressed to the regulations and to the way these are implemented by staff — who may be unfeeling, or in the case of institutionalized dying patients, merely frightened by the imminence of death into impersonal behavior. Patients have the right to refuse this treatment by staff, as well as the right to refuse to submit to medical therapy. They can refuse to sign papers, and to submit to discourteous or demeaning behavior on the part of the staff. However, the consequences of refusal to be an accepting patient may be such that it is easier to submit than to assert. The sick individual in an acute-care setting need only submit for a few days; then he can go home. He may decide not to rock the boat for such a short stay. As can be seen in the interviews which follow, dying patients are well aware of their dependent position, and are more likely to try to gain their goals by persuasion and agreement than by exercise of any right of refusal.

The AHA has recognized the right of the patient to refuse treatment, and presents guidelines for staff behavior in the event of patient refusal. The guidelines* are presented below.

It is suggested that the following points receive consideration by hospitals and members of their medical staffs in the case of persons who, for reli-

---

*"The Right of the Patient to Refuse Treatment;" Reprinted by permission of the American Hospital Association.

gious or other reasons, refuse to consent to medical or surgical treatment recommended by the attending physician:

1. When the patient is an adult of sound mind, a written refusal is recommended to absolve the hospital, the physician(s), and all other personnel from liability, if any, for failure to furnish the recommended treatment.
2. When the patient is legally too young to make his own decision, the written refusal of the parents or the legal guardian, if available, should be obtained.
3. When an adult patient is legally incapable of making his own decision, written refusal should be obtained from someone authorized under law to act for him, whether the authority rests on relationship or personal or official appointment. (By law, a power of attorney generally expires upon mental disability of the principal.)
4. Before obtaining a written refusal of treatment, the attending physician(s) should explain the medical consequences of such a refusal to the patient or other person refusing consent to the recommended treatment.
5. When consent for the recommended treatment is refused, the attending physician(s) should undertake to obtain a consent for an alternative method of management.
6. The hospital and its medical staff should establish a system whereby the attending physician will report promptly to the hospital any refusal of consent to treatment that might in his opinion have probable medical consequences that would be adverse and substantial.
7. The hospital should ascertain that its response to a refusal, whether action or nonaction, is consistent with current state and federal law.

The courts and legislatures of various states have placed restrictions on the right of a patient, or someone on his behalf, to refuse medical or surgical procedures. The legal pronouncements among various states differ in important particulars.

It behooves every hospital to obtain legal advice on an ongoing basis as to the hospital's obligation under state law when such a refusal occurs. Otherwise the hospital will be unable to respect the right of a patient to refuse treatment to the extent permitted by law or to avoid or reduce any legal problems to the hospital itself. Such advice should deal with:

1. Both adult patients and minor patients, including those in either category who may lack mental or legal capacity to consent or refuse consent for themselves.
2. The effect, if any, when the probable medical consequences of the refusal to consent are substantial but not necessarily fatal.
3. The effect, if any, of a refusal based on religious belief or any equivalent personal conviction.

4. *The effect of a refusal when another authorized person gives a consent.*
5. *The types of refusal that may be entitled to unquestioned observance, and whether the hospital or the attending physician has any duty to report any type of refusal to an official agency or court or to take other action.*
6. *Those persons who have a legal right to consent or refuse to consent for themselves or other persons.*

The refusal of treatment may in the case of a terminal patient be the refusal of life-saving treatment, and there are questions arising almost daily in the courts as to the right of others (in the person of the state) to intervene and order life-saving treatment for a reluctant patient. Cantor (1973) has analyzed the public interests which might be involved. He lists preservation of society; sanctity of life; public morals (on the basis that rejection of life-saving treatment is a form of suicide); protection of the individual against his own imprudence; and protection of third parties (e.g., survivors, fellow patients, physicians) as areas of contest, but perceives that principles of self-determination (liberty), bodily control, and the protections surrounding personal privacy take precedence (1973). He says

> *I have little difficulty extending my basic position — that a physician must legally respect a patient's decision to reject treatment — to the terminally ill patient. The same considerations of bodily integrity and self-determination apply. They assume added importance where the patient faces a loss of faculties and dignity before inevitably succumbing. (Cantor 1973)*

Although there is general support for the right of a patient to refuse treatment, the right to choose not to prolong dying is not so well recognized. Veatch (1972) presents four alternative policies related to the decision to refuse or stop treatment. The first alternative is the current position of no public policy; this means in fact that the decision is made on an *ad hoc* basis by the individual physician when the patient is in a terminal condition. Although the physician *may* consult peers or family, the decision is his. A second alternative is followed by a number of hospitals: committees of physicians make decisions as to the allocation of scarce resources, thereby impinging on treatment decisions. Veatch suggests that "the committee mechanism perpetuates the view that the medical professional by his training has somehow acquired expertise in making the moral judgment about when it is no longer appropriate to prolong dying" (1972); Veatch is no more comfortable with this form of medical decision than he is with allowing the decision to remain in the hands of the individual physician. A third alternative can be found in personal letters, living wills, or various kinds of instructions from individuals as to how they wish to be treated in situations requiring artificial means of life support. While these documents would appear to put the decision in the hands of the patient, in fact they are usually so ambiguous as to leave the decision in the hands of the physician; also, they are not legally binding. The fourth alternative is legislation, and there are a good many legislative proposals dealing with options in dying. Veatch considers legislation "based on the already existing right of the patients to refuse treatment is probably most worthy of consideration as a public policy" (1972). For competent adults the exercise of this right is enough. For persons who are not competent, some agent must make the decision on the person's behalf. Veatch suggests an agent, appointed by the individual while he is competent, should have first priority; if this is not done the next of kin or court-appointed agents can decide. In spite of the ambiguity of the legal status of such documents, many healthy persons now make written arrangements for their terminal care. The best-known document of this type is the Living Will distributed by the Euthanasia Educational Council (reproduced in Appendix C). Criticism of this document addresses its ambiguity and vagueness of wording; the absence of direction about what to do in situations of conflict (if relatives disagree with the instructions); and lack of clarity concerning which life-support procedures should be carried out in various possible situations. In addressing these criticisms, Bok (1976) proposes a document which is a request rather than a plea; it makes provisions for acceptance and refusal of treatment; it is brief, clear, leaves space for specific instructions; and it encourages consultation with physicians. Her proposed direction, while it is a clearer and more comprehensive statement than the Living Will, shares with that document the lack of legal standing. It is not a contract, but a request.

The medical profession has made its own efforts regarding the issue of "how best to manage hopelessly ill patients" (Critical Care Committee 1976). The Critical Care Committee of the Massachusetts General Hospital — charged with study and recommendation concerning treatment of the hopelessly ill patient and utilization of critical-care facilities — has recommended the establishment of a permanent committee on optimum treatment of the hopelessly ill patient, and a classification system for patients based on the medical therapeutic effort. The committee is advisory in nature; a request for review must come from the responsible physician.

The classification system and recommendations suggest an effort to attain professional consensus concerning life-saving treatment; input from family and patients may also be sought.

> Whenever a question arises about the appropriateness of treatment of a patient with an irreversible illness the situation should be reviewed at unit rounds. Such questions may arise from the patient, the family, the responsible physician, the staff of the unit or its director, or consultants called by the responsible physician (Critical Care Committee 1976).

Experience with this system of committee consultation and patient classification by therapeutic effort provided high correlation among nurses and physicians as to how patients should be assigned, and requests for Optimum Care Committee consultation were rare. The authors suggest that the main benefits of the consultation were

> clarification of misunderstanding about the patient's prognosis, reopening of communication, re-establishment of unified treatment objectives and

rationale, restoration of the sense of shared responsibility for patient and family and, above all, maximizing support for the responsible physician who makes the medical decision to intensify, maintain or limit effort at reversing the illness (Critical Care Committee 1976).

It is, however, difficult to see how documents such as the Living Will or Bok's (1976) directions for care would be given consideration; in any case, the decision apparently remains with the physician. It is, of course, entirely appropriate for institutions to consider allocation of scarce resources in therapeutic deliberations. It is equally appropriate to consider the expressed wishes of patients and families. The very real concern to save life felt by most physicians and nurses is necessarily in conflict with patient decisions to refuse treatment. It is extremely difficult in the clinical setting *not* to move to the life-supporting effort, in spite of rational objections on the part of patients and families and rational objections on the grounds of economy. This attitude is, on the whole, protective of patients and should certainly not be discouraged. However, the right of self-determination should also be protected in the weak and vulnerable terminally ill population. Alsop (1973) writes, ". . . a dying man needs to die, as a sleepy man needs to sleep, and there comes a time when it is wrong as well as useless to resist."

The Right to Excellence in Care

The definition of excellence in care must arise from the needs of an individual patient, and is tied to his perceptions. Technical care of the highest quality is a necessary but not sufficient criterion for excellence. The patient as well as the practitioner must be satisfied that the care is appropriate, and the procedures and technique correctly implemented. Correctness implies attention to expressive as well as instrumental detail. The right to excellence in care is related to the right to information, both because informing is part of care, and because the patient cannot judge his care if he lacks information as to what it should be.

Also related to excellence is availability and accessibility of care. Fried (1976) has pointed out that a claim of right invokes entitlements; a right confers not just what it would be desirable to have but it also bestows the ability to demand on the person exercising the right. Implicit in a right to excellence in care is the right to availability of care, and Fried asks whether a right to health care implies a right to *equal* access to health care. He suggests that the slogan of equal access to the best health care available cannot be translated into reality without submitting to intolerable controls or expense (Fried 1976). He states that the right which has been recognized in the past is not the right to health care as such, nor even a right to health, but a right to a certain standard of health care that was defined in terms of what medicine could reasonably do for people (Fried 1976). Because what medicine *can* reasonably do for people is not required in most situations, it is wise not to opt for an all-inclusive right to health care if this means an *equal* right to whatever health care is available. Fried (1976) opts for a decent minimum that *should include humane and, I would say, worthy surroundings of care for those whom we know we are not going to be able to treat. Here, it seems to me the emphasis on technology and the attention of highly trained specialists is seriously mistaken. Not only is it unrealistic to imagine that such fancy services can be provided for everyone "as a right," but there is serious doubt whether these kinds of services are what most people really want or can benefit from.*

Obviously Fried considers care to be medical care, and the highly trained specialist in fancy services is the doctor. However, the point that he makes is a good one. Excellence in care should be evaluated in terms of the patient's need rather than in terms of whether he is receiving all of the benefit of all possible technology. The services needed by those who will not survive in spite of a given technology may be provided by specialists equally highly trained in another field. Fried suggests the necessity of identifying what health care can and cannot provide, measuring the cost, and then deciding how much care — and what level of care — should be underwritten as the standard to be available for all citizenry. Mechanic (1976), on the other hand, does not believe that the public is so demanding of equality of access to all possible care; people are satisfied with "reasonable access to needed services and assurance that people who share a common entitlement will be treated fairly within the context of whatever program exists."

In many aspects of their care, patients with a terminal prognosis have the same needs as patients with short-term illness. Weisman (1972) identifies further psychosocial needs that also need attention from care givers. He states that the secondary suffering related to terminal illness includes impaired self-esteem, feelings of endangerment, annihilation anxiety, and alienation anxiety.

Impaired self-esteem is demonstrated by statements of worthlessness, quiet withdrawal from usual interests, unusual tendencies to do what the staff seems to expect. The gathering depression and self-derogation can be mistaken for cooperation; the terminally ill person seldom expresses guilt and retribution, except at time of diagnosis, but especially not toward the end of life. He may feel taken over by the disease against which struggle does not avail. The person becomes the disease.

Feelings of endangerment are shown by unnecessary regression, such as extreme denial, projection, magical expectations about recovery, and hallucinatory experiences. The patient may respond to the danger of the situation by false optimism, careless disregard of symptoms, and excessive preoccupation with peripheral problems.

Annihilation anxiety is fear of dying and disintegration, often associated with impaired reality testing. The patient complains about everything. Everyone becomes "they" — staff, family, friends. The patient fears becoming a thing or a number. Fear of losing sanity means fear of becoming nothing. Alienation anxiety stems from fear of separation from key supports and rewarding activities. Much of personality is attached to things; persons die not only *from* illness but *to* many activities, which generates a sense of being alone. Alienation occurs in the presence of major and minor losses, partial grief, total bereavement. Individuals with terminal illness may be preoccupied with trivia, as if attachment to something routine and smaller than life-size will preserve contact with the world. Loneliness and depression are felt.

While there may be a reasonable consensus as to the psychological states and behaviors of terminally ill persons, there is no agreement as to what constitutes good treatment which should be delivered to everyone. Responsible medical and nursing practitioners may perceive the pronouncements of behavioral scientists concerning truth-telling and self-determination to be naive in situations in which there is a very real patient dependence on staff. Also, physicians and nurses frequently disagree as to the relative importance of instrumental and expressive therapies.

In the presence of the questions as to what constitutes good care, and lack of information among terminal patients as to what their expectations are, it is difficult to identify any *right* to excellence of care. At the barest minimum, excellence includes safety, trust, support, and a sense of control for patients. Continuity, confidentiality, and education are required. Jellinek (1976) has pointed out the erosion of patient trust in physicians and staff which grows out of standard practice procedures in medical centers. The existence of these practices speaks against the probability that any right to excellence exists. Gross negligence can be addressed by patients through the courts if they have the necessary strength, time, money, and sources of information about their options. Anything short of gross negligence is so difficult to identify and document that rights become meaningless. Sullivan (1973) contends that there is " a dire need for a mechanism whereby his [the dying patient] preferences can be enforced" and "the polestar of any legislation must be the dying person's right to make the decisions concerning his relationships."

Some legal rights do exist, and consumers of health services are becoming aware of their rights and are seeking compensation for injuries caused by professionals. The following information concerns what an injured patient must prove to win a lawsuit against a physician or a hospital.

> To prevail . . . the patient must demonstrate four things: (1) that the doctor or hospital had a duty of care . . . (2) that the duty was breached . . . (3) that damages to the patient resulted . . . and (4) that the damages were caused directly by the breach of duty. Only by proving all of these in court can the plaintiff prevail. (Annas 1975, p. 199)

Annas further reports that only about one in 226,000 patient visits to doctors results in a legal action, and the majority of hospitals go through an entire year without having a claim filed against them. However, legal action can be brought for the denial of essential services (e.g., emergency care) or constitutionally protected services (e.g., abortion); against an insuror to challenge the denial of payment; for invasion of the right to informational or bodily privacy; for breach of confidentiality; for denial of access to medical records, etc. (Annas 1975, p. 206).

All patient-consumers must realize that unless they complain about condi-
tions that they don't like and take strong legal action when their rights are
violated, hospitals will have no incentive or rationale, other than general
principles, to change their policies to reflect consumer wishes. (Annas
1975, p. 207)

In the hospital, as in other settings, the exercise of rights appears to be inextricably tied to the ability to defend them. Whether terminal patients or their families really have that ability remains a question. The interviews reported in this
book suggest that if expectations for physical care are met, pain is controlled,
and staff are pleasant, patients will report they are satisfied with care that is not
perceived by a professional to attain excellence.

Constraints on Patients' Rights

In spite of the laudable concern for the rights of patients currently expressed by
politicians, administrators, and caregivers, the effort to give the best care to the
most people at the least cost requires some abrogation of individual rights. Medical, surgical, laboratory, and even nursing procedures must be carried out as staff
is available to do so, rather than when patients are biologically or psychologically ready. On nursing divisions, evening and night shifts are staffed only to the
extent necessary to carry out physician directives concerning medications and
treatments. Professional nursing requires knowledge, skill, and time; personnel
policies dictate how much of any of these factors will be available to specified
categories of patients at specified times.

Another hospital policy impinging on the rights of patients is the policy that
dictates discharge or transfer when treatment is no longer expected to result in
the cure or at the least the inhibition of the disease process. The right of any patient to the technologies of cure is limited by the willingness of the institution to
maintain him in the acute-care environment. Patients may be discharged from
the institution or from the intensive-care unit. They may be transferred from a
familiar ward to a private room nearer the nursing station. Patients must become
accustomed to new people in a new space at a time when they need consistent
relationships. Feelings of fear and abandonment are commonly noted at times of
change.

Rules for visiting may inadvertently reinforce the fears, loneliness, and feelings of abandonment experienced by dying patients. Although visiting hours are
becoming more flexible in many institutions, particularly on pediatric divisions,
many still stipulate strictly who can visit as well as the number of visitors and
the length of time they may stay (Kneisl 1968). A statement carried without
critical comment by several newspapers quotes "a panel of surgeons" as stating
that visitors are sources of infection. Hospitals are criticized by the panel for an
"open-door policy" for visitors who often "make their visit a social event." The
presence of fathers in delivery rooms and spouses in operating rooms following
surgery is blamed by implication for higher hospital infection rates (*Detroit Free
Press*, 23 October, 1977; *St. Louis Globe Democrat*, 19 October, 1977). To cou-

ple rising infection rates with relaxed visiting rules is to ignore the effect on the patient environment of physicians, nurses, and other personnel who work with patients in street clothes and do not necessarily stay home from work when they are ill with colds or fevers. The relaxation of rules for clean techniques in caring for patients is more surely related to the incidence of nosocomial infections than the continued presence of family and friends.

Hospitals are complex bureaucracies in interaction with other complex bureaucracies (federal, state, and insurance bureaucracies), and the range of regulations with which they must comply is great. The existence of such regulations makes it necessary to impose constraints on the behavior of patients, who must be kept safe from a dangerous environment while they are being treated (frequently with dangerous equipment or drugs). The complexity of the environment leads to a necessary curtailment of some personal autonomy of patients. However, there is no doubt that much of the curtailment of patient independence is for the convenience of the staff rather than the protection of the patients, and is not necessary. The identification and discard of rules, procedures, and other constraints on patient behavior which are not required for patient protection might make patients more willing to accept those which must be retained. Acceptance is even more likely if the retained constraints are implemented in a courteous manner.

References

Ad Hoc Committee of the Harvard Medical School to Examine the Definition of Brain Death. A definition of irreversible coma JAMA 205 (6):337, 1968

Alsop S: Stay of execution. SR/World (18 December 1973), pp. 20-23

American Hospital Association. Patient's Bill of Rights. Chicago, AHA, 1973

Annas GJ: The Rights of Hospital Patients. New York, Avon, 1975

Annas GJ: Rights of the terminally ill patient. J Nurs Admin 1 (2):40, 1974

Barnes B: Organ donation and transplantation. In Grollman E (ed), Concerning Death: A Practical Guide for the Living. Boston, Beacon, 1974, pp. 253-264

Bok S: Personal directions for care at the end of life. N Engl J Med 295 (7):367, 1976

Callahan D: On defining a "natural death." Hastings Cent Rep 7:32, 1977

Cantor NL: A patient's decision to decline life-saving medical treatment: Bodily integrity versus the preservation of life. Rutgers Law Rev 26:228, 1973

Collaborative Study. National Institute of Neurological and Communicative Disorders and Stroke: An appraisal of the criteria of cerebral death—a summary statement. JAMA 237 (10):982, 1977

Critical Care Committee of the Massachusetts General Hospital. Optimum care for hopelessly ill patients. N Engl J Med 295 (7):364, 1976

Fried C: Equality and rights in medical care. Hastings Cent Rep 6 (1):29, 1976

Fulton R: Death and dying: some sociologic aspects of terminal care. Mod Med 40 (11):74, 1972

Glaser BG, Strauss AL: Awareness of Dying. Chicago, Aldine, 1965

Herter F: The right to die in dignity. Arch Found Thanatol 1 (3):93, 1969

High DM: Death: its conceptual elusiveness. Soundings 40 (4):438, 1972

Jellinek M: Erosion of patient trust in large medical centers. Hastings Cent Rep 6 (3):16, 1976

Kaas LR: Death as an event: a commentary on Robert Morison. Science 173: 698, 1971

Kneisl C: Thoughtful care of the dying. Am J Nurs 3:550, 1968

Mechanic D: Rationing health care: public policy and the medical market place. Hastings Cent Rep 6 (1):34, 1976

Morison RS: Death: process or event? Science 173:694, 1971

Silverman D, Masland RL, Saunders M, Schwab R: Irreversible coma associated with electrocerebral silence. Neurology 20 (6):525, 1970

Sullivan MT: The dying person—his plight and his right. N Engl Law Rev 8:197, 1973

Veatch RM: Choosing not to prolong dying. Med Dimensions (December 1972), pp. 8-10, 40

——: The whole-brain oriented concept of death: an outmoded philosophical formulation. J Thanatol 3:13, 1975

Weisman A: Psychosocial considerations in terminal care. In Schoenberg B, Carr A, Peretz D, Kutscher A (eds), Psychosocial Aspects of Terminal Care. New York, Columbia University Press, 1972, pp. 162-172

Williams R: Management of the sick with kindness, compassion, wisdom, and efficiency. In Williams R (ed), To Live and to Die. New York, Springer-Verlag, 1973, pp. 147-149

Chapter 4

Patients' Perceptions

People who are dying live until the moment of death, and usually feel, think, and respond to the present and future, to the illness, and to those around them. They may strive to control and manipulate the persons around them, so as to prevent significant others from leaving or withdrawing love; they may pretend to avoid feelings of loss and despair.

The primary concern of the dying may not be with death, but with pain in life. Fear of dying is a part of the time when the person still lives and is faced with loss of bodily functions, with uncontrolled pain, with anxiety about anticipated failure of control. If there is no felt need to be in control, the individual may not fear death, but show only realistic concerns for self and loved ones. However, refusal to admit dying may be intensive; patients may be angry and bitter, and try to retaliate. They may berate themselves, feel self-pity, and cling or demand. They may consider the final act of control, suicide, to end life and pain. Resolution involves accepting loss; saying goodbye to loved ones with full resources of the self, with sadness, grace, and equanimity (Sobel 1974).

Aged men and women who see themselves abandoned and rootless on earth often wait impatiently for death, as may terminally ill people of any age. For some who are ready to resign from life, it is a wait for release to be taken away. Others desire the new life, the transfiguration, the reunion with loved ones under perfect conditions. Most people do not "fall apart" as death approaches. The dying person is also a living person. General personality, behavior, and patterns of living are not suddenly suspended because death is in prospect (Datan and Ginsberg 1975).

Fischer (1967) and Hammerschlag (1964) were among early observers of behavior in terminal patients. They report individual differences in response to the threat of illness: helplessness, disability, pain, and the experience of separation depend on personality differences, which in turn derive from past experiences. The patient's responses to life-threatening illness may be considered maladaptive by staff if reactions are stronger than the danger appears to warrant, if they persist when the threat no longer exists, or if appropriate responses to danger are lacking. Schoenberg and Senscu (1970) suggest that autonomous, independent individuals resist the patient role and do not submit easily to staff directives.

The feelings experienced by terminal patients were delineated by Fischer (1967) and Hammerschlag (1964) as follows. For the patient with a life-threatening disease, *fear* can be realistic or exaggerated. The patient's fear of dying may be displaced from other sources of anxiety, such as fear of separation, abandonment, loneliness, mutilation, loss of control, loss of identity, and expression of infantile behavior. Many patients regard fear as a sign of weakness, inferiority, or immaturity, and are therefore reluctant to verbalize it. The fear then expresses itself in physical symptoms, fearful dreams, or emotional withdrawal.

In chronic disease or any illness with repeated and prolonged hospitalization, the patient is placed in a *dependent* position that causes him to feel childlike and helpless. Many patients react with resentment as feelings of weakness, inferiority, shame, and smallness are reawakened. How the person handles these feelings depends on how his dependency needs were met in earlier relationships. If he felt secure in early life, he may find it easier to trust medical and nursing staff. Out of the fear and shame of dependency the patient may present a facade of independence and rebellion: if his illness is too severe he will become apathetic and depressed, clinging to others and exaggerating minor complaints. He may be unaware of how the deprivation of self-sufficiency influences his behavior and he may suffer severe loss of self-esteem.

A fundamental characteristic of the dependent patient is his tendency to perceive the doctors and nurses as parents. In order to remain in their good graces, he is likely to be compliant and ingratiating, as loss of parental figures' approval is a threat to security. He views the doctor and nurse as potentially punitive and is reluctant to voice complaints or make demands. If he disagrees with treatment, he is inclined to feel guilty, even if his reaction is appropriate.

Like fear, *anger* can be an anticipatory response to threat of pain, damage, or loss of function. In the hospital, expression of anger is likely to be discouraged even more strongly than fear. The fearful, compliant, ingratiating patient is likely to be rewarded; the angry, demanding, complaining patient elicits punitive or retaliative behavior. In the dependent patient, anger often stimulates feelings of guilt and fear of retaliation. It is frightening for the patient in a dependent position to express anger toward medical staff upon whom he depends for survival and care; in order to control his anger, he may withdraw from self-assertive behavior and become emotionally inaccessible. He may express great relief when his anger is acknowledged and accepted, and the patient who is encouraged to discuss angry feelings is less likely to develop feelings of guilt and depression, or to regard the environment as hostile.

Damage to self-esteem is initially a result of the patient's reaction to his primary disease and is closely related to: (1) illness and loss of capacity to function, (2) loss of self-sufficiency and independent feelings, (3) fear, (4) guilt, (5) inability to gain gratification, and (6) interpretation of the attitudes and feelings of significant figures (family, nurses, physician) toward him. Everyone aspires to be loved and appreciated, not aggressive or hateful and not dependent or helpless. The failure to fulfill these aspirations can cause serious reduction of self-esteem and consequent depression. Both Fischer and Hammerschlag suggest that, generally, health-care personnel tend to underestimate their influence on the patient's attitudes and feelings about himself, although this is not supported by the interviews that follow.

Guilt is related to fear of punishment, based on the child's belief that the all-powerful parent sees, hears, and knows all. The doctor is likely to be cast in the benign parent role by the helpless patient; but he is also likely to be cast in the punitive role. The guilty person (the patient) may feel dirty, bad, unworthy and anticipate punishment, feelings which may cause anxiety and lowered self-esteem. He may feel guilt over his hostile thoughts and feelings as well as his overtly angry behavior, and he may view disease as punishment for past sins and indiscretions that are usually minor or not even explainable when they are explored with a therapist. Feelings of envy, jealousy, and dependency also contribute to guilt feelings.

Loss of pleasure from life activities results from chronic or terminal illness. Pleasure buffers or neutralizes the pain and frustration which are inevitable in life and which especially accompany loss of health and function. The person who recognizes his life span as limited is reluctant to engage in pleasurable activities; this reluctance is encouraged by institutionalization, as in most hospitals opportunity for pleasurable activity is limited, routinized, and peripheral to the therapeutic program.

The term "dying" is at times inappropriate for the terminally ill patient; he may have a fatal illness and yet currently enjoy good physical health. The process of dying is temporal, and at different stages of illness the patient's needs and requirements of care differ. As stated previously, persons are likely to face death the way they faced life. Schneidman (1963) identifies the following orientations to death: (1) the postponer (who wishes not to die and exerts his will to live); (2) the acceptor (who is resigned); (3) the disdainer (who is disdainful and does not believe death will take him); (4) the welcomer (who sees death as a relief); and (5) the fearer (who greatly fears death).

Regardless of the patient's orientation, Schneidman believes that the defensive process of *denial* is common to some degree in all patients with a fatal illness. The mechanism is one of avoidance, which is integrated into the adaptive system of the person and serves the temporary function of negating intolerable or painful stimuli and rendering him unconscious of them. Denial consumes energy and avoids reality but makes life more tolerable; thus the defense should be respected unless there is clear evidence that the patient would be better off without it. Stripping the patient of this defense is likely to cause further depression, emotional disorganization, and more withdrawal from reality, causing him to be less accessible to medical staff or family.

Denial, however, may lead to unwise behavior in patients; for instance, they may expand a business, or engage in strenuous activities; they may identify with physicians, thinking only *other* patients are ill; or they may isolate themselves from the source of accurate information, the physician, and not take medications or keep follow-up appointments. They may avoid making wills, or financial provisions for families.

Feelings of grief and depression gradually emerge as a patient recognizes the potential loss of loved ones. To protect himself from painful feelings of separation and loss, the patient tends to withdraw from important relationships. Unable to cope with their feelings of loss, friends, family, and medical staff also withdraw. This mutual withdrawal or disengagement causes isolation and loneliness, reducing the patient's capacity for living during the last days. Because depression is so common in hospitalized patients, suicide must be considered a potential behavior. The period preceding discharge from the hospital — when "everything possible has been done" — is when the patient is potentially suicidal, because unrealistic hopes and fantasies of cure have been deflated. The suicide attempt may be related to a wish to punish a family member or physician. It may represent the need to relieve intolerable guilt or regain control. It may be viewed as relief from pain, isolation, loneliness, or loss of valued function or body part. Some patients cannot endure the waiting and want to get death over with (Schneidman 1963).

Webster (1973) states that the patient who is ill and facing the possibility of death from the illness is likely to be considered as a dying patient by staff for therapeutic purposes, although the actual dying process may take months or even years. It is this perspective of the dying process that is utilized in the identification of patients for the interviews which follow.

The focus of this chapter is on the care of an individual who is dying and who must spend most of the time he is dying in a regulated setting. Thus we are more concerned with defining dying than death.

It is, of course, not easy to obtain information about dying — particularly from persons who *are* dying. The meaning of death varies with the individual and with the setting; the problems of generating legal and clinical criteria for the state of "death" have been discussed earlier, and are of concern when there is no congruence among staff, patients, and families as to when the process of dying begins to be the event of death. When death *has* occurred, the caring responsibility of the nurse must shift from the corpse to those survivors who have needs that they cannot meet alone. As the pronouncement of death is a medical act, the nurse can only react to that pronouncement. The issue in medicine may well be the development of criteria to determine death; the issue in nursing is to develop criteria to determine dying. If care of the patient who is dying demands nursing therapies which are different from therapies utilized in the care of the patient who will live, it is necessary to be able to determine who is dying. The literature indicates that staff do indeed make this differentiation because staff behaviors are perceptibly different when the prognosis is negative.

There is, however, a certain ambiguity even in the term "negative prognosis." Physicians are reluctant to officially indicate that any patient is in a terminal state, although Sudnow (1967) found that the expression is usually reserved by staff for those patients who are expected to die during their present hospitalization. Glaser and Strauss (1965) suggest that staff consider patients to be dying when there is no further treatment that will stabilize the condition for an extended period of time.

In research terms, the reliability of the findings in studies of the process of dying is questionable. Descriptions of the process are likely to be narrative in nature — case studies of a single patient or a category of patients, derived from interview data. Observational data, when present, are likely to be the product of clinical assessments — that is, the observations of therapists who are providing care to patients. The clinical insights of the therapist add a great deal to the significance of the findings; those same clinical insights are a source of observational bias.

The data in this book derived from interviews with dying patients are subject to the same sources of error as any interview data: the tendency of the subject to report what the investigator would obviously like to hear and the tendency of the investigator to ask questions in such a way that a desirable response will be elicited. Structured interview schedules control for such error to some extent, but given the situation of the subjects and the topic of the discussion one wonders how much significant information can be obtained with a highly structured set of questions. If the research interest is in some epidemiology of dying, short responses to a structured question set may provide the necessary information. If one wishes to understand the needs of an individual who is dying, it is necessary to allow some variation in the information-gathering procedure.

The problems of caring for the dying are confounded by the ambiguity about what constitutes appropriate behavior for both the giver and the recipient of care (Elder 1973). In an effort to identify whether patients and nurses were in agreement about patient needs and appropriate patient and nurse behaviors, taped interviews were obtained with patients whose diagnoses predicted terminal prognoses and with the nursing personnel involved in their care. The difficulties of obtaining access to subjects when research questions address the topic of death is well known (Kübler-Ross 1969; Crane 1970), and this investigation was hampered by the same problems as other investigators have experienced. However, once access was obtained, nursing personnel were without exception helpful and interested.

In this study, the requirements of the various committees devoted to the protection of human subjects were such that it was not possible to pose to the patients who were interviewed the questions directly related to dying. Further, physicians generally did not care to identify which patients they considered to be terminal. Under these circumstances, it was difficult to develop and utilize an interview schedule that would provide the desired information about normative behavior in terminal, hospitalized patients, and their nursing needs. The dilemma was resolved to some extent by defining a "dying" patient as one who was identified by the professional nurse in charge of his care as manifesting irreversible symptoms of a progressive disease. However, this definition generated some problems of its own; when subjects were selected in the absence of the investigator, it became clear that for many nurses a patient is dying only when he is almost dead. In at least one institution visited, all of the patients selected were within several hours of death, and even when they were conscious and reasonably coherent did not, understandably enough, care to be interviewed.

Schusterman (1973) points out in her critical review of the literature that the majority of investigators believe that patients should be informed of a negative prognosis but in any case are likely to be able to determine their condition from physiological and environmental cues. The institutional committees, however, required the deletion from the interview schedule of all questions that explicitly addressed dying or death. The compromise which was acceptable to all of the committees involved was to refer throughout the interview to "patients like you"; for instance, if the subject was hospitalized for treatment of cancer, all of the questions were asked in terms of patients hospitalized for the treatment of cancer. This led to some difficult circumlocution; some subjects responded immediately with, "What do you mean, patients like me?" In fact, a good many of the patients interviewed volunteered the information that they might not get well or that the current treatment was "a last resort." When patients indicated they were at risk of death, the questions were asked about (other) patients who were at risk of death.

The majority of the patients quoted below were hospitalized with malignancies of one kind or another; although mobility was quite limited for many, almost all of them were ambulatory to some extent. They were predominantly of lower socioeconomic status and rural background. There is no assumption that this sample is representative of any specified population, as the concept of random selection in this context is without meaning. Those persons who were resident in selected institutions, who in the opinion of the nurse in charge manifested irreversible symptoms of a progressive disease, and who were willing and able to talk with the investigator provide the data in these interviews. Obviously it is not possible to know whether other patients would respond in the same way to the same questions posed by a different interviewer at a different time.

The study patients responded to questions about nurses: what nurses did for them, what they would like nurses to do for them. They responded to questions about how "patients like you" *should* behave in the hospital, and how they *did* behave. They responded poignantly, and at some length, to questions about their current concerns and sources of support. Another report is available with attention given to the statistical implications of the results (Castles and Keith 1979) and the study is summarized in Appendix A. The intent in this chapter is not to interpret the meaning of chi square, but to let patients speak for themselves about their concerns.

PATIENTS' PERCEPTIONS OF NURSES

What Do Nurses Do for You?

The responses to the question "What do nurses do for you?" are characterized by extravagant praise of nurses functioning in a cheerful manner in instrumental roles, directly dependent on medical directives to dictate their activities. As will become evident, regardless of the nature of the question and in spite of the praise of nurses, there was a recurrent implication in the responses that there exists between patients and nurses a reciprocal responsibility in which benefit to the patient occurs only if he cooperates with the nurses.

An elderly veteran of World War II knew immediately and exactly what nurses did:

> R (Respondent): Bring me pills, bring me pills and what they're for I don't suppose they know.

Two of his colleagues were more expansive in their remarks, but less specific about nursing activities:

> R: They're a bunch of little angels.

> R: They are devotedly attentive. They don't always even wait for the signal light. Sometimes they stop in and inquire if there's anything I need or want. You can't beat that for dedication.

This sample of patients was apparently almost entirely ignorant of independent nursing functions, and thought that only physicians could prescribe care.

> R: Well, they help me every time I ask, every time I ask them. Now they ain't been able to help me this time because they're waiting on the doctors, for his information.

> R: Well, they give me medicine and stuff, whatever the doctor prescribes for me.

Some patients were comprehensive: nurses do everything. Some qualified their responses: nurses do whatever you need, but not very much was really needed. Patients tended to deny their dependency or need for help. One of the patients who responded most globally — "they wait on you hand and foot" — provided an interesting side-remark indicating pride in the fact that the nurses had no reason to complain about *her* behavior. The general trend of the responses indicates that nurses do what needs to be done, even if the patient doesn't want it, and are *more likely to do it for the cooperative patient*. Cheerfulness and "niceness" are valued traits in nurses.

> R: [They do] everything that you ask them, and so many many more that you don't [sic].

> R: [They are] very considerate, cheerful. They've always made me feel real welcome and always made me feel like I been a good patient.

> R: Well, if I have a hurting, they see that I'm taken care of. That hurting, all you have to do is go up to the desk and tell them. Now the other night I took cobalt . . . and I told her that I was sick at my stomach. And she said, "Well, we'll fix that," and so she give me a shot, and that was the end of it.

R: See that my food was right on the table, get my linen, and they're
       cheerful — which I think means a lot.

R: They wait on me hand and foot, I think. They really do.

R: Of course, after the operation, in the recovery room, I was on my
       feet. They get you on your feet first thing. Whether you can stand it
       or not, you're on your feet . . . I was able to get around, so most of
       the things they did for me was answer my calls for a shot to help kill
       the pain. Like that, but most of the time I was able to take care
       of myself.

R: If there's anything you want, and you're cooperating, if possible
       they'll get it for you. But if you don't, I've seen other patients that
       don't cooperate, they don't get any cooperation from the nurse
       hardly at all either. Now that's my opinion of nurses.

R: Well, they see that I'm clean, cleaned up, and they give me my medi-
       cine when it's due. Oh, they're wonderful here.

I (Interviewer):   What else do they do?

R: Well, I never ask for anything, but I know they'd do it for me because
       they're wonderful here.

The demand for a cheerful disposition in nurses is explicit, although at least
one of the patients perceives that nurses have a difficult task because they can't
escape the patients' statements and behavior, and several express the feeling that
patients should be helpful to staff.

R: They got to listen to you when you cry, and whenever anybody lets
       out steam it's on the nurses, it's not on the doctors.

I: Do you think this is hard for nurses?

R: I think so.

I: Don't you think it's one of the things they *should* do for patients,
       let them blow off steam?

R: It's a hard job, especially when you get emotionally involved with
       these people, and you can't help but get that way.

R: I really truthfully think the patients could help the nurses a lot, too.

I: Do you think they should?

R: I do. I mean, it'd be good for them to get up and stir around a little
       bit, and you know, such as taking their bath and getting some exer-
       cise, and you know, straightening up the room a little bit, and just
       kind of keeping their place kind of straightened up around their bed
       and the desk and so on.

An occasional maverick reports a fault.

R: On the whole, the nursing staff in general, boys, young men, as well as the women, are just delightfully friendly, but there's a few that we call "sour-puss" or "there's old smiley." And this is something that really annoys me. When they come to work and they're working with people, they could try to be a little pleasant. There are two or three on each shift that you really want to trip on their way past. You know, they're really not . . . they're very efficient, but they're just not nice to have around, they're just not pleasant to you.

What Would You Like Nurses to Do for You?

If nurses are perceived as cheerful providers of physical care, this is apparently what they should be. The responses to "What would you *like* nurses to do for you?" are not easily distinguished from the responses to the previous question about what nurses do. Patients reiterated their disinclination to be any trouble to a busy staff and their determination to do all they could for themselves. They indicate their wish to be well cared for, to receive what is needed yet maintain independence, and to be distracted by the cheerfulness of the nurses from their feelings and concerns.

R: Just what they're doing. Just be theirself and do their duties is all. I don't want them to cater to me or anything.
_____

R: Just have those pretty smiles that they have morning and noon, and if you ask them for anything, they'll see that you get what you're supposed to.
_____

R: Oh, just things you couldn't do yourself.

I: Like what?

R: Like taking enemas and stuff like that.
_____

R: Just like they do, but I don't think they should be taken advantage of.

I: Can you talk about that a little bit?

R: I mean, for instance, once in a while you'll find a griper, you know. That isn't my . . . for instance keep the light on continuously for a nurse. I don't think that's necessary.

I: Why do you think people do that?

R: Well, I don't know. I suppose that's the way they feel. Maybe they're spoiled or something.

I: Maybe they're scared? And they want somebody with them?

R: That's possible, but back in Room 639 we're just like a big family back there and the nurses have made it that way. I mean, they come back and share our fun with us too. And I haven't found a nurse here

I: that I could say anything against. Not a one. Even the one that drops ice down my back.

I: Well, I think I'd complain about that!

R: She said she thought I needed to be woke up. I said, "Well, I'll get you back."

R: Well, really, there isn't much they need to do for me.

I: There isn't anything more that you'd like to have?

R: They give me my medication, I just had it at nine o'clock.

Two points are clearly important: the patients would like nurses to be *available*, and they should be *informative*.

R: One thing — what do they call that room out there?

I: Recovery room?

R: Recovery room, yes. I would like them to come in regularly without me having to look for the button or something, because that's a time when you sort of panic when you come down from the operating room . . . if somebody would just look in every five or ten minutes as they pass by, I'd appreciate that.

I: Just knowing that somebody's around?

R: Yes, I don't need somebody to sit there, oh, four or five hours, just come in once in a while. The other thing I like . . . they don't do this and this is what I resent. When they give you a needle, and when they give you a barium enema, when they give you a pill, I think they should tell what it is, and what it's for, even if I don't understand the whole thing. Like downstairs I was absolutely amazed. They gave me some kind of rectal examination, and after it was over, the lady there showed me how it worked and why they did it, and how it worked inside of me. And I was absolutely enamored with the whole process. At least if I ask them what it's for, let them answer me. Some patients may not want to know, but if you ask "What is it for?", I don't like them to tell me "Well, you'll have to ask your doctor," or "We can't tell you." Oh, I resent that. They did that in the other hospital — "Well, you'll have to ask Dr. _____," or "Well, we can't tell you what we're giving you," and I said, "Well, I want to know, or you're not going to give it to me." And then because I created a stink, Dr. _____ came in and told me what it was all about.

In one patient, an unconscious shift in pronouns provides a poignant insight.

R: I think they should work at their job and take an interest in the patients, and not shun them all the time, but go by and see them once in a while, see if they need anything, and if they do, why, try to answer their questions and tell them what they can do and what they can't do, and let them know just where they stand. Instead of staying away from me all the time where you can't find them. They do sometimes, you can't get a hold of one. I'd like to be able to see one come by once in awhile that I can ask a question or something like that, something that I need to know or want to know.

Another manifests his distress with obviously limited treatment objectives.

> I: O.K. They bring you pills and meals and provide a bed, and I asked you what else you would want them to do for you.
>
> R: I don't know, because it's quite obvious they don't know what to do. The doctors don't know what to do. How can they expect nurses to know if the doctor don't know?

Patients would like their nurses to be friendly and understanding; indeed, one suggests curriculum changes (a little more psychology) to help develop such understanding.

> R: Sometimes [nurses] misunderstand. Well, that makes the patient contrary or something. In other words, I think they could be domineering . . . I've seen them where there could be a better understanding of the nurse and of the patient how they feel. I think maybe all of us. I don't know how much schooling nurses take in psychology, or anything, but I think it could be a little more.
>
> ----
>
> R: [Friendliness] isn't a subject that can be put down in black and white because there's circumstances that are just different. Here where I'm not known, it's just a little different than places where I am known, and they think so much of my husband and everything. It just makes a lot of difference.

What Do You Look for Most of All in a Nurse?

It is evident that these patients did not separate what the nurses actually do from the affective component of care: they responded to questions about what the nurses *did* in terms of whether they were friendly and cheerful. When they were asked what they looked for most of all in a nurse, responses were in terms of both behavior and personality. It is clear that for these patients nursing is not to be separated from the personal characteristics of the nurse. The most valued qualities are kindness and friendliness; in one patient this is manifested by the nurse in her willingness to provide cues for his own behavior.

> R: Well, I don't know any more than information . . . I don't know how to adapt myself to this kind of life. I'd like some information. Be

able to ask 'em what I'm supposed to do and what I'm not supposed
to do, so I'll know how to do my part.

To be kind, to be gentle, to be pleasant are major factors. The nurses should
really care.

R: Well, any kindness, you know, because patients are sick, and if you
     spill something, or like that, and if they tell you to clean it up, I don't
     think that's right.

I: So they're kind to you, and that's what you look for most in the
     nurses who take care of you?

R: Yes, well, I really don't look for it, but it's there. I'm not really *look-
     ing* for anything, but it's still there, and it shows a lot.

R: A good disposition. A good disposition. Somebody that's happy all
     the time. I don't like somebody to come into the room with a mouth
     hanging down about a mile, you know.

I: You like somebody cheerful, to cheer you when you're down?

R: Yes.

R: Well, that is kind of hard to explain. The most thing I look for, if I
     have a bandage or something that is bothering me, she'll be willing to
     go in and change it.

I: So, a willingness to care for you . . .?

R: To care for the patient, right.

R: Personality.

I: What kind of personality do you like?

R: I like somebody that's kind, and friendly, and then if she kind of
     hurts you it doesn't hurt.

Courtesy to, respect for, and interest in the patient as a person are identified
as valued qualities in nurses, although there is perhaps some difference of opinion as to how the nurse shows respect. It is important for the patient to be
identified by name and not to be talked to as though he were a child. Including
the family in such teaching and support is also recognized as helpful.

R: Well, I'll tell you what I look for, I look for a nurse to be courtesy
     [sic], not too mouthy and not too talkative, consider her patients,
     and devoted to her patients, and as far as come up and baby the guys,
     and sweetheart this and sweetheart that and honey this, I don't go for
     that, but I go for just plain Clay, or Mr. J., how are you?

R: Calling you by your name, and explaining things. Yes, I guess it's
     more identity.

I: It's hard to keep it? Your identity?

R: Yes, and I'm the type that hangs on to my identity jealously, you know.

R: You can tell whether they actually take a genuine interest or whether they . . . it's more or less a personal interest. And both of them are nice, and when they take that personal interest I think it's a lot nicer. They call you by your first name.

I: I was going to say, what do they do when they take a personal interest? They recognize you by name?

R: Yes, and they'll speak to you out on the streets, and they'll do little favors for you, like if you need something out in the town, they'll make sure you get it, or they'll run little errands for you, and speak to your family.

The plea to be treated as an individual, as a person with all the characteristics of any other adult, is plain. The nurse is expected to keep her troubles to herself, to focus on the patient and his problems.

The need to know that nurses are available, are keeping watch, and will provide immediate attention is reflected in the responses to this question, as in the responses to all of the questions.

What Have Nurses Done That You Remember as Meaningful or Important?

It is obvious in the responses that meaningfulness is directly related to the provision of personal, individual attention.

R: A nurse come by, and she talked to me, and she said to me, "Now I know you're lonesome, and we want to help you every bit we can. We don't want you to be lonesome or anything like that. Now if there's anything possible I can do for you, you tell me." Well, I said, "Right now my back's hurting." And she went and got some kind of a backrub stuff, ointment or something, and rubbed my back. Then she asked me if there was anything else. Yes, my water bottle was empty. So she grabbed up my water bottle. I couldn't get me a drink, it was empty. And went and filled it. And little things like that . . .

I: Are very important?

R: Just changed my whole outlook on staying in the hospital. I was about ready to go home if she hadn't done that, I think I'd have just walked out of that hospital and gone home.

R: This nurse asked me if she could rub my back for me or make me more comfortable, and I know her back must have hurt a lot worse than mine did. Cause she'd been running like crazy all day.

> *R:*   I hadn't been there but a few days, and she came back and introduced
> herself to me, and all of us, and told us her names, and says, "I'm
> charge nurse today. And I'll be glad to help you. If there's any prob-
> lems let me know and turn on your light." And there's never been
> another charge nurse that did that. They've been nice, but none of
> them came back and introduced themselves.

Although a wide range of specific nursing activities was reported to be particularly helpful, the importance of nurses' treating patients as persons, as individuals, continues to be identified.

The caring behavior of other patients is reported along with the behavior of
the nurses.

> *R:*   Well, I couldn't get down to the nurses station, and the patients that
> was in the other room went down there and told them how I was
> hurting, and the nurses all run right down. And so the patients really
> help one another, and they help the nurses too.
>
> *I:*   You think that's a good thing?
>
> *R:*   I think it's a grand thing.
> _____
> *R:*   I had this here stomach operation, and had these machines going back
> and forth in your stomach, through here and out the stomach here
> and I was very weak. No one knew it; I didn't know it myself, the old
> gentleman next door to me told the nurse and he said that boy don't
> seem to be doing right, so she come in, and she seen right then what
> was wrong and she called the doctor and the doctor put two machines
> on.

One of the patients who was interviewed was entirely convinced that the
doctor dictates all care activities. He could identify no meaningful nursing
activity separate from the physician directive. However, for the majority of the
patients who could not recall any most meaningful or important nursing activities, it was because *all* activities were said to be important and all the nurses
were helpful.

Is There Anything Nurses Could Be Doing to Make You Comfortable Which They Are Not Doing?

The responses in this instance are a sequence of negatives; this is somewhat
depressing, as the institutions visited were certainly not overstaffed and even
to the eye of a nonclinical investigator extremely sympathetic to nursing
there was *some* room for improvement. In line with a general view of nursing
as a subordinate branch of medicine, and a belief that nurses are overworked
and are doing all they can do, patients generally did not themselves identify
anything lacking—although to the experienced ear they were damning with
faint praise. For example, a prompt response to the light would be appreciated—

but only if sicker patients were not deprived of service. If staffing could be improved, more help at meals and more help with exercise would also be appreciated.

R: I don't know of a thing. Now, an instance, I had to come to the toilet here one night, and I didn't think a soul saw me come. Well, I was in no hurry — I just sat there and smoked a cigarette and paid a little overtime [sic] and here come that girl right down there and thought maybe I was in trouble, see. She said, "Are you having trouble?", and I said, "No, I'm just dawdling around and smoking a cigarette." But now, she saw me leave, and I didn't even know she had.

I: They keep an eye on you?

R: Yes, they do.

R: No, I wouldn't know of anything because they're wonderful to me.

I: O.K., now tell me about that, when you say that they're wonderful to you, what do they do that makes you think they're wonderful to you?

R: Well, they're always in a good humor, they're never cross . . . I don't have to ask them to do too many things for me really, but I know I could ask them for anything and they would willingly do it.

R: No. They're trying to make me as comfortable as possible . . . Nope, no, just that . . . they said they'd get to that as quick as they could. Probably in there waiting on the doctors in there. Said they'll be back quickly, then they'll do what they're going to do, I guess.

R: Actually, facts are facts, and most institutions are understaffed and . . . there just isn't enough help.

I: But say there was enough staff, what could nurses be doing that they're not doing?

R: Maybe patients that can't feed themselves correctly, and you find that they're not eating properly, but the trays possibly are taken away quickly, and they say that they are finished, but you know they're not filled.

When nurses could not respond as patients wished, the nurses were usually not considered to be aware. Also, while independence is valued, a *supervised* independence is, realistically enough, preferred.

The minority who responded in the affirmative were most articulate about verbal behavior which they defined correctly as depersonalizing and non-professional.

R: Yes, I think there's one thing that's a psychological thing more than a physical thing. I think they should attempt to look at you as an individual rather than, you know, that "group down in that room" or something like this. They're inclined to, even the pleasant ones, are inclined to treat us as nonpersons. They talk about things as though you weren't sitting there. They talk to one another about things just as though it doesn't matter. It's just like you go to a restaurant and there are rather wealthy people sitting there, they will sit and talk about the most intimate details and you don't count, you're not part of their group. And I don't think they should be discussing private things in front of you as if you're a nonperson. And another thing, too. Like last night on the third shift, down here I was awakened by hilarity. I didn't mind — it was pleasant to hear. But obviously they were not paying attention that there were patients closer to them, and that they were waking up really sick people. I'm not that sick but it annoyed me on behalf of the other patients, that they were acting as if there were nobody here except them. They can talk, they can talk softly, they can go into the alcove, they can play cards, if they want. I don't care what they do, as long as they pay attention to the lights.

I: And be quiet when people are trying to sleep?

R: Right.

R: Yes. They could keep their mouths shut. I don't like for them to talk to me about other peoples' disease.

I: Have you ever told them you'd just as soon they didn't?

R: No, I don't want to hurt their feelings. I just think they got to have someone to talk to and I keep my mouth shut. But I'd appreciate, you know . . . if they wouldn't talk about other people to me. I hate to think they're talking about me to someone else.

If You Could Make an Anonymous Suggestion to Improve Nursing Care, What Would It Be?

Although they had difficulty identifying anything nurses could be doing which they were not doing, many patients were able to respond to the above question with some definite suggestions. Whether they became more comfortable in the situation as the interview progressed, or whether the interview questions triggered questions in their minds about their own experiences is not known, but many of the individuals were quite willing to make anonymous suggestions to improve care, some of which were quite specific. One subject reports inexcusable behavior; another looks back to a time when "the human touch" was more likely.

R: We have some older ones [nurses] who will let their feelings show when they're treating an older patient, who missed the bedpan, you know, and they get carried away, and say . . . well, I know I'd get awful mad if they'd say it to me. In fact I'd walk out of the hospital if it would ever be said about me like some of the things they've said about other patients.

I: *About* or *to?*

R: To and about.

I: What kinds of things?

R: Just, for instance, there awhile back we had a patient, oh he was approximately 70 years old, and he wasn't able to walk or get out of bed, he was sick, and he was . . . he'd want to use the bedpan. Of course, he did press his light a lot, and wanting little things, but he was sick. And one time he didn't get on the bedpan and he messed the bed. And the nurse came in and said, "If you'd quit shitting your bed, you old son of a bitch . . ."

I: Did anybody ever report that?

R: If it was me I would have got up and said something, but it wasn't involving me. I felt I should keep my mouth shut because I never did know what they were going through. Might have been a bad day for them, or something.

I: It could never be that bad.

R: Well, that's what I thought.

R: I think a lot has to do with the way they [nurses] look at themselves. I find the old-fashioned nurse, that got involved with her patients, was something that's been lost by the professionalism that's come and taken it's place . . . We've lost that human touch. But there was something they did in the old days that I didn't like. They thought they knew what was better for you, and I didn't like that either. Like the old schoolteacher and the old nurse, she knew what was good for you, and I didn't like that authoritarian figure at all. So if we could just be less prima donna-ish and stick to the human touch, but not go back to the real old ways, I'd like that. And it doesn't have to be anonymous. Anyone who knows me, already knows what I think.

Poor staffing and dietary deficiencies are also addressed.

R: [How] to improve the care? One is to get more help.

I: Get more help?

R: They really do need that. Because at night sometimes there's just two nurses to take care of this whole floor . . . They're in a tizzy, and I don't think that's fair.

I: To the patients?

R: Or to the nurses.

R: I can't understand why they feed you so many times a day. About five times a day, and there don't seem to be no diet or anything. And all that stuff, I can't eat five times a day, and they just get on me for not eating. And when I'm home, even though I'm a big man, I don't eat like that.

R: Well, when they serve a meal, keep the utilities [sic] out of the deep freeze.

I: Your knives and forks you mean, they're cold?

R: They are, they're out of the deep freeze. And they serve a warm dinner with a cold knife and fork. You still be here at supper?

I: Yes, I might be.

R: Check it, they serve around 4:30. It's the damnedest thing, you take a knife out of the deep freeze and put it on a baked potato, your butter'll turn cold in two minutes.

What Is the Most Annoying Thing Nurses Do or Say?

In this instance depersonalization which occurs to patients committed to institutional care is the major component of responses. Sometimes the behavior described is physical — a treatment — and sometimes it is an inferred attitude; but in all cases the patient has felt humiliated.

R: Well, the most thing I think that I can see or remember is that we have a lot of nurses [that] seems to me like takes for granted that a patient should know and understand this deal here as well as they do, and because you don't they seem to get irritated at you. They don't like you to ask them silly questions, they don't like you to demand them things that's not their duty, which I haven't so far, but I hear it going on. Each nurse has their duty, and sometimes if you ask them something that's out of their line they just act like they don't appreciate it, and [it] kind of irritates them. Which the patient don't know. I don't know who is who, or who's responsible, I don't know who to ask and if I ask the wrong one why it's just a mistake; they come tell me so and tell me who to ask, or somebody.

I: Without being unkind about it.

R: Yes. Like if a nurse comes in and you say "good morning," sometimes she may say "good morning," and you'll say "good morning" and other times you say "good morning" to a nurse and she just won't say a word. Now that kind of irritates me.

R: The most annoying thing that I can see that the nurses does to me is come in and holler, "Well, how are ya baby, how are ya, honey, this morning." Course some men like that, and I guess if he don't mind that's all right. But that's the most annoying thing to me.

R: [Nurses] cautioned me to tell them [x-ray personnel] not to try to force this white stuff in my rectum, because there's a block in it. Well, I told this [male x-ray attendant] and he said, "Well, I'll turn it over to the big boy." And I said, "All right, fine." So he come and put it in there, you know, and it just leaked out of there, and I was just laying there like a log and he said, "You ain't trying to hold it," and I said, "I'm a-doing all I can." So he put it back in there again and just squashed it out. He said, "You ain't trying to hold it." And I said, "You're a goddamn liar." I cool him off because I couldn't do anything, there's nobody knows the matter to hold it.

I: Did he let you be?

R: He quit that then. Now there's one thing that made me mad. When they got through they wanted me to get up and put my robe over that goddamn chocolate clothes that come clear down here to the floor. I said, "You got a bathroom?" and went in there and didn't even have a tub. But I couldn't go any further. I just pulled them damn things off, and I got myself some paper towels and wiped off as best I could, and I went to this boy, and I says, "You got all clean things to put on?" And he says, "No." And I says, "I'm going right down through there nude then," so he says, "Wait a minute." He got me a little old shirt of a thing, and I put my robe on over it. But that, why couldn't they have a bathtub up there? There's a lot of people what have mishaps. That's the silliest thing I ever saw in my life.

R: I hate a nurse giving me an enema. I don't mind an orderly, but I hate a nurse doing it.

R: I hate to see nurses get in a group, a bunch, and giggle and carry on. I know everybody does it. I've done it myself, but hate to see them do it. And I also hate to see partiality in nurses. I mean, well, there was one lady here I felt sorry for, she had the blues so bad, but this other lady, she had a good personality, and everybody liked her. And all the nurses hovered around her bed. And this other lady was in the same room and everything, and she never got any attention at all. And it hurt her, it really did. You talked to her and you could tell, it just hurt her. I don't like to see that.

Patients are also annoyed by regulations and routines, and constraints on their behavior.

R: Well, if you want to go outside or something like that . . . now there ain't nothing wrong with me all that bad, but they won't let me go outside . . . You do what they want you to, or else.

I: Well, you want to cooperate in your treatment.

R: I don't want to get throwed out.

I: No, but it does seem a shame on these pretty days, to have to sit in, if there'd be a way you could get out.

R: Well, me and this guy here, we got those IV poles on us, there ain't nothing wrong with us. We can pack them along with us. Don't bother us none. Nobody need help us, but they still won't let us go out.

I: Would they let you go out if somebody went with you?

R: They ain't no need anybody to go with us, you know; we wouldn't want nobody to go with us, anyway.

I: You know it might be a legal problem.

R: Well, they was letting us out for a while there. But I guess some big shot didn't like it . . . I guess some big shot didn't like it that runs the joint.

I: They wake you up to take temperatures? What time do they wake you up?

R: Well, it was 5:30. Of course, that isn't too early but when you don't sleep very good at night . . .

R: Like I said, I just want to be let alone. Or get out in the fresh air. Kind of help myself. I had a little freedom at home; we ain't got no freedom here whatsoever. We can't get out.

Nurses who smoke annoyed one respondent who says, "I just don't like the habit." However, this interviewer felt more concern about the reports of observed rough handling of other patients.

R: Well, one time I saw . . . they talked a little bit rough to one patient in the hospital, something like that, but what they was trying to do is to quiet the patient down. He was unruly and everything, and they was trying to quiet him down. That was the only thing. As far as nurses that's the only time I ever saw one talk back to [a patient]. But the only reason they was doing it was trying to quiet the patient down because he was unruly.

R: Personally, I can't think of any. I had a roommate one time who I thought was treated kind of unfairly, but . . .

I: What did they do to her?

R: I would classify it as unnecessary roughness.

I: They handled her roughly physically? Or verbally?

R: No, physically.

The lack of individualized attention was identified, and nurses were expected to know the patients' needs. Further, patients sometimes felt that nurses or others did not want to work, or at least not do anything extra. The excuse of understaffing is not necessarily accepted by patients, who may see that some personnel are not very interested, committed, or efficient.

> R: Well, I don't know what to say in that respect. That is, the nurses, they're just human like the rest of us, and they have their business to take care of and all they do is bring the pills and a glass of water and that's it, pills and a glass of water. But so far as bending my knees, and legs and exercise, they don't. Now that, that could be an annoyance.
>
> I: I imagine.
>
> R: You see if I could just get enough exercise into these knees daily or twice or three times a day, maybe that would tend to wake them up.

However, here, also, there was a chorus of patients who do not find anything to annoy them in the behavior of their nurses, or if they were able to identify a little something, they excused the nurses because the units were understaffed.

How Often Do the Nurses Come in to See You?

Avoidance behavior in staff is described by all investigators and is universally deplored. Patients in this sample were asked how often their nurses came in to see them, and whether they would like to see them more frequently. While not particularly averse to being visited more frequently, so long as the care of sicker patients did not suffer, they generally did not report avoidance behavior.

> R: Oh, they're in and out of here all the time.
>
> R: Well, they're just in and out all the time with the patients, you know, over here, and they're real busy. I mean they're in and out of the room just as often as they can. If you put your light on or something, they come and see what you need.

However, some patients inadvertently provided evidence that personnel were not present very frequently and a few said so explicitly. Further, nurses apparently would visit the patient only if a task had to be done.

> R: Well, me they don't come to see very . . . If I'm awake they come to the door to check on us to see if everybody's all right, but being as I'm not sick of course they don't check on me. But when I had this surgery, they were in quite often.
>
> R: Well, I get them at 12:00 and at 6:00 for shots, then of course for

blood pressure and all, so I really don't know. It seems like they come quite often.

R: Oh, when I'm real sick they come in to see me real often, and when I'm not sick, when I'm like I am now, I'm up and around and everything, oh, probably at least every hour and maybe oftener.

R: Well, they comes in, you know, and check the bed sometimes, or something like that, but other ways they don't never come.

Do the Nurses Come Often Enough?

Although many of the patients were dependent on the nurses for the alleviation of many physical needs, they generally did not perceive the necessity for nurses to be seen more frequently. When they were asked whether the nurses came in often enough, patients reported that they did, and in any case they came when they were summoned.

R: Oh, I don't think it's necessary, if a man doesn't have any fever, doesn't have any pain, it's not necessary for a nurse to be coming in.

R: No, I think they're doing just fine.

R: If I do, I could just turn that light on, you see.

I: And they come?

R: They come.

I: O.K. You think you see enough of them, they get in here often enough that . . .

R: Well, I wouldn't *mind* seeing more of them. It seems like the day goes pretty fast. You have the cleaning woman to talk to, and there's other people . . . I've been here so long there's other people who put their head in the door and holler at me, and ask how I'm doing and chat a little bit.

They wouldn't "mind" more frequent interaction if nurses were less busy, but do not see this as necessary. When the physical care is given, patients wish only to see the nurse when their medications or treatments are due, or when they think they need someone — otherwise, it "doesn't do any good." Patients also sense responsibilities to staff and for each other; they try to spare staff any unnecessary activity, and also to spare staff for sicker patients. Ambulatory patients are somehow not perceived to be in need of attention from the nurses.

R: No, not when I feel as good as I do. I think they should be taking care of those who really need it.

R: I'm sure there's somebody else in the hospital probably needs more attention than I do. I'm able to walk on my own two feet.

Only two patients responded clearly and immediately that "a little oftener would be better" — one patient explained that this would be better so he could have a little more water. The other thought that if nurses came more frequently it would not be necessary to call. He did not think it was correct to bother the nurses.

Do the Nurses Sit and Talk with You?

Although the general report was that the nurses were seen frequently enough, most of the answers to "Do the nurses sit and talk with you?" were some form of "no." However, many patients were not interested in having the nurses do so. Apparently they perceive a social component in sitting down to talk, and conversation was not understood to be a nursing duty. There was also the usual concern for overworked staff.

> *R:* They'll come in, the head nurse, and greet you like they do, and ask you how you are and what kind of a night you had, and visit with you a little bit as they make their rounds.
>
> *I:* Do they come in and just sit down and talk with you like I'm talking now?
>
> *R:* They don't have time.
>
> *I:* Would you like that if they could?
>
> *R:* Oh, I don't know. I think everything's fine just the way it is.
>
> *R:* I'm not too much of a talker, no ma'am. It would be all right, I guess, if we would talk on the same subjects or anything like that, but I don't know, I'm just not too much on conversation — never was.
>
> *R:* Well, I'll tell you, I wouldn't ask anybody to come and sit and talk with me because I don't have anything to talk about. I'm 88 years old, you see, and I'm no good, and I think it would be a crime to have to tie a nurse down from such an important job.

Some patients specifically want an information interaction, either to ask questions or to answer them. Those who do wish company are still concerned about the work load, and also the condition of the patient; sick people should not be bothered with conversation — but if the nurse is needed she should be available.

A fortunate few do have nurses who sit and talk with them at times — sometimes about the nurses' problems.

> *I:* Do they sit and talk to you?
>
> *R:* They do. They really do.
>
> *I:* You like that?

R: Yes, I sure do, I like that.

R: Oh, yes, quite often they'll come in, and we'll discuss family problems
     and their problems and their schooling, such as this.

R: Yes ma'am, they do.

I: Do you like that?

R: I do that. I think that it's very enjoyable that the nurse is friendly
     enough to come in and sit down just for a minute. It shows that she
     cares for the patient she is taking care of.

PATIENTS' PERCEPTIONS OF PATIENTS

How Should Patients Like You Behave?

Although the patients sampled were predominantly of rural background, the
independent character popularly ascribed to farmers and small-town citizens
was conspicuously lacking in most patients' perceptions of how hospitalized patients should behave. The predominant theme of the responses was the perceived
necessity for cooperation with the requirements of the disease condition and the
requirements of the health care system (Castles and Keith, 1979). Nurses were,
on the whole, willing to allow some idiosyncratic and system-threatening behaviors in patients; the patients themselves demanded that they comport themselves in obedience to the directives of the staff, and that they not demand more
than a necessary minimum of staff time and effort. The role of the patient is
described by patients almost unanimously to be cooperative, obedient, and nonthreatening. Only if one is very ill and helpless is it considered appropriate to
demand the services of busy nurses, or to complain if such services are not available. Otherwise, expected behavior apparently is based on the realization that
nurses do not have enough time to care for everyone.

In response to the question "How should patients like you behave in the
hospital?" there was general agreement among the patients that cooperative,
nonaggressive behavior was required. This point of view is exemplified in the
following selected responses.

R: To try to have a cheerful attitude and try not to call the nurse unless
     you had a question or a need. They're busy people. And then not to
     try to bawl a nurse out or something like that if something doesn't
     exactly suit you.

I: What should you do though if something doesn't exactly suit you?

R: Well, I don't know. I wouldn't want to report a nurse to the head
     nurse and get her in trouble if I . . . unless it was something that was
     necessary, was something that just kept on, you know.

R: I think they should be . . . they should cooperate with the nurses.

R: Behave, that's the word. Well, some people they get in the hospital
      and they think, "I can't lift my finger to do this and I can't lift my
      finger to do that." Well, you can, and I think you should. You should
      help the nurses as much as you can, not only for their sake but for
      your own sake.

That cooperation is both necessary and possible is believed even by those patients who perceive that people bring to any situation a history that will to some
extent dictate present behavior.

R: I don't know if they can control their behavior so much. I think a pa-
      tient when they come into the hospital is like a boy when he goes into
      the Navy, or the Army, or whatever. Whatever they had before is
      what they are now. And we're not going to change them. I don't
      think they can help their behavior much. What they can do is be, one
      thing, cooperative with the people in the hospital.

When reasons were offered for the expected cooperation with the medical
and nursing staffs, the rationale was realistic and somewhat grim: patients understood that if they behaved in pleasant and cooperative ways, staff would be
pleasant and cooperative with them; they also expressed fear of retaliation for
noncooperative behavior.

R: Well, I think a lot more can be accomplished by kindness than by bel-
      ligerency.

I: You think you can accomplish more . . .?

R: I think you can. I think that if I were to come up to you and would
      try to be pleasant, you would go out of your way to help me more
      than if I'd tear into you and give you double hell.

I: So they should behave in a cooperative way?

R: Right. Because if you don't, some of them can be pretty damned
      mean to you, too.

I: It might be safer to cooperate, is that what you're telling me?

R: Yes.

R: Like I say, I think the main thing is always obey the nurses. Like I
      said at first, if you cooperate with the nurses they'll cooperate with
      you.

A norm of patients' being helpful to other patients and treating them with
respect and consideration is also identified. Further, in spite of the stresses imposed by critical illness, the patients considered their behavior to be under their
control; only a few would allow idiosyncratic and system-threatening behavior.
However, allowances would be made in some situations; those persons who

were not really competent either to identify or to control their behavior were excused from the usual requirement of nondemanding cooperation. Persons who are very old, very ill, or in great pain are not expected to manifest those cooperative behaviors (supportive of the staff) which others should maintain.

Is It All Right to Yell and Complain?

When inquiry was made relevant to probable mental states (e.g., sadness or anger) and specific behaviors (e.g., complaining) that might accompany these feelings, it became clear that — to the patients — anger was a more acceptable response than sadness, although here also situations were identified in which behavior could be beyond the control of an individual because of pain or other mitigating circumstances. However, even when patients could be coaxed into admitting that vociferous complaint was appropriate, they did not consider this a useful response. Typical answers to the question "Do you think patients like you should yell or complain?" include the following.

R: Oh no. I don't think a patient . . . no I don't! Unless they are in pain or have something to yell about or have reason to complain . . .

I: Well, don't you think you have reason to complain?

R: No, I don't.

I: If you can't keep your meals down?

R: Oh well, that ain't the nurse's fault.

R: Well, I just don't see any use in it. Of course, if you need to do a little complaining, I guess it wouldn't be too bad, but I don't see no necessity for it, so . . .

R: Absolutely not. You have to live with those patients for the next ten days or two weeks or whatever . . .

I: If you're in a private room and not disturbing other patients, do you think it's all right to yell and complain?

R: I don't think it's going to help the patient, I think they're out of their mind to do it. I don't think it's going to help anything.

I: Why not?

R: Well, it wouldn't help me, and maybe I'm looking at it from my viewpoint.

I: That's what I want.

R: Let me say something my grandmother said once when I was a youngster. She said, "Jealousy, hate, and self-pity has to go through you before it can touch anyone else, and it only disturbs you in the process."

R: Well, I think it's all right for them to, but . . . I just think it is de-grading to them. I think.

I: You don't think because they're scared they need to yell?

R: Yes, I think that's why they do it.

I: But you don't really think it's an appropriate way to behave?

R: No, definitely not, I mean they just aren't grown up, that's all there is to it, and being scared; you never can tell how you're going to die . . . they should act decent to their nurses and doctors, and their nurses and doctors will act much more decent to them.

R: No ma'am, I do not.

I: Why not?

R: First place I think it marks a person as somewhat of a sissy and in the second place it's disturbing to others.

Is It All Right to Be Sad?

Although there were a few exceptions, there was general agreement that sadness is to be concealed — to some extent because of its effect on the other patients. There is, however, frequent acknowledgment that it is not easy to be cheerful.

R: I try not to be. If I'd let myself I guess I could lay here in bed all day and cry. But what good does that do me to? You have to look on the bright side.

I: Can you do that?

R: You have to. It's not whether you can, you have to.

R: I didn't put it out of my mind, I'm not a denier, I don't deny I have a problem. I don't deny I have cancer, I don't deny I might never see my son. But once I accept the fact that I might not, I say all right now, take a deep breath, say "to hell with it," and get busy, do some-thing, put it out of your mind.

R: No. If I was sad I'd want somebody to come in and talk to me, it could possibly brighten my life and make me happy again.

I: You wouldn't approve of a patient who just turned his head away?

R: No, I would not.

R: You drag yourself down, is all, if you go around feeling sorry for yourself. There's always somebody worse off. If you get that way, don't stay that way. And it can be a hard struggle to get back out of it, too. But there's always somebody else just a little bit worse. I didn't believe before I came here, but I do now.

Is It All Right to Be Angry?

A few patients cautioned against anger for fear of retaliation, but generally the expression of anger was more acceptable then complaints, or expressions of sadness, especially if the person has been wronged. Anger about the disease was likely to be denied.

> R: The louder you are, the nastier you get, the less anybody's going to pay attention to you.

> R: I think it's foolish.

> I: Why?

> R: Well, I'll answer you by asking you a question. What good did anger ever do anyone? I mean, unless somebody really wrongs you or hurts you, that is.

> I: I don't know. You don't always think in terms of how much good it's going to do you . . . if you're hurt or wronged and you're angry. You know, what if one of the doctors or the nurses is careless with you and hurts your feelings and you think they have . . . you think maybe they've done something that would impede your recovery; or you're angry at the diagnosis, and you figure, what have you ever done that you have to have cancer. I can see that somebody could be angry.

> R: Well, I think there's someone else to look to for something like that and that's the dear Lord himself. I mean, the doctors and nurses didn't bring the cancer on us.

> I: But they're there, you know. And they don't have it and you do. Generally speaking, the people who take care of you are reasonably healthy, and they're out and you're in. I can see myself being angry just for that reason.

> R: Because it's happening to you, you mean?

> I: And not to them, and they're free to go and you're not.

> R: Well, in my case, I'm not saying that I don't ever get angry, because I wouldn't be normal if I didn't, but angry that I have cancer, no I'm not. In fact, I think I'm thankful it's no worse than it is, and that it can be cured. I think it's done me good.

> I: How?

> R: Well, I've learned so much since I've been here, and seen other people suffer, and I realize how lucky I am . . . that I have a family at home, a good family, a good husband and children. There's a lot of these people in here that are alone.

> R: What for?

> I: Well, just because you're angry.

R: People shouldn't get angry.

I: Why not?

R: Well, the first thing, it speeds up your adrenal gland. First thing you know, you have spleen trouble.

R: No, it wouldn't be right. It wouldn't be right to take it out on the nurses, just because I'm homesick and want to go home.

R: Well, I, I got to put it this way. They, they don't put up with it. No use doing it.

I: You're likely to get in trouble if you are angry?

R: Yes.

It is clear that the responses to these probe questions are consistent with earlier responses concerning normative behavior: courtesy and cooperation are rewarded by staff and there may be staff retaliation for aggressive behavior.

How Do Patients Like You Behave?

In answer to the question "How do patients like you behave?" these patients reported they were behaving in the best possible way, and that their good behavior would be rewarded by staff.* Good behavior is equated with compliance, with "being nice."

R: Very well, really. The majority of them do, I think. There's a few you couldn't make happy regardless.

I: When you say "very well," can you explain that a little bit?

R: Well, they don't complain too much, you know, and want too much. Some of them want so much, they just seem to want to keep somebody busy doing things for them. I think the majority of people are pretty considerate about stuff like that.

I: Considerate of the nurses?

R: Of the nurses. I mean, they're here to do things for us, and they do, too, but they're not just our slaves.

R: I don't know, to me the most of them that I have seen have been exceptionally nice, they've been . . . hate for the nurses to have to

---

*Since the nurses who were giving them care did *not* report this cooperative behavior, there is some question about what is being communicated. If patients perceive they are cooperative, and that cooperation will be rewarded, and nurses believe they are not cooperative yet only reward cooperative behavior, both will be bewildered by the outcomes.

> wait on them and that sort of thing. They're so used to doing it themselves.

R: The only thing I've seen around here, I think they behave quite well. I've seen no animosity or belligerency around here from the patients to hospital staff at all.

Patients who do not behave well are not doing as they "should" — although there is some notion that if they are treated well, and kept informed, they will behave well.

R: Most patients adjust to the situation if they're told frankly by doctors and all what they're trying to do for them, what they expect in the way of results, or that they don't think they have too much chance, that they are critical. If they'll tell you, you will adjust to that to where you can pretty well handle it.

Again, the rewards of good behavior are clear.

R: Well, that's a pretty hard question. You have the old one who thinks he's got more rights than anyone else, and won't have them telling him, and then you have the good one.

I: How does the good one behave?

R: Well, he does what they said, kids around a little, and first thing you know, he's still a-living, he isn't just a-laying there 24 hours a day and just breathing. He's still living.

Some idiosyncratic behavior was identified.

R: Well, I think they fall into several categories. One is the noncomplainer who won't ask for a thing, she's scared to death of authority figures all her life or his, and they'll never ask for things, even sometimes when they should. Then there's the other kind. Chronic complainer, demanding figure, male or female again. But I think most of us fall in the middle. Just like us.

And sometimes patients behave in ways which annoy other patients.

R: This girl I'm in here with now, she goes to the sewing machine and sews 8 and 9 o'clock at night. The other night she got up at 12 o'clock and went in there, and shut the door and got that machine just a-roaring. Well then, we just got this light up here, we haven't got none over our beds. And this light up here, she turned it on, and that would wake anybody up, because it seems like it would be a fire or something.

I: Did you tell the nurse?

R: No, ma'am, I didn't.

I: Why didn't you?

R: Well, I didn't want to cause this girl any trouble.

R: Well, some just aggravate you half to death. The others try to make everybody happy where they go.

I: What do they do to aggravate you?

R: Always griping 'bout this and talking down this one and talking down that one, or telling somebody to turn this off or turn that off. They expect to have the whole hospital run to their thinking. Such as radios and TVs and things.

PATIENTS' PERCEPTIONS OF SELF

What Aspect of Your Illness Is Most Distressing to You?

In a study which was designed to compare patients and nurses on various parameters of the care of dying patients, it was necessary to inquire whether patients were, as nurses are reported to be, more concerned about the fact that they were dying than they were about the conditions of the disease.

Because institution review committees were reluctant to allow the mention of death, patients were asked, "What aspect of your illness is most distressing to you?" As can be seen, they were not particularly well deceived by the circumlocution.

R: I say if I got it I got it, and that's it. When my time comes to leave this good earth I'll leave it. I went in the Navy and I was the only one in the whole platoon wasn't afraid of nothing, because I figure when your times up, it's up. If somebody could help you, they're going to help you. It doesn't distress me at all.

R: What the turnout would be of it. What it would be. You know, something lingery that I couldn't get over or something like that. And that's the worst kind of a dread on my mind.

R: Worrying about finding another cancer.

R: Well, I think you'ved picked yourself a peculiar interviewee. I have faced operations since I've been eleven . . . So I've faced death for a long time . . . So I'm not afraid.

I: You're ready?

R: Um-hum. I've always been ready. It's my philosophy.

R: That it's incurable.

I: That it's incurable. Have they told you this?

R: Well, no, but they haven't found a cure for it yet. That's a known fact.
_____

R: Well, the fact that cancer is such a deadly thing, you know. There's no cure for it, and they don't pretend, they don't tell you they cure it. They tell you they prolong your life. They're experts, you know, but there is no absolute cure for it. And the worst thing that I . . . the fact that it can break out in another area, somewhere else in the body . . . That's the part I'm worried about.

I: That's what bothers you the most?

R: That's what bothers me the most. And I think if I was to live I'll always have that thought, of course . . . I'm learning to live with it though. I'm a Christian and I'm learning to live with it, and it's not like it was at first. There at first I just couldn't see how it could happen to me, and why it did happen to me, you know. I sure hope . . . I'd like to live to see a cure found and what causes it.
_____

I: Can you tell me what bothers you most about your illness, about your sickness; about [using the patient's phrase] being at the end of your rope?

R: Oh well, I can't eat anything. I can't eat anything and if I do eat anything I just throw it right up. I don't always throw it up. Sometimes I do and sometimes I don't. And I can't tell you why that is either.

Along with the explicit recognition of the probable outcome of the illness, physical and sociopsychological aspects of illness were about equally reported as distressing; whether these factors are amenable to nursing intervention is addressed in a later chapter.

Pain was reported to be an important distress factor, as was being away from home. Limited mobility is a lesser concern, although it is mentioned. The need for comprehensive information about the condition is identified, and a few patients discussed the difficulties they encountered with employers and friends who were afraid of the disease.

R: Well, what distresses me most, which I try not to think too much about, except I write letters all the time, is that I have two children at home. And their school starts the 28th of this month. And their daddy's doing a wonderful job, but he's trying to hold down a job of his own and take care of them.
_____

I: You feel the most distressing part of it is the fact that your friends don't understand it and drop away from you because they're afraid?

R: Yes, not even that. Your employers. People don't want to hire you even though we're able people, you know, and got the physical strength and stuff. You mention the word "cancer" and they'll shun right away from you, they won't have a job for you. That's the biggest distressing part too, that you're unable to work, and you have to stoop down to welfare.

I: You're perfectly willing to work, but people won't hire you, because of your . . .?

R: The illness, yes. But after a period of time, like five years, now, I get to where it doesn't bother me, if they feel that way. I just take it as their ignorance and not mine and forget about it.

R: It's the pain.

I: Pain. Were you in a great deal of pain?

R: Yes, I've been in a great deal of pain. And once the pain's gone I don't feel too bad, but the pain just about tears me apart.

R: I'm worrying if I have the pain. No, I don't have pain now . . .

I: But you're afraid you will have?

R: Yes.

I: But that distresses you as much as anything does, that you can't use your hands?

R: Well, really it does more so than anything. Of course I'd like to be able to, I'd like to be able to get up and around, but if I could use my arms and hands I could do a lot of things, say write or something, but I just can't do nothin!

Can You Share Some of the Things You Think About Now?

One would expect that when personal mortality becomes a concrete issue, the thought of death would be uppermost. In this group of patients, however, in answer to the question "Can you share some of the things you think about now?" the thought most frequently reported was the desire to get out and go home. Families were paramount, and if death and disease are mentioned it is in terms of fighting them, of not allowing them to interfere with planned activities.

R: Oh, yes, home is the most important thing. The rest of it, as for cancer, I know I've got it, and I'm here for them to cure it.

I: You're going to get yourself cured and get back?

R: Get back home. Because my husband's 86 years old. And his days are numbered.

I: Do the two of you live alone?

R: Just me and him.

I: How is he taking it?

R: Well, he's taking it a lot harder than I am, because he don't think that I'll ever get well.

I: What makes him think that?

R: Well, he don't know too much about it [but] he thinks they should do surgery and get it over with, but they explained to me that they could not do it. Otherwise it'd spread all over my whole body. This way they think they can get a 100 percent cure. Contain it, and take it all out, and I'll be 100 percent well, and that's what I'm working for.

I: And you're going to work hard at it?

R: You ain't a-kidding. I'm going to work hard at it.

R: Well, it's a normal human being's thoughts. You consider about your family, and the support of them, and your vacations, and just everything. As far as the disease itself entering, I don't let it bother me. I don't give it a thought. I've got it, and I'll have it unless they find a cure for it, and it's a critical disease, and I don't let it bother me at all.

R: Oh, I think about my family, I have a brother and I think about him, he's not been well and that upsets me a little at times, and as I say the most of it is that I'd like to go home, I'd like to be able to walk, and I could go back home.

Although patients continue to plan, there was some immediate and explicit mention of death and of fear. However, the responses generally reflect an effort to control the situation in some way (for instance, arranging how the family farm is to be bestowed), as well as a feeling of hope.

R: I would like to live. I've worked hard all my life, and now I could finally go to Europe with the money I've saved instead of putting the boys through college and stuff like that. I sort of resent the idea of having to die now when I could enjoy a little bit, but I'm not afraid of it, and I don't intend to [become afraid].

R: Well, I think I went through a lot of punishment. Still, the future . . . I've got one of the best families in the world — two daughters married, no fussing . . . they come every Sunday and then we have a big dinner . . . that's quite a bit to leave, you know?

I: Yes it is.

R: And I had to tell them what I wanted done if I did pass away, and that's a little hard to do. . . . and I've got good machinery, and I've got a lot of tools in the shop, and I'm going to leave them that there for them to work with, and without a doubt everything'll go right on smooth. But I kind of hated to tell them, because I was afraid I'd scare them, see?

I: How did they take it?

R: Well, didn't say a word, but you could feel it kind of worked on them. Of course, it worked on me a little, but I couldn't tell them after death.

I: So you went ahead and made your plans, no matter what happens?

R: Yes. I couldn't tell them after death, I had to tell them beforehand; it was hard but I got it done.

I: Do you feel better now that you've got it done?

R: You bet I do.

I: Kind of a relief?

R: You bet, it would have worried me to death if I come down here and think about I had never told them what I wanted done or nothing.

I: And now that you have told them and that's kind of off your mind you are able to go ahead and make plans for the future?

R: It don't scare me at all, after I told them that something's gonna happen. But I just want to be prepared, see?

The desire to know what will happen is evident, as is expressed in an excerpt from one interview.

R: Well, the first two times I was in here, I was scared. I probably would put it thataway.

I: What were you scared of?

R: You don't know what's going to happen when it comes out, or what they're going to find. . . . When they explain to you, you're not scared like before. If they'll come in and explain to you. You don't fear the operation, and you know just exactly what they're going to do.

Another patient expressed a wish to die at home, and the fear that if he stayed in the institution he would indeed die.

R: Well, well I think about going home. Naturally, I, I got a much better place to die than in the hospital like this. I've got a home. I got it fixed primarily for my usage . . . so that I can get my wheelchair to the door quite easily and like that.

I: You say you have a better place to die than here?

R: Yeah. Home.

I: Do you think you're going to die here?

R: If I stay here long enough I will. . . . Like I say, I have a much better place to die at home than I do have here in this hospital.

> *I:* Why are they keeping you here?
>
> *R:* I don't know. That's one thing, I never have had a chance to talk with the doctor, if there is a doctor in my case here. But there is one. I spoke to him, I think, and that's all.

The subjects in this study usually identified a strong religious background. They report themselves as in some way safe in the hands of God, or of fate, or of the physician. Even those who believed they were in the hands of God were likely to derive hope from the pronouncements of the doctors, from medical science. The inclination to be sorry for others who are no doubt in worse shape continues to occupy some patients' minds.

> *R:* Of course I think about home and all that, and I look forward very much to my visitors, from Our Lady of Lourdes. Father, he comes to see me too, he's just like sunshine when he walks in. But yes, I think when I go up on the third and fourth floors and look around and see some of the other patients, and the shape they're in, and how courageous they are, you know. Still trying to stay cheerful, then I go back to the same thing: how much I've got to be thankful for.

Would You Like to Talk to Anyone About Yourself, Your Illness?

Those who study the process of dying are in agreement that dying patients need to talk about their fears and concerns about death and what they are leaving, and that the people they want to talk with are the people who are giving them care. For institutionalized patients, this means that staff are the recipients of the confidences. Clinical writers (e.g., Greene, 1974) are less likely to agree that all dying patients want to talk about dying and death; however, the nursing literature (Quint, 1970; Epstein, 1975) supports "listening" as particularly necessary in the care of the dying. The need to talk is explicitly identified by some of the patients interviewed.

> *R:* Somebody that would, that knows something about it, too, not just anybody. There's a couple of nurses here that I can talk to. But they're always so busy you hate to ask them if they can talk to you.
>
> *R:* Sometimes if you ask a nurse a question, she'll say maybe "I'll see," and "I'll be back later," and it slips her mind and . . . and sometimes they may forget and you have to ask three or four times.
>
> *R:* They told me it showed some more cancer cells, and I would probably have to have more treatments. But to wait a few days and see. And during those few days, why I felt very low. I thought, "If I have to have some more treatments down there . . . and up here too . . ." Then one of the little nurses, she came back and sat down beside me. She talked to me, and was real sweet, trying to cheer me up.

I: Did it help?

R: Yes, it helped. Of course it did.

R: I'd say yes, I imagine a nurse would be more comforting, you know. I think they'd know more about what they was talking about, you know, be more comforting to you than a member of the family.

Others did not always see the need, but did on their own initiative spend some time in talk with the interviewer.

R: No, I can't say that. It'd be up to me because nobody knows that much about it as I do. It's my trouble. And I'm bothered with it daily. And so I don't know how anyone could predict anything in my case to do what I haven't tried to do myself.

I: But just to share some of your feelings about it? Get it off your chest a little? You don't think that would be useful once in a while?

R: Well, I do once in a while, just like the few words I've told you about these bowels.

I: Well, would you like to talk with anybody in particular about how you're feeling, how things are going for you?

R: Not unless to you.

I: Thank you. But I'm thinking about the nurses who are here, the doctors who are here . . . or your folks, or whoever.

R: Yes, my mother was here yesterday. My sisters was just out, and my brother.

On the other hand, some were equally explicit that they did not wish to discuss their illness, or show any emotion about it.

R: No, I wouldn't want to do that. I don't like to talk about my illness.

I: You don't?

R: Except like in a case of this kind. Because I don't feel like it's something that should be talked about.

I: Even to the nurses?

R: Well, if they ask me how I'm feeling I'll tell them, but otherwise I don't say anything.

R: No.

I: Wouldn't that be helpful to you?

R: No, because really I don't want to think about it that much. It doesn't make me sad or anything to think about it, but I just don't want to think about it.

I: So you don't want to talk to anybody about feeling bad about leaving your sister?

R: That's it. No, I don't want to talk about it. That's, that's all [starts to cry]. That's something I can't cope with. I can't talk on that. I hate so bad to leave her.

R: No. I don't like to share my troubles with somebody else. I . . . just myself.

It was further expected that conditions and feelings would be known and understood by the staff without much discussion.

R: No, well, I'd say they know pretty well, know the situation pretty well, I think.

Patients indicate that at times they need to avoid talking, to be distracted, or even deny. But they also indicate that they want a thoughtful and informed listener when they are ready to talk. Doctors are identified as the persons with whom patients would like to talk.

R: There are times when you just really don't care to discuss it very much at all. I think it just depends on how you feel.

I: So when you are feeling like you'd like to discuss it, who would you like to discuss it with?

R: Well, a lot of times the doctors think I'm just full of questions, and then there's times I just go along with what they're saying and don't ask so many questions, hardly. It just more or less depends on the way you feel. Because there are times you feel like talking about it, and there's times you don't.

However, the role of confidante is to provide information.

R: It perhaps would, yes, yes, it would probably help. If I found any-one, someone with authority or something like that. It don't seem as though . . . I've had a pretty hard time getting any information here. They're pretty silent. I've only just sat here and waited, and that's about it, until yesterday. It was yesterday they told me what they had found and all. I've had several tests, and they don't give me much idea of what they had found or anything about . . .

I: You would have appreciated a little more information?

R: I would, yes. I would. I would have appreciated something to let me know about what I might expect or something like that, rather than just a-sitting wondering, a blank, with nothing to think on, you know. Just like I was when I come up here.

R: Well, as I said a while ago, only one in particular I feel . . . is my doctor . . . I do think in the hospital a patient and the doctor does not have enough time to really talk. I feel you should have confidence in your doctor, and if a patient . . . and the doctor does not have time to answer some of the simple questions that the patient asks, to me, I don't have as much confidence in that doctor . . .

I: You want the entire information?

R: I think it's wrong in all hospitals. . . . I think that patients should be allowed . . . to me it's taking away his constitutional right. In other words if we're all free and equal, and if you're sick, you should be able to read your own report the doctor makes. We don't have that right.

Once again we find that patients may be supported by other patients, but "wanting to talk" was for some patients equated with having a psychological problem, which they did not care to admit.

R: Not necessarily. The doctors here, you know, they're very capable, and I haven't had a mental problem or anything like that. I just think, "Now I can no longer do this," like walking and hunting or something like that. . . . But I don't let it get me down mentally, as to think that a person needs to talk to a psychiatrist or anything like that.

I: Well, not necessarily a psychiatrist. I was thinking about maybe the nurses or your family.

R: I talk freely with all those people. My minister lives next door, and we visit back and forth and talk, and he keeps up with my story. And so I talk freely with the nurses and with the doctors, anything that comes up.

R: I'm not depressed about it or anything, and it kind of gets me when people imply that I am, it does do that.

PATIENTS' PERCEPTIONS OF PAIN

Would You Like to Have the Pain Medicine Offered Before the Pain Starts?

In contrast with what is usually reported in the literature, this group of subjects did not believe they wanted access to pain medicine before the pain began. One should hurt and *then* get medicine, not get the medicine to prevent the pain. They were very aware and afraid of the addictive characteristics of narcotics, and perceived pain — to bearable limits — to be preferable to addiction.

They were also very aware of a schedule of administration, and the necessity for a physician's order to change that schedule. The following are a few of the typical responses to the question "Would you like to have the pain medicine offered before the pain starts?"

R: No, because I wouldn't know if I was going to have pain or not.

R: Well, not that dope there . . . I don't believe in drugs too much because I had the experience up here on morphine. It was just like going out on trips. . . . I'd rather have the pain a little more severe than going out because it was worse.

I: So they cut you back to where you could handle it?

R: To where I could handle it. But I think a party can stand pain more, and I found out myself, because I'm really chicken when it comes to all this pain. And it's just like I knew that I could stand pain, I'm going to do it.

R: No, in overall answer, no, I think if you're in a hospital under orders from a doctor, it ought to be administered from the desk. Yes, I think it would be dangerous.

R: Well, no. I wouldn't know when it's going to start.

I: You'd rather wait and ask and then have it right away?

R: I'd rather wait for the pains to start and then ask them to give me something.

However, a more elastic schedule would be appreciated — such that medication could be given for severe pain, even if it wasn't quite time.

R: I would like the doctor to have it so that if I come to where I need it worse than some other time, like if there was something they could give you regardless of it being the time for the shot or something, you know, if it go uncontrollable, that it would calm it down.

Conversely, a schedule should be established so that a person who wants to wait past the four hours could do so.

R: I'd rather have it on demand, if I want it sometime, go five hours without the pain, I'd want to stay without the medicine. And I think it would be better, if the patient is physically able and everything, just to let him call when the pain comes back.

Very few patients wanted medicine offered before it was requested. When they did, it was because the nurse was thought to recognize the need before the patient could, and also because it showed that nurses were concerned.

Do You Get Pain Medicine as Soon as You Ask?

When asked the above question, patients with pain who asked for medication generally got it in a reasonable length of time. There was an occasional remark that the medicine should have been given more frequently, but the blame for this is ascribed to doctors rather than nurses.

> *I:* Do they bring it to you as soon as you ask for it?

> *R:* Right.

> *R:* I get it as soon as I ask for it. There has been times when I thought I didn't get it close enough together. I realize how the doctors feel about any narcotics, because like I said, I worked in a hospital myself. But I do believe in receiving it under control so you can rest at night.

Patients understood and did not resent that the medicine was ordered to a schedule. Resignation rather than resentment was evident when medicine was not prompt.

> *I:* Do you get something as soon as you ask?

> *R:* Well, they say, "No. Can't give you any 'til seven. That's the time." Depends on the doctor. This morning he didn't order no pain medicine.

> *R:* No, just whenever the doctor orders. I'm not the doctor. I don't know what I need. I think it's the doctor's place to tell you what you need. That's what I'm up here for, for the doctor's care.

> *R:* Well, they're not as prompt as they could be, but then they generally bring it. Eventually.

SOURCES OF SUPPORT

What Is Most Helpful to You in Trying to Keep Up Your Spirits?

The public has been exposed to two images of the nurse in the last decades: on the one hand, the dominating dispenser of medications and treatments, ruling with starched efficiency over a domain inhabited by such lesser persons as patients and nursing assistants, and whose decrees can be vetoed only by physicians. On the other hand, she is seen as the patients' advocate, the only person who is there in the night to relieve pain and alleviate anxiety, the only member of the health team who is willing and able to stand with the patient against his physician, or at least to negotiate with physicians to provide patients with information or alleviate treatments.

Because patients are still afraid of physicians, and also are usually ignorant of what nurses *can* do, they probably endorse the first description. Nurses, however, see themselves in the second role and are likely to believe they *should* assume the responsibilities implicit in the latter description and feel guilt when they do not or cannot.

Behavioral scientists apparently are also in agreement with the latter description. When their study results indicate nurses do not function in such a manner, the assumption is that they should be doing so. In spite of their ignorance, patients also are reported as likely to feel in some way hurt and betrayed when nurses (and doctors) are not interested, available, and protective.

The provision of some kind of emotional support to patients — however this may be defined — is perceived by sociologists, psychologists, and nurses as a nursing responsibility of equal importance with the provision of physical care.

However, there is a real question whether when pain is controlled, medications are prompt and accurate, treatment is given as scheduled, and diet is as good as an institution diet can be expected to be — that is, when safe, good physical care is given in a courteous manner — patients might find emotional support in other than institutional sources.

The question "Can you tell me what keeps your spirits up?" was asked to provide information as to whether patients would report nurses as primary sources of emotional support. Two categories of support were identified: (1) institutional factors (personnel, other patients, a feeling of security engendered by being in the institution), and (2) extrainstitutional factors (family, religion, or personality factors). Quite evident in all the responses is the effect of encouragement to continue, and the importance of being remembered by friends. The ambience in which one is ill is important, but it cannot be entirely structured by staff. It is also clear that, in spite of what patients say, spirits are probably not high. Dying is depressing to self and others, and it is not always possible to alleviate that depression. The most important factor is that family and staff continue to be interested in the patient as a person.

EXTRAINSTITUTIONAL SOURCES

The two primary extrainstitutional sources of support are religion and family. In the religious responses it is sometimes difficult to separate the effect of interaction with others around the religious ritual from the effect of beliefs; but beliefs are apparently paramount.

> *R:* Oh, you think about the hereafter and those things, and try to put yourself through God, and if it's His will you'll get well, and things such as that.

> *I:* You think about possibly not getting well, and the hereafter, but you are a believer and you do trust in God? And you find it supportive for you?

> *R:* So far it has been, yes.

R: Well, I don't know. I have a lot of faith in God. I'm sure that helps.

I: Can you tell me about that? About how it helps?

R: Well, I believe that God will help me, and I just say my prayers and have lots of faith that things won't be too bad.

I: Can you tell me how the prayers help. Are you relieved or . . .?

R: I feel closer to Jesus.

I: With the prayers?

R: The more I pray, and the more I read the Bible . . . I feel closer, and that's a comfort.

I: Would you say this is your best support in this bad time?

R: Yes, I would.

Frequent motifs are: continue to hope, try not to worry, trust in God.

R: Well, there's really not much you can do except just hope and pray and try to remain optimistic, try not to worry too much.

R: Well, I just try not to think too much. I just turn it over to God and let Him worry.

I: You turn it over to God. You mean your worry about your illness?

R: Yes. I just don't worry about it.

I: How do you do this?

R: Well, I just always put my faith in God, and let Him pretty well run my life . . . if He's willing for you to get well, He does perform miracles, so I always feel that way. I suspected even before they told me. My husband came home two days early, two nights early from work, so I knew there was something else, but they wouldn't tell me what was wrong. This was at the other hospital. I was there a month, and then they told me about this hospital here, and sent me over here. When I got here they told me that as far as they were concerned there was nothing wrong with me until their tests were confirmed, and then they came back and told me that it was confirmed. And they told me they had one drug that had been in use for less than a year, a little over six months, and for this particular type which was a fast-acting type. And they said frankly they didn't think it would do me any good, but they were going on as if it would cure me. And that was in '69, December of '69.

I: And that's how you're going on too?

R: We have different drugs now that we didn't have then . . . they're saving the new drug until the old drug wears out on me.

I: So it just keeps moving along pretty well, one drug wears out and by that time there's another one to try that helps?

R: Seems like that's the way it's been working all along.

R: Well, I just look ahead. Something on the happy side of life. I have a lot of faith in God, and I just don't let it get me down. I just keep going. I go on like all these ailments is . . . like it's someone else that has them. I just keep going on from day to day, have faith in God. There's a reason behind everything.

I: So you do pray. Can you tell me about that, what it does for you?

R: Oh, it just makes you feel different. I don't know. You don't let yourself dwell on how you are or anything, you know.

I: What do you pray for?

R: Oh, I pray to get well, if it's God's will. But whatever he has for me, that's . . .

I: What I'm getting at with this question is to find out from you, if I can, what helps you through this bad time, and the reason I want to find that out is to know if nurses could be any help to you.

R: Well, I guess, I suppose they could, you know. But I think the main thing is God, to help you through these things, and you put your trust in Him.

I: And the nurses are not that important to this?

R: Well, no, really, because you're really not that close, you know. Of course they can help a lot, I admit.

I: How can they help?

R: Well, just talking to you and things like that would be a help.

R: All I know is that inside I talk to myself, more or less, when I find out I've got something going on. I have a great deal of faith.

I: What do you mean by a great deal of faith?

R: Well, I believe in a Being. I believe that faith — or whatever you want to call it, religious faith or whatever type of faith, brought me here.

I: Many of the people that I am talking with here are religious people, and talk with me about how helpful prayer is to them. Is this one of your sources?

R: No. I am not religious in what they call the institutionalized religious sense. I don't . . . I was born in one faith and am another now. And I pray in a different way. . . . And I read the Old Testament a great deal, and to me, the power — I call it the power, because God is not necessarily in the image of man — she might be black, you know, but whatever it is I think it has a great deal to do with what I am. But when I pray it's a different type of prayer than a so-called religious person who prays by rote.

R: Prayer and belief in God, and things like that, everything a Christian should believe in is what's keeping me going.

I: So your religion is your strongest source of support during this bad time?

R: Yes, it is.

For those fortunate enough to have families, there is no doubt as to the importance of continued interaction with family members. Thinking ahead to visits or thinking ahead to going home was a major source of support. Planning for future family activity, while it may not be realistic, is supportive.

R: Well, I think possibly visits from my family might have helped more than anything. And of course I had a lot of friends to come in and see me. And reassuring myself that things are getting better. I'll get out one of these days. Kind of like being in the army. If you have to be in there, you have no choice, but boy, the day you can get out, that's the day.

R: Well, I just think that I'm going to get well and go home, and if I don't stay up here and do it, I know I won't. And I think that's what keeps it up. Looking forward to getting well and going home. Cause as I said, him and me's just up now where we can enjoy one another, because it's always been that we had to work so hard for one another, and now we've got our own home. And I sorta hate to be away from, on account of we got our own home there and he really needs me to take care of him.

Planning or "looking forward" helps in not thinking about "it," and there is a pervasive and urgent desire and hope to be able to lead a normal life.

R: Well, encouragement from people, not only in the hospital but out of the hospital, everywhere. Almost everywhere I go they say, "Well now you're walking on that leg certainly a lot better than you were a week ago, or last time I saw you," see, and things like that. And a lot of times people that I know will say, "Well, I'm going to make a trip over to so and so, would you like to come along?" And they take you, and things like that.

R: I guess waiting to get back to my work.

I: Waiting to get back to your work?

R: You see, in a drugstore like I'm in, everybody knows you. It's a large drugstore. We fill about 125 prescriptions a day to 150, so you get to know those people. In fact, I got about 60 get-well cards the first

R: day I was in here. People I never expected from, you know, customers . . . and 22 employees in the store. I got one from every one of them.

I: So you're eager to get back to that and that keeps your spirits up, thinking about that?

R: Right. Not only that, my boss calls me up once a week, asks me how I'm getting along. Says, "Your job is waiting for you as long as you live." So that really makes me feel good.

R: Well, I think it's more or less the wanting to live. That you have family, and you still have hope that they're going to find it. And you want to get the whole thing. . . .

I: So you generally keep your spirits up by planning for your family?

R: Planning for my family and the future. I never want to go back.

I: You look ahead?

R: I look ahead.

I: All the time, no matter what?

R: Yes, I did this now, with my wife. I've fought this sickness ten years with her. She was in and out of the hospital for about twelve solid years. I brought her in. Of course now she's doing the same thing for me. My family's the big thing. That's what I live for, is my family.

A few individuals are cheerful fighters by nature, and meet this event as they have met all other events of their lives.

R: I'm just not a giver-upper, if I think there's chances of anything. I've seen some of the most hopeless deals and come through and win just by hanging in there. You got to have a spirit.

R: My friends through the years have given me credit for a cheerful disposition and a keen sense of humor. And if I'm worthy of that compliment, I would say that's perhaps the basis.

Frequently the question "What is most helpful to you in trying to keep up your spirits," triggered tears or a long, long silence; for some, the burden is not alleviated — not by prayer, and not by families, although some effort was made to respond in a manner that might be pleasing to the interviewer.

R: I tell you . . . keep my spirits up? I don't get nothing, I guess. It's boring, that all there is to it. . . . I'll sit around and smoke my cigarettes. That's what I usually do.

I: Your bad habit keeps your spirits up, too?

R: I got no other use in life.

I: Are you a religious man?

R: I don't go to church. I don't know if . . . I believe in God, but I don't go to church. I don't know if you'd call it religious or . . .

I: I'll call it religious if you do. Do you find that prayer helps you now? . . .

R: Oh, when I get shook-up it does.

I: When you get shook-up?

R: Yes, yes. Everybody does, I guess.

I: And does it help?

R: It probably does. I guess it helps.

I: O.K. How about family?

R: You mean my family?

I: Do they help you?

R: Oh yes, maybe too much.

I: Do they cheer you up?

R: Yes, they help me too much. Like before I got sick, they get outside and follow me around. And now all of this and that, don't do this, don't do that. And it . . . kind of baby me along, and I ain't used to that.

I: You don't like it?

R: No. I don't like it. I wish it was back the way it was. That's the way it goes, though. I let them have their way. Make them feel good.

I: But when you're down, they are a source of support for you?

R: Oh . . . yes.
___

R: No, I just, I don't know what's been helpful to me except . . . I don't know.
___

R: There ain't anything. There ain't anything that would keep my spirits up because I'm in too bad a shape. I'm too old. I'm in too bad a shape and there's no, there's nothing that would keep me in . . . I'm just at the end of my rope and that's all there is to it. And to tell the truth, the quicker I pass away, the happier I'll be.

INSTITUTIONAL SOURCES

A few individuals did identify what might be considered institutional sources of support: reassurance from the doctor, patient–nurse relationships, other patients' interactions.

R: Well, I think it goes back to the same old thing as a while ago, the nursing staff and the patient relationship. I think it goes back to what we said a while ago, the nurses and the people in the room with you. In other words, if you have a nurse . . . maybe you're low in spirits, comes and sits down and talks. Or another patient. If you feel bad. We have a tendency in here to ask one another once in a while how he feels, and so on.

R: Reassurance from my doctor.

I: Reassurance about what?

R: That I was getting along beautifully. My improvement.

I: Then your doctor was a strong source of support to you in your illness?

R: Oh, yes, yes.

R: Oh, just listening a bit . . . somebody talking, maybe it's just stories but then it's still interesting . . .

I: So having somebody to chat with . . .?

R: That's right.

Concluding Comments

In this sample of patients, religious beliefs and family relationships are clearly the major sources of emotional support — to the critically ill patient — even though one individual (not quoted) managed to combine all possible institutional and extrainstitutional sources in her response: religion, family, the doctor, the nurses, the other patients, and her own disposition to be busy, happy, and make the best of things. While one can wish her situation were more typical, she must be regarded as a fortunate, but rare, exception.

References

Castles M, Keith P: Patient concerns, emotional resources and perceptions of nurse and patient roles. Omega 10, 1979

Crane D: Dying and its dilemmas as a field of research. In Brim O, Freeman H, Levine S, Scotch N (eds), The Dying Patient. New York, Russell Sage Foundation, 1970, pp. 303–325

Datan N, Ginsberg L: Life-span Developmental Psychology. New York, Academic, 1975

Elder R: Dying in the U.S.A. Int J Nurs Stud 10:171, 1973

Epstein C: Nursing the Dying Patient. Reston, Va., Reston Publishing, 1975

Fisher S: Motivation for patient delay. Arch Gen Psychiatry 16:676, 1967

Glaser BG, Strauss AL: Awareness of Dying. Chicago, Aldine, 1965

Greene WA: The physician and his dying patient. In Troup S, Greene WA (eds), The Patient, Death and the Family. New York, Scribners, 1974

Hammerschlag C, Fisher S, DeCosse J, Kaplan E: Breast symptoms and patient lelay: psychological variables involved. Cancer 7 (17):1480, 1964

Kübler-Ross E: On Death and Dying. New York, Macmillan, 1969

Quint J: Personalizing institutional care of the dying. Arch Found Thanatol 2 (2):60, 1970

Schneidman E: Orientations toward death. In White RW (ed), The Study of Lives. New York, Atherton, 1963, p. 201

Schoenberg B, Senscu R: The patient's reaction to fatal illness. In Schoenberg B, Carr A, Peretz D, Kutscher A (eds), Loss and Grief: Psychological Management in Medical Practice. New York, Columbia University Press, 1970, pp. 221–237

Schusterman LR: Death and dying. Nurs Outlook, 21:465, 1973

Sobel D: Death and dying. Am J Nurs 74 (1):98, 1974

Sudnow D: Passing on: The social organization of dying. Englewood Cliffs, NJ, Prentice-Hall, 1967

Webster F: Perspectives on death and the dying patient. Hospital Progress 54 (12):32, 1973

Chapter 5

Institutional
Caregivers

Behavioral studies damning to institutional caregivers are thought by Crane (1970) to stem largely from a conflict concerning treatment, which — when it involves dying patients — involves and may challenge norms and values such as sanctity of life, humanitarianism, the most appropriate allocation of resources, advancement of scientific knowledge, and altruism. Depersonalization is, unfortunately, a common means of dulling the impact of caring for dying patients, but a number of investigators (Quint 1970; Kübler-Ross 1969; Lasagna 1968) point out that permitting staff to discuss their problems openly facilitates avoidance of this and other negative behaviors.

To generate more insight into nurses' responses to specific interview questions concerning the care of dying patients (see the next chapter), we will present some research material about professional roles, the orientation of care, and questions of ethics and policies.

PROFESSIONAL ROLES

Physicians and nurses are the major caregivers in the institutional setting. This is not to denigrate the activities of social workers, chaplains, and others employed in institutions for the comfort and care of the ill; however, patients are institutionalized so that they may avail themselves of the skills of medical and nursing personnel. They are hospitalized for medical problems, as defined and treated by physicians; nurses both implement medical therapies and perform independent nursing tasks. The activities of other caregivers are necessarily secondary. In both of these disciplines the service ideology is paramount; devotion to the interests of others is required by the professional ethic. Service is perceived as taking place in the context of individual relations between practitioners and the clients, and the relation is of a certain kind. It is based on what has been described as mutual trust, but is in fact the trust of the client in the skills and the interest of the practitioner. The relationship is one of superior and subordinate. Although the client is purchasing the services of the practitioner, the practitioner dictates which services are rendered, and how and where they are rendered. No valid standards exist for the use of clients in evaluating services, since every relationship is different and therefore every service is different. Trust in the technical competence and individualized interest of practitioners is the only comfortable recourse of the relatively powerless patients. The belief that cure follows compliance with medical and nursing directives makes the relationship endurable for some clients, but not for all.

In discussing hospital-based care by a health team, Georgopoulous (1972) states that it is necessary to have mutual understanding of one another's roles and tasks among participants (in his discussion, the patient is not explicitly considered to be a team member). Good coordination is essential for work efficiency and patient care. Such coordination becomes as a rule the responsibility of nursing. This leads to the effort of balance between the performance of clinical and coordinative functions by nurses.

> *Nurses are the only major professional group whose members are present at work at all times, thus being capable of ensuring continuity of effort. But the more nurses assume coordinative functions, the less time and energy they have to devote to patient care functions. Traditionally, nursing has served as repository of residual and supportive functions in the system — functions that are essential to coordination but not necessarily to professional nursing practice. As nursing specializes further (very likely in the manner and pattern of medicine), however, it will no longer be willing or able to carry out coordinative activities and still discharge its professional responsibilities to the patient and the organization. New ways of handling coordination problems will have to be sought out, for such problems will become even more acute rather than diminish. (Georgopoulous 1972, p. 23)*

A high level of commitment, loyalty, and involvement and a sense of satisfaction in members are critical to efficient functioning of the organization, since a high level of effectiveness depends upon both technical and social efficiency, and the social efficiency is based upon the organizational members.

Organizational members must perform their roles reliably and achieve and maintain high levels of performance. They must also maintain and continue to update their professional skills and knowledge.

> *In the process of doing their work, moreover, members are faced with the problem of how best to accomplish particular tasks or meet specific task requirements, and how to allocate their energy and time among the various tasks and functions which make up the organizational roles they*

carry out. Additionally, they must coordinate their work with that of other members, because of the specialization of roles and functions and the interdependence and cooperation requirements which characterize the work, and this entails problems of communication and feedback, planning, interpersonal relations difficulties, decision making and authority. . . . Similarly, members must cope with the complexity, uncertainties, and stresses to which they are exposed in the work situation, and handle the conflicts, frustrations and strain that these generate. . . . Finally, in the process of resolving these problems, individual members must protect their own identity and psychological integrity and well being. (Georgopoulous 1972, p. 33)

For nurses, it must be added, there are also the problems of protecting their professional identity and developing their nursing activities out of their body of knowledge and nursing skills, rather than merely reacting to physician, patient, and administrative demands. When these problems are confounded by the fear of death common to patients and personnel alike, it is to be seen that the nursing care of institutionalized dying patients might not meet the need requirement identified by Georgopoulous (1972, p. 35) that "From the point of view of its members as individual human beings with personal interests, needs and goals, many of which must be satisfied at work, it is important that the hospital be an attractive and rewarding setting."

Although the subservience of personal interests to the basic goals of the institution is an accepted norm, the costs of such commitment to the organization are not equally shared among the different groups of members. The high-status physicians, administrators, department heads, and supervisors are likely to be more satisfied with their personal goal attainment than the staff nurses and other lower-echelon employees.

During a lengthy period of socialization, physicians learn that quality medical care is "customized, individualized care under the direction of a competent practitioner" (Scott 1972, p. 152). In the face of tremendous technical knowledge and the multiple skills required to treat patients, Scott (1972, p. 152) suggests that physicians are "increasingly confronted with the choice of becoming incompetent generalists or competent specialists," with the majority choosing the latter role. The treatment of seriously ill patients necessitates the coordination of a team of such specialists — plus specialists from other disciplines — to function as what Scott (1972, p. 153) calls a temporary system: "a transitory system of relations among a team of physicians and other medical personnel brought together around a particular patient and existing for the duration of that patient's illness." When it becomes evident to the team that the illness is incurable and will result in death in some uncertain but near future, the specialists whose competency has been defeated drift away from the team, and from the patient. The question of who remains to manage the care when cure is no longer possible is not answered from an awareness of customized, individualized patient needs. The patient may be returned to the family practitioner, if there is one; otherwise, he is left to the therapy practiced by the medical personnel staffing whatever institution has accepted him for care.

TABLE 1. A PARADIGM OF MODAL TASK ORIENTATIONS

MODEL	TARGET	EXPECTED OUTCOME	CRITERION
Professional	Client needs	Reduction of client problem	Appropriateness, principles
Bureaucratic	Institutional integrity	Satisfaction of job requirements	Policies
Craft	Task itself	Product appearance, esthetic quality	Beauty, elegance
Technical	Specific task purpose	Task completion	Efficiency
Service	Client demands	Client satisfaction	Compliance
Entrepreneurial	Task performer	Profit	Selling maximization

From Mauksch: In Georgopoulous (ed.), Organization Research on Health Institutions. Ann Arbor, Institute for Social Research, Univ. of Michigan, 1972.

Greene (1974, p. 94) suggests that it is unlikely that "our culture will permit the physician to make a living administering to dying patients." There is not likely to be a medical specialty in thanatology.

Mauksch (1972) provides a paradigm of models of task behaviors in hospitals which is useful as a framework for the examination of physician and nurse behaviors in the general hospital setting. He identifies six ideal types, and suggests that pure versions are rare. Mauksch suggests that although the "service model is more likely an appropriate framework for tasks performed by certain personnel categories, it is by no means absent from any level of status, including physicians" (1972, p. 169); also, while not explicitly ascribed to by hospital personnel, the entrepreneurial model is not absent from the institution setting. Mauksch suggests, and observation of staff behaviors support him, that this expanded set of models might be necessary to account for the behavior of personnel in the institutional setting, and is closer to reality than the usual professional–bureaucratic dichotomy. The existence of this diversity of task orientations in all of the persons participating in the care of the dying patient may make the nursing role of coordinator (described by Georgopoulous) impossible.

The (usually benevolent) despotic and avoidance behaviors ascribed to personnel in the institution have been, to a great extent, identified by non-clinical investigators. Researchers are usually *not* involved in the immediate physical and psychological care of the dying. Those who are required to implement the findings have some reservations. For example, Greene questions whether the practicing physician can be expected to care for dying patients with the understanding and attention currently dictated by nonmedical experts in thanatology, and suggests realistically that "one becomes and remains affiliated with dying patients only to a certain depth; one then either bounces back or finds some other field of interest" (1974, p. 86). He points out that 80 percent of the most frequently referenced authors writing about dying patients and their needs since 1955 are primarily interested in psychological or social variables, and the majority are not persons who have been responsible for the unsuccessful treatment of the illness from which the patient is dying. Greene expresses well the realistic and appropriate caveat which is a focus of this book: whether the physician (and we would add the nurse)

> . . . can or should be expected to attend to his dying patients with the depth of understanding and participation which present findings suggests are most beneficial for patients. There is about the land a great deal of morally and politically motivated demand that all individuals be granted the right to health care and immortality, or the right to mental health care and happy immortality, and if that mortality must ensue it should be made at least contented — all presumably by physicians. For even the most perceptive, sensitive, and well-meaning physician who has cared unsuccessfully for the patient with cardiac failure, septicemia, carcinoma, or trauma, attention to his dying patient is very different than it is for the transient observer or participant in the dying days of the patient's life. (Greene 1974, p. 91)

Greene believes that the physician should understand and alleviate the suffering of the patient, but points out the difficulties imposed by families, patients, and his own feelings in talking with the patient as though he is dying. He is uncertain about whether "the physician should be expected to administer to his dying patient, I am not sure who should do this. Perhaps more is to be expected of the family, of nurses, or of specially trained paramedical personnel (whoever they are)" (Greene 1974, p. 92).

To the physician, care may indeed be "unsuccessful" when he cannot cure the disease from which his patient suffers. Cassell (1976) differentiates between the disease of an organ of the body and the illness experienced by the whole man (see also Coe 1970). He uses the term *illness* to stand for what the patient feels when he goes to the doctor and *disease* for what he has when he leaves. The disease afflicts an organ; illness is something a person has. The patient is a person with both an illness and a disease, and he is healed to the extent that both are made better. The nondisease elements of the illness include loss of connectedness (existence is defined by relationships) and the patient's realization that he is not indestructible. Cassell states that illness disturbs intactness inasmuch as it threatens the individual's connectedness to his world. The group is also threatened, as they are forced to recognize the possibility of the same threat to themselves. If illness is characterized by loss of connectedness to relevant groups, and the perception of vulnerability, certainly the patient who is dying from his disease must manifest these components of illness. Medicine can cure disease, but may not be able to treat illness as it is defined here. When *disease* cannot be cured, even the most perceptive of physicians may define their efforts as "unsuccessful."

If one accepts Cassell's notion that illness and disease are not synonymous, curing and healing may be different functions. The dying patient is ill, and cannot be *cured;* he may be *healed* to the extent that he is helped to maintain his connectedness to his world.

The domain of nursing is described by nurses to be holistic man and his environment. The independent functions of nursing are oriented toward healing, rather than toward cure. Physicians who treat the disease of the dying may not be able also to treat the illness and generate healing as this is described above, and should not be expected to do so. If they do not "administer to [the] dying patient," the authority to do so must be relinquished to those who have the necessary skills. Nurses state explicitly that they have such skills and wish to exercise them. It is obvious that they cannot do so in institutional settings if they do not control their practice. So long as physicians, patients, and hospital administrators believe that patients "belong to" the physician, that long will nurses be inhibited in the practice of nursing and necessarily orient themselves to the bureaucratic and technical models described above in the performance of their tasks. However, even if the ambiguous boundaries of medicine and nursing were clearly identified and recognized by all, there remains some doubt as to the extent of the contributions which can be made by either group to patients who are dying in an institution. The recognition that individuals should be treated as individuals, which permeates much of the literature on the subject, is surely a simple matter of human courtesy rather than a medical or nursing therapeutic ploy. This is not to suggest that therapeutic nihilism is appropriate; it is only to point out that nursing need not be responsible for meeting *all* of the needs of the patients, the physicians, and the organization, even if nurses are willing to assume the role of coordinator.

The role that nurses play in the care of the dying depends to some extent on whether or not they practice in an acute-care setting. Illich (1976, p. 97) reports the costs of terminal care to range from $500 to $2,000 per day. He states, and deplores, that 12 percent of the graduate nurses in this country are employed in Coronary Care Units, which require three times the amount of equipment and five times the number of staff as other units (1974, p. 106). He attacks the medicalization of dying, and while many of his opinions are explicitly based in his politics, the evidence he marshalls is not. Economy and humanism may both be served by the development of nonmedical therapies for persons with incurable diseases. Because it is not likely that such therapies can be developed or will be approved by physicians, nurses who care for dying patients may wish to organize and record their activities, and the outcomes of their activities, as a means of developing and testing nonmedical therapies.

The orientation to nursing intervention provided by the concept of holistic man in his environment lends itself to the perception of the dying patient as an individual who remains responsible for himself and his decisions. If the role of the nurse is not to be limited to the provision of good physical care — which is, in itself, an extremely important component of nursing — patients must have the opportunity to share equally in therapeutic decisions with physicians and nurses. This equality is not likely to occur in an intensive-care setting, where the machinery of the medical, life-saving technologies is so evident and the explicit goal of the unit personnel is preservation of life. In this setting, the role of the nurse is very likely to be similar to the role of the physician, and the care of holistic man necessarily gives way to activities related to his body, in order to save his life. Therapeutic activities with dying patients cannot occur until the life-saving activities are perceived as inappropriate and are relinquished. Quality care is always care which is appropriate to the condition of the individual.

A burgeoning literature reiterates that health-care professionals are dedicated to the preservation of life, and find it extremely difficult to function when cure is no longer a possibility. They are overwhelmed by the demands of the dying person and his family, particularly when all possible medical measures have been taken. Their anger at their helplessness may be directed toward the dying person and his family. The family, impotent and helpless, rages at health workers, who return the rage in counterdefensive reaction. Staff feelings of inadequacy, anger, or guilt may be handled by avoiding contact with the patient or his family. A death may be brusquely announced to the family; their weeping is then misperceived as a personal attack on staff or as regret about the care rather than as a reaction to loss (M. Robinson 1970). Staff are vulnerable because of unresolved personal fears of death, and professional goals related to protecting life and their strategies of self-protection are not therapeutic for dying patients or their families. Efforts by nurses and others to develop therapeutic methods of interaction with dying patients have resulted in a growing trend toward the development of a nursing specialty in the care of the dying.

One such specialist (Ufema 1976) describes her role as that of a staff nurse who specializes in the care of terminally ill and dying patients and their families; she describes the reactions of fear and rejection from other staff until they became familiar with her work. She feels the more knowledge and experience nurses have in care of the dying, the less frightening it appears. She suggests that inhumanity — not death — is the enemy.

She identifies the following responsibilities of the nurse specialist who works with the terminally ill and dying patient and his family.

1. *Assesses terminally ill patients to determine their perception of illness.*
2. *Gives total nursing care to selected patients to formulate a nursing diagnosis, determines need for future interaction, and gives care that other team members cannot.*
3. *Intercedes for the patient with staff, family, or friends as the patient voices this need.*
4. *Assists nursing staff to plan and implement care with the patient's participation, suited to the patient's needs.*
5. *Teaches hospital personnel about the dynamics of thanatology.*
6. *Functions as a team member with Social Service and pastoral care on behalf of the patient and family.*
7. *Forms a patient group to help patients work through their feelings.*
8. *Continues to learn about the dying process, from literature, seminars, and conferences but especially from dying patients.*

Drummond (1970) reports some institutional trends in the specialty of thanatology — specifically, the Foundation of Thanatology, developed in 1968, and devoted to scientific and humanistic inquiries into death, loss, grief, and bereavement. It is a nonprofit organization that is designed to serve inter-disciplinary needs of workers in the health professions — theology, psychology, and social science — through an educational and publication program. Drummond also discusses the American Nurses' Association commitment to care, cure and coordination, and suggests that while cure is of little importance in this situation, coordination between nurses and other members of the health team is vital, as clear communication among all members inhibits deception, avoidance, and inappropriate remarks to patients. However, in spite of the ANA emphasis, coordination and communication cannot be accomplished by the nurse, alone, and no one else seems to perceive the necessity. The physician believes he is co-ordinating care when he communicates the medical orders to all team members. Thanatology is now being embraced as a speciality by members of many disci-plines, none of whom are able to meet physiological and safety needs of pa-tients, or willing to assume the responsibility for 24-hour care. Thus continued care of the dying remains in the hands of nursing personnel employed by acute-care and extended-care institutions.

ORIENTATION TO CARE

The Sick Role

The sick role was conceptualized by Parsons (1951) as a special case of deviant behavior: it is deviant because the sick person does not meet the group norms for performance, and special because of the involuntary nature of the failure to meet the group norms (Coe 1970). The sick individual is considered to be an unwilling victim. Although he is considered unable (because of his illness) to function in his usual roles, he has certain rights. His rights include release from his normal duties, and assistance and care from others. He is obliged, however, to want and to try to get well as quickly as possible, and to both seek competent help and cooperate in the process of getting well. Legitimation of the sick role is provided by the physician, who validates the fact that the individual is ill, and may legitimately abdicate his usual responsibilities.

Parsons (1951) considers the physician–patient relationship analogous to the parent–child relationship, in that when adults are ill they resemble children: they lack the capacity to perform adult functions and must depend on the stronger parent figure, the physician. Because of this close correspondence between the sick person and the child, Parsons and Fox (1952) suggest that the illness must be treated away from the family setting. This protects the family from disruption and facilitates the therapeutic process, both motiva-tionally and technologically. In a discussion of this concept of the therapeutic relationship, while explicitly stating that the patient and the child are not the same, Wilson (1963) sees the parallels in the process of inducting a new member into society and returning an absent member to full function. The subordinate position held by the patient is clear in Wilson's analysis of the four major features of the therapist-patient relationship (1963, p. 287). *Support* is provided by the therapist, who is nurturant toward patients' needs for dependency; this is a temporary support and is contingent on the patient's efforts to get well. The therapist is *permissive;* he allows the expression of feelings and actions by the patient which would not be allowed in a nontherapeutic interaction. This permissiveness is also temporary, and is justified because the patient, like a child, cannot help himself. The therapist *controls rewards,* which are offered for trying to get well. The major reward is approval. As a condition for the provision of support and permissiveness, the therapist withholds his full interpersonal response. The patient does not have access to the true feelings of the therapist. The potential for being therapeutic depends on the therapist's maintaining independence from personal involvement in a relationship which is perceived as only professional by at least one party to the interaction.

Parsons' model is interpreted to postulate two distinct states, health and illness; clear boundaries for the sick role; and simultaneous recovery along physical and psychosocial dimensions (Brown and Rawlinson 1977). In spite of clinical understanding of illness and recovery as process, the Parsons model continues to be accepted, and patients continue to be regarded as subordinate in some way. Bloom (1963) describes the Szasz and Hollender types of doctor-patient relationships: (1) *activity-passivity*, compared to parent-child relationships, in which treatment occurs regardless of the patient's contribution; (2) *guidance-cooperation*, comparable to the parent-adolescent relationship, in which the therapist guides and the patient follows directions, exercises some judgment, and cooperates; and *mutual-participation,* modeled on an adult-adult relationship, in which the physician helps the patient to help himself. Bloom says that one model is no better than another, only more appropriate to a given situation. He perceives guidance-cooperation as the usual model, with few patients able to sustain the mutual-participation relationship. When staff interactions with terminal patients were observed by us, activity-passivity relations were more frequent, with staff unable to sustain mutual-participation.

The "sick role" as a perspective for viewing patient behavior may have heuristic value to sociologists. When it is used by clinicians as an orientation to care, patients are perceived as passive and dependent, and families as intruders. Castles (1973, p. 109) has reported as follows.

> . . . *clinical practitioners in nursing are not at all uncomfortable with the concept of the patient as dependent, passive, and childlike. A young nursing student admitting an elderly woman to the division calls her by her first name. A practical nurse giving a bed bath to a middle-aged man is visible from the hall. She washes his exposed buttocks vigorously while carrying on a conversation with the patient in the next bed. The medication nurse says to an adult woman, "Now let's take our medicine, we want to get better, don't we?" Nurse clinicians and educators may deplore but are unable to prevent such practices. When nurses unconsciously assume patients are indeed dependent, passive and childlike, the usual rules of*

*modesty and courtesy between adult and adult are apparently not con-
sidered applicable.*

Patients who have been independently functioning adults before their admission to an institution are transformed into dependent, passive individuals
by nurses who act as authority figures and relegate patients to subsidiary roles
(Blaylock 1972; L. Robinson 1968). To practitioners who make the assumptions
inherent in this orientation to care, ideal patients cooperate with the therapy
and the therapists without complaint. They are expected to do what they are
told, because physicians and nurses know what is best for patients. When
patients are viewed from this preconceived attitude that illness generates dependency and regression, the patient who "retains his adult expectations of
himself and demands to be treated as an adult by the persons caring for his
physical needs is only too likely to be considered recalcitrant" (Castles 1973,
p. 112).

Because it is an important nursing function to encourage independence in
patients, the assumptions inherent in the sick role inhibit quality in care: "it
appears detrimental to the nursing process to think of the patient as dependent
and childlike, a social deviant who must be 'returned' to the assumption of adult
role requirements" (Castles 1973, p. 112). An orientation to care which makes
more optimistic assumptions about the dignity and the ability of people even
in illness, is suggested below.

Game Theory

Game theory considers decision-making in certain situations: there is conflict,
incomplete information, and decision-makers are not in control of events.
Decision-makers do not have the same goals, and the various outcomes in the
situation have different values for all persons involved. In this situation of interdependence, the consequences for each participant depend both on his own
behavior and the behavior of others — over which he has little control. Shubik
(1964, p. 8) maintains:

> *The essence of a "game" in this context is that it involves decision makers
> with different goals or objectives whose fates are intertwined. The in-
> dividuals are in a situation in which there may be many possible outcomes
> with different values to them. Although they may have some control
> which will influence the outcome, they do not have complete control
> over others.*

Although the theory is concerned with the ideal behavior of a rational person,
it is not necessarily limited to the concept of a number of rational players using
optimum relevant information to make best decisions. "Free" or open gaming
accommodates the possibility of irrational moves by players; all of the rules
are not specified and known in advance.

In the game of ill health, the patient, the family, the doctor, and the nurse are all players—each controlling some resources, each with different goals. The salient consideration is that all are *equal* players in the game. The assumption is that in spite of illness, patients and families function as rational adults, utilizing old strengths to meet new problems. Their strategies have equal importance with the strategies of the health professionals. This orientation to care is based in decision-making in a situation of conflict, rather than on the perception of childlike dependence and vulnerability in sick individuals. Patients and families have the status of players, rather than counters to be manipulated.

Obviously this theory is to be differentiated from the transactional kind of gaming described by Levin and Berne (1972). The superficial and manipulative activities involved in the "doctor–nurse game" or the "patient–nurse game" are carried out because of assumptions of inferiority on the part of some participants. Powerless individuals caught in a situation they cannot leave endeavor to obtain some control by persuasion and manipulation of the more powerful groups. Relationships are not authentic, and the goals of the caregivers are personal, not related to the health of patients, and not made explicit. This "games-people-play" orientation makes even more negative assumptions about patients than the current interpretations of Parsons' sick-role model. Game theory as it is presented here as an orientation to care is based on the economic theory developed by Von Neumann and Morgenstern (Shubik 1964). The model has been adapted to other areas of practice, but it remains a model for decision-making in situations of conflict and incomplete information.

Professional and lay behavior in illness is probably best described by the *two-person, nonconstant sum game*. A *person* is defined as an individual (or a group) with similar interests. The players—the "two persons"—could be the physician–patient, the nurse–patient, the physician–nurse, the nurse–family-patient, the physican–nurse–family–patient; any combination of players is possible because, although the model is described for two persons, it can be generalized to any number. In the economic model, chance is recognized as a player. In illness, chance is exemplified by the disease process, or the illness, which is never entirely under the control of the rational decision-makers. *Nonconstant* refers to the fact that no player is committed to any one strategy; plans of action may be changed at will in response to the action of other players or the progress of the illness. In a *sum game*, the winnings of one player are not equal to the losses of another; everyone can win or lose something simultaneously, in that *cooperative solutions* may be found. In a cooperative solution, gains are realized by all players, and the only conflict is about shares (Castles 1973). Illness is always a situation of conflict and negotiation. Even when there is agreement or coalition among the professional and lay players as to the strategies to be employed and the values of the possible outcomes (and such agreement is surely unusual), the basic conflict between the other players and chance—as exemplified by the progress of the disease—remains. The values attached to the possible outcomes by professional and lay players are seldom congruent. Dying patients may be more concerned with comfort and family visitors than with the change in laboratory values that are of such importance to their physicians, and there is no consensus as to when the use of life-saving measures is appropriate. If the games orientation, as contrasted with the sick-role orientation, does nothing else, it makes explicit the assumptions of health personnel that their values are shared by their patients, and when this is *not* the case, the professionals' values are in some way the "correct" values.

Ideally, the conflict in the health game is between chance (the disease process) and a coalition consisting of the family, the patient, the physician(s), the nurse(s), and any other health workers required by the game. The preferred outcome is the patients' return to health. Actually, the interests of the players seldom coincide so nicely. The information held by each player about the patient's illness is one source of potential disagreement. Coe differentiates between the lay and professional approach to illness on the basis of the understanding and knowledge of each.

1. *Laymen and specialists have widely divergent understandings about the events of illness. Although the layman's understanding of diseases is, in our culture, certainly strongly dependent upon the scientific knowledge concerning diseases and is informed by its general perspectives, lay understanding is scientifically quite imperfect both in detail and in its broad outlines.*

2. *The person who has a disease not only understands it differently, but regards it from a different perspective than does a medical scientist. He is emotionally involved in a way that other people — and particularly specialists, who have an abstract scientific understanding and methodology as tools to confront an illness — can never be. In short, while the physician exercises objectivity in evaluating the meaning of symptoms, the patient's perspective is a subjective one — he is the one who feels the pain. It is his life that is affected by the illness.*

3. *For the most part the specialist sees a case of disease in terms of knowledge he already possesses — although even after they have been fully trained, physicians certainly learn from their patients; the layman ordinarily finds that his perspectives about disease change markedly as a result of his experience with it and particularly because of what he learns from the specialists whom he may consult about the disease.*

4. *The basis for deciding what action to take with respect to a disease is often quite different for the patient than for the professional. The physician has his detailed knowledge of pathology as a basis against which to evaluate what he is doing. Particularly, he is able to make a prognosis or an estimate of the probabilities of a particular patient's situation in view of what he can understand about the disease that the patient may have and about the patient's general physiological condition. Moreover, he has professional standards against which to judge his ability and effectiveness in diagnosis and treatment. (Coe 1970, pp. 96–97)*

In spite of the differences among players, the game theory orientation includes the patient and family in a way that the sick-role orientation cannot; it makes them active and equal participants in decision-making. When cure or rehabilitation does not have the same value to patients, physicians, and nurses, the patient's high value on stabilizing the situation will not be ignored.

Patients today are better educated about both their own civil rights and the positive outcomes of the treatment of illness. Democracy has to some extent infiltrated the health-care system, so that the old respect for medical authority is lacking in both patients and nurses. The civil rights of patients threaten the omnipotence of the physician, and of institutional rules and regulations. It is no longer enough to present patients with decisions about their care — they wish to have the necessary information to participate in those decisions. It seems foolish for physicians and nurses to continue to interact with patients from the framework of the sick role when those same patients are resorting to the courts to retain their rights of decision. Implicit in the game orientation is also a change in the status of the nurse who is an *equal* player. From this framework, nursing strategies of care will no longer be relegated to the bottom of a long list of medical strategies.

The ability to accept the gaming framework as an orientation to care demands qualities of maturity, competence, and knowledge in all players. The relationship must be one of mutual participation of adults. Medical and nursing staffs must concede as equally important with their own, patients' strategies and goals; similarly, patients must relinquish the unpredictable rewards of the sick role. Nurses, physicians, and the public will all need to be educated into this recognition of rights and responsibilities.

Neville (1972) says "A cheap way out in the conflict of values is to believe one side really does not count, or is secretly served by being subordinated to the other. The truth is, we must balance and choose, with inevitable loss." The sick role with its automatic assignment of dependency and subordination to patients may be functional to the institutional goal of accomplishing a given number of instrumental tasks in an allotted period of time. It is surely not an appropriate model for professional nursing. Game theory with its assumptions of equality and rational behavior articulates more nearly with the nursing commitment to holistic man, who can balance and choose and accept the inevitable loss.

ETHICAL DILEMMAS

Nursing, like other secular service guilds, is faced with the ethical difficulties generated by societal pluralism. At one time, most Western communities shared similar beliefs about the existence and activities of God; the authority of God, as reflected in the pronouncements of the Church of ones' choice was the final court of moral appeal. Today, however, even believers will claim only that God commands us to "act lovingly, to be concerned with human need and well-being" (Fletcher 1974, p. 127); Fletcher further suggests that only an "ethics rooted in human well-being can or should survive the pressures of man's struggles and advances" (1974, p. 127). He speaks against trying to cope with current bioethical values questions simply by applying the rules of traditional value systems. People who decide value questions in this way are, in effect, handing the decision to an external authority. Nursing — with its roots in military and religious soils — has been guilty of this withdrawal from accountability for professional behavior in the past. The authority of the medical directive, the hospital administrator, or hospital policy are all advanced as reasons not to carry out nursing interventions dictated by nursing knowledge or to keep silent in the presence of activities that violate professional values.

In nursing, as in medicine, good is described in terms of the health and well-being of patients. Even when clinical relationships are authentic or genuine — that is, growing out of and manifested by shared caring and concern (Fletcher 1974, p. 144) — ethical dilemmas arise in the clinical setting. There is no *ethical* dilemma in a clear choice between what is perceived as right and what is perceived as wrong. There may be pragmatic difficulties if the choice goes one way rather than another, or personal problems in implementing the decision, but an ethical dilemma occurs only when a choice must be made between conflicting goods — when either choice means that some rights are abrogated, or some basic needs are not met.

Fletcher (1974) describes this focus as "clinical" ethics — decisions are made on the basis of good to the patient, and not predicated in advance on some concrete law of care. He suggests that the "heart of a responsible ethic is this question: what, of what can be done, should be done; what of what should be done can we afford; and what of what we can afford are we prepared to pay?" and differentiates between "obedience to abstract principles and service to concrete human needs: one is dogmatic, the other compassionate" (Fletcher 1974, p. 121).

Ethical codes in nursing and medicine are written in terms of human needs, but the fact that the codes exist at all suggests codification of the guidelines for behavior in clinical situations that dictates decision based on rights and rules rather than on individual perception of human needs. Fletcher answers the question of what to do when rights are in conflict and one right has to be set aside with the concept of the greatest good for the greatest number: "Human need comes first and the general welfare of widest need prevails" (1974, p. 125). Pappworth disagrees with this and suggests that "morality rests on what is right in itself towards the individual immediately involved, not on justification by result even though that may possibly benefit a great many others" (1967, p. 185). Fletcher mentions Typhoid Mary as an example: her right to travel freely and live and work as she chose was forcibly restricted for the good of those persons whom she would otherwise have infected with typhoid. On the other hand, nobody suggested shooting her, although this would have been safer for the many and more economical. Fletcher says the validation of human rights is found in human need although the reasoning becomes involved here. It might be suggested that a basic human need is to have certain rights respected *or* that a basic human right is that certain human needs be respected. Certainly needs are not synonymous with rights. The right to withhold treatment does not equal a need to withhold treatment, and the need of a dialysis patient for a healthy kidney does not give him the right to take a kidney where, when, and from whom he chooses. However, "The sanction for our humanistic ethics lies in need; need is the court of appeal" (Fletcher 1974, p. 125).

All rights are subject to moral weighing; sometimes they pass the critical test of human needs and sometimes they fail it. The "right to life," for instance, is qualified by justifiable homicide. The "right to die" is gaining acceptance as the need for human dignity and compassion in terminal illness must be explicit in cases involving the use of resuscitative medicine and various artificial life-support systems. Legislators continue to talk about the "right to health" in terms of national insurance and an equal distribution of medical care. The right of control of one's body has long been recognized in the requirement of the patient's consent to surgery. The same right of self-determination plays a growing role in the abortion debate, in refusals of transfusions and transplants, and in patients' decisions against medical prolongation of life. Human rights are acknowledged under the pressure of human need; changed human needs may then suspend or even cancel them, and "only an ethics rooted in human well being can or should survive the pressures of mans' struggles and advances" (Fletcher 1974, p. 127).

Nurses represent a heterogenous population and do not share common personal values. The professional values which are expected to dictate professional behavior are found in the American Nurses' Association Code for Nurses with Interpretive Statements (1976; see Appendix B). The eleven items of the Code cover

> . . . several areas of responsibility and obligation: the obligation to respect human dignity and individuality; to safeguard patients and the public from variety of threats; to assist in quality assurance activities; to collaborate with other health professionals; to maintain competencies, and to contribute to the professional body of knowledge. Presumably it guides and even dictates decisions relevant to specific practice problems (Castles 1978).

The Code is obviously humanistic in intent; while in its Introduction it demands that nurses should comply with its dictates while functioning as nurses, consideration for personal values in conflict with the Code is found in the Preamble and in the gloss to item 1. However, although a nurse may withdraw from a situation in which she is opposed to the delivery of care, patients may not be left unattended. The professional obligation to assure patients of the best possible care takes precedence over the personal values of the nurse. Personal values also influence professional decisions. Castles (1978) discusses ethical dilemmas inherent in two common nursing decisions: (1) the decision as to what kinds of care will be given to whom, and in what order (the triage function) and (2) the decision to prescribe or implement placebo therapy. She suggests that as the requirement of the Code is only that care be dictated by human need (item 1), personal values affect decisions when nurses are required to ration inadequate resources in some reasonably equitable manner.

> Conflict in the rights of individuals necessarily leading to triage . . . can be found in the decisions of a night duty charge nurse on a division housing several seriously ill persons. In order to accommodate the victims of a multiple automobile crash in the intensive care unit, several persons are

moved from the ICU to her division. What are her options in the fact of general need and short staffing, if she wishes to adhere to the mandates of her professional code? Does she mobilize the best resources of the division around the life support needs of one or two severely damaged persons? Does she do the best she can for the many, ignoring the greater needs of one or two? Does she do an excellent best for a reasonable number, shorting the many somewhat, and not providing nearly enough for the sickest persons? Obviously equality of care is not feasible, nor is the determination of care by human needs. Some form of triage is necessary when demand exceeds supply; personal values will pay a major and usually unexplored part in the decisions . . . (Castles 1978)

Item 1 also addresses the self-determination of clients, their involvement in planning their care, their right to be given the information necessary for making informed judgments, and their right to be told the possible effects of care. This item would appear to rule out placebos, although clinicians endorse their use as being in the best interests of patients. The Code, therefore, is not prescribing usual practice. Nurses who do not believe in deceiving competent adults, even for their own good, are supported by the Code; they must then address the issue of whether it is ethical either to carry out medically directed placebo therapy or to inform the patient that his physician has prescribed an inert substance.

In the interpretive remarks concerning item 1, there is a paragraph addressed specifically to the care of the dying person:

As the concept of death and ways of dealing with it changes, the basic human values remain. The ethical problems posed, however, and the decision-making responsibilities of the patient, family and professional are increased.

The nurse seeks ways to protect these values while working with the client and others to arrive at the best decisions dictated by the circumstances, the client's rights and wishes, and the highest standards of care. The measures used to provide assistance should enable the client to live with as much comfort, dignity and freedom from anxiety and pain as possible. The client's nursing care will determine to a great degree how this final human experience is lived and the peace and dignity with which death is approached (ANA Code, 1976).

This language identifies nursing goals specifically (arrive at the best decisions; enable the client to live with as much comfort, dignity, and freedom from anxiety and care as possible) but is ambiguous as to how goals are attained (ways to protect these values while working with the client and others) or which goals might take priority. The responsibility of the nurse to monitor all of the therapy is clear, as "client's *nursing* care will determine how this final human experience is lived and the peace and dignity with which death is approached" (ANA Code, 1976). The behavior of the nurse will be based on some combination of medical directive and personal values. The Haemmerli case (Culliton 1975) in Switzerland is an example. Dr. Haemmerli and his staff care for many comatose, elderly patients in their institution. In these patients, although cerebral function is failed, spontaneous respiration continues. The patients are fed through nasogastric tubes, and when there is staff consensus that coma is irreversible, nutrients may be discontinued and the feedings will consist of salt and water. Death usually occurs within a few weeks.

> *It is, in fact, death by starvation; it is (as far as anyone knows) painless to the comatose patient. After the staff members make the collective decision to discontinue nutrition, the doctor talks with the family. However, the decision remains a staff decision. The value expressed here is that therapy which is not likely to succeed is pointless; Haemmerli suggests that prolongation of life possibly should not constitute the overriding purpose of medical practice, although the medical rhetoric generally supports this purpose (Castles 1978).*

Following Haemmerli's trial (and acquittal) on a charge of murder, the Swiss Medical Academy issued guidelines regarding the cessation of life-prolonging treatment for dying or comatose patients. Haemmerli has been quoted as saying that "renunciation of treatment or its limitation to alleviate sufferings is medically justified if putting off death would mean for the dying an unreasonable prolongation of suffering and if the basic condition has taken . . . an irreversible course" (London [Ontario] Free Press, April 2, 1977, p. 3).

This physician's personal values concerning prolongation of life in the presence of irreversible coma are now reflected in his professional code. The nurses who feed saline instead of nutrients in response to the medical order may not be supported by *their* professional code. Castles (1978) asks what nursing obligations are to patients in irreversible coma.

> *Historically, and this is reflected in the ANA Code, nurses are patient advocates, patient protectors. The question is whether the patients are to be protected from those physicians and family members who wish to sustain physiological life in the apparent absence of psychological responses, or whether they are to be protected from those who would allow them or even help them to die. The professional Code is not entirely clear and helpful here, and personal values must dictate decisions.*

The Nursing Code is a humanistic statement, which identifies areas of ethical conflict in nursing care. It does not resolve conflict between personal and professional values, nor does it suggest how changing societal values may affect professional behavior. When personal values conflict with the dictates of the Code, and when practice activities do not reflect the Code, nurses must make difficult decisions. Some public attention is now being given to problems in *nursing* ethics, as these are separate from problems in medical ethics.

One of the most recent meetings concerned with this was the Hastings Center Conference on Ethics in Nursing, which addressed three major issues: the nature of ethical dilemmas nurses face in their practice; how ethics should be reflected in curriculum; and how an ethics curriculum might be organized and taught. Case studies of care related ethical dilemmas were considered. The first case study (Steinfels 1977, p. 20) was reported to address the question for what and to whom the nurse is ethically responsible. It is unclear as to why there is any question about this: the nurse is responsible ethically to herself and to her profession. Jameton (1977, p. 22) points out that

> . . . the practice of nursing gives rise to a variety of ethical problems either unique to the profession or significantly modified by it. . . . [the] professional nurse performs an unusual variety of roles—patient advocate, aide to the medical profession, hospital staff worker or administrator — as well as nursing professional. This combination of roles, very different from the physician's role, raises a host of ethical problems related to autonomy, coercion, role conflict and personal identity.

Since Jameton perceives that the main function of health care institutions is the care and comfort of the sick, and that "this is a paradigmatic nursing function; the nurse is the central figure in health care, not the physician," the practice questions he raises are relevant. However, he perceives the questions of "who should say . . . who should make this decision?" to be ethical, rather than practice questions; the responses to the case studies reported in this section of the Hastings Center Report are couched in terms of ethics, although they would appear frequently to be questions of practice rather than real ethical dilemmas for nurses. In one discussion of the nurse's responsibility when personal values are in conflict with a medical directive — for example, a "no code" order on a patient with no information as to the patient's wishes — it is suggested that the nurse should attempt either to change the institution policy if it supported the order, or to resign. Flaherty (1977, p. 28) suggests that the moral principles involved include:

> . . . the nurse's commitment to a high standard of nursing behavior that will enhance a patient's ability to cope effectively with her situation (that could involve helping her toward a peaceful death), to ensuring that the patient gives informed consent for any treatment, to providing for and respecting the patient's right to self-determination of care (that might include a decision to refuse care), to practicing with integrity and being accountable for her own professional behavior, and to safe-guarding the client and the public when health care and safety are affected by the incompetent, unethical, or illegal practice of any person.

Any one of these items, all of which are found in the ANA Code of Ethics, might suggest that the real ethical question here is whether the nurse should inform the patient that the physician has given the order not to resuscitate her if she arrests during an asthma attack and inquire as to the patient's wishes. However, this question is not addressed by the discussants.

Medical ethical codes have evolved through the centuries from the Hippocratic Oath to the various declarations and statements reproduced in Appendix B, and the guidelines based on them.

The International Code of Medical Ethics is addressed to duties in general, duties to the sick, and duties to each other. The "medical vow" that is the Declaration of Geneva incorporates and updates those portions of the Hippocratic Oath which do not invoke pagan deities. The Declaration of Sydney provides guidelines for physicians who must determine the point of death of a patient whose organs will be harvested.

There is already a library of volumes on medical ethics written by philosophers, sociologists, and physicians whose interests and background make the examination of medical ethics appropriate. Medical ethics are of concern here only as they impinge on the practice of nursing, and the care of patients who are institutionalized to die. The basic documents are provided for examination (see Appendix B), as are the nursing documents. In the following discussion of professional duties, as these are inferred from patients rights, the various documents are not further referenced, although in the aggregate, they form the basis for the duties. That is, these *practice* statements are based on ethical considerations rather than the body of knowledge of either medicine or nursing. The patients' rights are those identified by Annas (1974).

Inherent in the patient's right to know the truth is the professional duty to provide full information. *Who* should provide this information is a question of power and usual practice, rather than a question of ethics. It becomes an ethical dilemma for nurses only when the full information is not given, as usual practice is to consider this the prerogative of physicians. The question of whether patient good is served when nurses provide information which conflicts with, or is more than, the information provided by physicians has not been considered for all patients in all situations. More and more frequently, the responsibility of the physician to disclose to patients the risk in treatment of the disease is legal as well as moral. Courts have held that the duty to disclose "does not spring from customs of medical practice nor does it require expert testimony (Lieberman 1974)," as this may be considered unfair to the patient. However, the ruling that holds physicians to disclosure such that there can be an informed decision by the patient as to whether to undergo a treatment has been described as imposing an uncertain and unclear burden on the physician. Lieberman suggests that

> . . . the topics discussed by a physician with his patient should include . . . the diagnosis; the treatment's nature, expected duration and purpose; the method and means by which the treatment is to be administered; the risks and hazards involved, including temporary and permanent after and side-effects; any alternative forms of therapy; expected beneficial effects of the treatment; and the prognosis if the patient foregoes treatment. (Lieberman 1974)

These items are taken from the Food and Drug Administration regulations on patient consent for new drugs, and appear to be comprehensive enough to allow the patient to make his own decisions as to whether he wishes to undergo treatment. However, it might be considered that the mere provision of information, while it may meet legal requirements, is not enough to meet ethical requirements because the way in which the information is presented, and by whom, will also affect the decision.

The patient's right to confidentiality and privacy suggests that it is the duty of physicians and nurses to inform the patient, rather than his family, of risks and benefits of treatment, and of probable prognosis. Patients should be protected from student invasion, and from examination by personnel not involved in treatment. The scientific itch to learn something new is not an adequate rationale for impinging on the privacy of a dying patient, nor is the educator's responsibility to curriculum.

The right to consent to treatment means that patients are fully informed as to the consequences of the treatment, and may choose either to accept it or not. Given the present medical technology, the consent to treatment — particularly when it is given by a dying patient — may be in effect a consent to experimentation. The medical research procedure that is carried out for the advancement of knowledge deviates from standard practice because ethical codes in medicine all speak to the good of the individual patient as the primary intent of the treatment. Pappworth states clearly that

> *The use of patients who are dying as subjects for experiments is shocking and wrong. This should hardly need saying. Indeed in the case of the dying, the doctors should perhaps be hesitant even about the use of an untried therapeutic technique, even though the patient may agree, especially if he is afraid of dying, as he may agree to anything. I myself have seen the trial use of new agents in cancer where the suffering produced by the agent in question has been very much worse than the suffering caused by the disease itself. Where a patient cannot be saved, it is common humanity that he should be allowed to die in peace. (Pappworth 1967, p. 195)*

The professional duty to continue to provide palliation when patients refuse curative and/or experimental techniques is clear. What is less clear is the extent to which patients can be transferred away from intensive-care units and institutions whose organizational goals are curative goals. Physicians presently make that decision, either alone or in committee, but such decisions may conflict with the patient's right to choose the place of death.

Discussions of the right to refuse treatment are usually concerned with patient's refusal of curative techniques which staff wish to perform. They might equally well be concerned with patients' refusal to be treated as though their death were certain, so that they are not provided life-prolonging interventions by staff who espouse a "quality-of-life" ethic. The pendulum may swing so far in the direction of support for a certain quality of life, rather than professional commitment to saving life at any cost, that the right of an individual to choose the place where he will die may come to be exercised against professionals who do not wish to admit him to institutions for treatment. Presently, however, the patient's right to choose where he will die implies a professional duty to attend him at home, as he needs such attendance. His right to choose when as well as where he dies implies that such documents as living wills should be binding on staff and that intensive resuscitation should not be performed against the wishes of the patient. Annas (1974) suggests the patient has a final right, which is to dictate the disposition of his body. The usual practice of obtaining an autopsy permission from the family immediately following the death of the patient is an obvious infringement. Is there a professional duty to obtain from the patient information as to what he wishes to be done with his body?

There is always some question in the minds of thoughtful practitioners as to whether the ethicists can really contribute to decisions about moral problems in practice. However, whether the philosopher — who does not experience the trauma of caring for the dying patient, and who is not responsible for the consequences of care decisions — can help the practitioner in decision-making is really not questionable. When the philosopher pares the situation of all variables but one, in order to develop thinking about the essence of the situation, the clinician may point out that situations are never so pure and that decisions must be made in the presence of confusing variables. It is indeed true that the confusing variables are always present in the clinical situation, but the painstaking work of the philosopher in analyzing the reasons for decision-making and for making a judgment can provide rationales for decisions or at the least make explicit the effects of previously covert values. "Moral judgments are not matters of taste nor rationalizations of private interests, but are universal claims which, if valid, are verifiable, at least in principle, through open and objective public discussion" (Brockway 1976, p. 12). Care of the dying must be based on a general therapeutic ethic and an articulated code of values specific to each profession involved in the care.

However, the ethical dilemma is always the dilemma of an individual, whose personal values will contribute both to the decisions made and to the way in which they are implemented. The conflicting goods of societal and individual rights, of research and service requirements, of professional and patient needs, must be resolved by individuals. Conflicts arise from the clash of strongly held values — for instance, values of individual freedom and individual autonomy that dictate patient choice of treatment — with the sanctity of human life, a value which requires that professionals override patients' decisions to refuse treatment or to commit suicide. Dilemmas may be resolved with a modicum of guilt given the understanding that it is not the professionals' role to constrain clients' decisions on the basis of their own values; rather the role is to contribute the information and support necessary to client decisions based on client values.

EUTHANASIA

Euthanasia is defined (Heritage Dictionary, 1977) as: "1. the action of inducing the painless death of a person for reasons assumed to be merciful; 2. an easy or painless death." The derivation is from the Greek words for good and for death.

Euthanasia is an ethical rather than a legal concept: statutes do not address merciful homicide, although courts are occasionally required to do so. Merciful homicide has been, on the whole, judged mercifully.

It is not the intent of this discussion to add to the already unwieldy literature on euthanasia but rather to take from that literature information that will be useful to nurses who are caring for terminally ill patients. In the minds of most people the word represents the problem of whether a merely physiological life should be prolonged when death is inevitable, or if a painless death should be encouraged. The question is not phrased in terms of killing but rather of allowing to die.

Euthanasia is an ancient practice; history records examples of group euthanasia practices on the Greek Isle of Cos in the 1st century BC. Early Christians, however, were opposed to self-destruction and euthanasia and their belief that life must be prolonged at nearly any cost has prevailed. Discussion in health-care, legal, and theological groups today centers around two forms of euthanasia: direct (positive or active) and indirect (negative or passive). Direct euthanasia is defined as deliberately shortening life through a specific action; legally, this is regarded as murder. Indirect euthanasia refers to permitting death through the omission of certain acts: halting or withholding treatments that would maintain life, or administering large doses of analgesics which will prove fatal — practices which are not uncommon.

There is increasing public discussion of the use of resuscitators, drugs, organ transplantations, and machines to maintain kidney function; increasingly, lay people are protesting a medical practice which maintains biological life for prolonged periods with extraordinary measures when there is no chance that brain function will be recovered. Unnecessary prolongation of life in the presence of terminal illness may rob the patient of the support of humanity and compassion; the practice is also wasteful of money, manpower, and hospital space. This is not to say that death should always be hastened, or that measures that would promote life or cure should always be withheld. However, proponents of euthanasia suggest that a time comes when the body cannot be cured and the need is for comfort, tender care, and an opportunity to prepare for death (Hendin 1973).

Morison (1973) suggests that attitudes and techniques developed to combat untimely death are obviously not always appropriate when death may be defined as timely. When recovery is impossible, recovery-oriented techniques are merely painful. The need is for the development of new techniques or the rediscovery of old ones.

> [No] moral or legal obligation requires one to do everything one knows how to do in order to preserve the life of a severely deteriorated patient beyond hope of recovery. . . . the difficulties then, are not with the general principle but with how to arrange the details. . . . [The] obligation to treat the living is neither absolute nor inexorable. (Morison 1973, pp. 58-59)

Various religious and philosophic groups have reiterated that health professionals are not required to utilize extraordinary means; the difficulty is with the definition of what constitutes extraordinary means, as there is no absolute scale of extraordinariness. What is extraordinary may be judged only in relation to the condition of the individual, and the definition of extraordinary may be reduced to "inappropriate in the circumstances." Negative euthanasia— the withdrawal of treatment from a patient who, as a result, is likely to die somewhat earlier than he otherwise would—can be regarded as changing from an inappropriate to an appropriate regimen, with death considered to occur merely as a result of illness. A positive action (for example, giving a narcotic for the control of pain in such a dosage that it may be lethal) may also be accepted on the basis of the principle of double action: the action is correct because the conscious intent is to achieve some licit purpose. It is necessary to differentiate in such an instance between the awareness of the probable result and the intent (Morison 1973).

In spite of the increased attention paid by the lay press to "pulling the plug" and "death with dignity," and the less impassioned comments in professional journals, there is no consensus as to the merits of either form of euthanasia and certainly no agreement that direct euthanasia is ever appropriate. Dyck (1973) is among those who speak against acceptance of the practice. He says that the arguments for euthanasia focus on two concerns: compassion for those who are painfully and terminally ill, and concern for human dignity associated with freedom of choice. Many people consider it inhumane to keep dying people alive when they are in great pain or have lost the ability to communicate with others. An ethic of euthanasia is exemplified in ancient Stoicism, in the belief that an individual has the right to dispose of his own life, and that the dignity of the individual depends on his freedom to make moral choices— including the choice for suicide if at some point life becomes not worth living, either because of distress, illness, physical or mental handicaps, or despair. The moral life of Christians and Jews, however, has been guided by the Decalogue, the Ten Commandments. "Thou shalt not kill" constrains euthanasia. The injunction not to kill not only preserves the individual but also prevents the destruction of the human community. No society can afford to be indifferent about the taking of human life.

Dyck is also among those who believe there is a moral difference between permitting death and causing death. To cause death is illegal and immoral. To permit death by allowing the patient or his family to refuse interventions that prolong dying for an individual who is incurably ill is humane. He says that the courage to be, expressed in Judeo-Christian thought, is more than overcoming fear of death. It is the courage to accept one's life as having worth no matter what that life may bring, because life is regarded as worthy by God. One's life is not merely one's own; it is a gift bestowed by God and protected by the human community and by the ultimate forces that make up the cycle of life and death. In this cycle there may be suffering and joy, but suffering does not render a life worthless. Suffering people need the support of others and should not be encouraged to commit suicide by the community, the physician, or the family.

If the physician engages in euthanasia, he accepts that another person's life is no longer meaningful enough to sustain. Everyone in the community is potentially a victim of such an ethic, especially the very young and very old, members of racial or religious minorities, anyone who is defenseless, voiceless, or dependent.

Careful analysis of medical practices and attitudes of German physicians before and during the reign of Nazism warns against the consequences of euthanasia as a public policy. The outlook of German physicians led to their cooperation with the policies of mass murders, which began with an attitude that the severely and chronically ill were not worthy of life — their life had no meaning. Gradually this attitude extended to the socially unproductive, the racially unwanted, and non-Germans. However, others point out that what was practiced during the Nazi regime can hardly qualify as euthanasia, and they suggest this is not a valid argument (e.g., Fletcher 1973A, 1973B).

Dyck perceives that the fallacy of euthanasia is that the physician encourages death in someone who could, with intervention, survive. Additionally, patients who are very ill are ambivalent about life but grateful for it when they recover. Physicians are human and can make a mistaken diagnosis or place research interests or a need for organs to be transplanted above the welfare of a single individual. Thus Dyck addresses the possibilities of abuse. He reiterates a cardinal principle of medicine, to cause no harm to the patient, and believes that relief of suffering does not include the attitude that the life of the suffering person is not worthwhile. The person who is suffering may find great moral, philosophical, mental, and emotional worth to his final days and to his suffering.

Stoic philosophy declares that life and selfhood belong to the individual to dispose of as and when he chooses. Judeo-Christian philosophy declares that life and selfhood are not at the disposition of the individual. Dyck (1973) suggests that the ethic of *benemortasia*, a good death, will include the following concepts:

> An individual's life is not solely at his disposal; every life is part of the human community which has as its ultimate goal the bestowing and protecting of its member's lives.

> Dignity of personhood, which includes freedom to make moral choices, includes the freedom of the dying person to refuse noncurative, life-prolonging interventions when he is dying, but does not allow him to take his own life, or allow others to do so.

> Every individual's life has some worth; there is no such thing as a worthless life.

> No individual or human community can presume to know who deserves to live or die.

Lach and Lamerton (1974) are in substantial agreement with this point of view. They argue that life can be precious even for patients with a fatal disease; the community should not regard terminally ill persons as victims to be abandoned to their unhappy fate. Euthanasia is considered to be the cry of despair of those who are afraid of life because they have never come to terms with it, but men and women of faith accept that death is a friend and gateway to everlasting life. Great attention should be given to the care of the dying, as the important time is not the hour of death but the weeks and months preceding it. Preparation for death takes study and time, which should be given. They believe the campaign for voluntary euthanasia to be founded on fallacies:

> It is a fallacy that persons with incurable diseases have no motive for continuing to live, that impaired life is useless, since even those with major physical disability find life sweet and can be useful.
> It is a fallacy that the incurably sick, because they are in pain, are unable to contemplate anything beyond present sufferings and death. Actually they may find security and peace, when cared for in a benign environment, such as an hospice.
> It is a fallacy that euthanasia reduces strain for the old and the sick; actually, it is a source of more strain. Almost everyone will need nursing some day, because bodies lose function, and all will feel they are burdens. The anguish of being a burden is increased if individuals must decide whether to tell physicians to let them die, to sign their own death warrants. It is a fallacy that euthanasia is an act of mercy. Sick animals are killed as an act of mercy, but people are not animals, and every human life has infinite value. (Lach and Lamerton 1974, pp. 2-3)

No religion would argue against stopping treatment, or even against starting treatment, for a patient facing miserable death if that treatment merely served biological prolongation. The basis of Christian opposition to euthanasia is not that life has paramount value, but that it is up to God to dispose of it. Even people who are in favor of euthanasia admit that doctors do misdiagnose terminally ill patients and even comatose patients do get well spontaneously and live many years thereafter (Elliott 1974).

Epstein (1976) believes that no rational decision for euthanasia can be made at this time. Society is morally confused; neither society nor professionals have faced the implications about human relationships, and the legal and medical professions are as confused as the rest of society. No one is prepared really to deal with "death with dignity;" this country has yet to enable all of its citizens to live with dignity. As long as we deny the fact that whole groups of people are systematically denigrated, we cannot trust ourselves to make any decisions about who shall die and when they are ready for death. Who can answer for another, or even for themselves, the question of when life has become too much of a burden, when suffering has been too great, when death is better than life, or when life is hopeless? Often the ill person, family member, and professional will vacillate in their decisions from day to day.

Epstein (1976) believes that perhaps the most frightening aspect of euthanasia is that in contemporary society whole groups of people — Blacks, Chicanos, Orientals, Jews, the aged, retarded children, the poor — are considered unworthy of society's goods and unworthy of education. Such people are still considered by some to be less than human — or at least to be "outsiders" and different. In the presence of any support for euthanasia, how remote is the judgment that all of these people would be better off dead? The argument that euthanasia will put the person out of his suffering Epstein considers unfounded, since Saunders and others who operate hospices have demonstrated that terminal patients can be kept relatively comfortable until death (Epstein 1976).

However, the humanistic philosophy declares that to let someone die a slow, ugly, dehumanizing death is harder to justify morally than to help him escape such misery. Humanistic ethics places humanness and personal integrity above biological life and functions. Fletcher (1973A, 1973B) states that it is no longer valid to argue the relative values of negative and positive euthanasia because in modern medicine passive (negative) euthanasia is frequently practiced when decisions are made to give no resuscitation, to stop administering intravenous fluids, or to give large doses of narcotics to ease pain. In any case, there is no moral difference between passive euthanasia (letting the person die) and active euthanasia (e.g., giving the person a lethal dose of medication). In fact, the suffering will be less with active euthanasia. Whenever the professional, family, or patient considers even passive euthanasia, they have decided that death is no greater an evil than the patient's continued existence (Rachels 1976).

The humanistic ethic holds that being human, personal, and mentally aware is more important than being biologically alive. Thus when a person's brain is dead or permanently injured, there is no real point in maintaining life biologically.

There are four forms of elective death:

1. Voluntary, direct euthanasia: chosen and carried out by the patient; actually suicide.

2. Voluntary, indirect euthanasia: when someone — the physician or a family member — gives a lethal dose of medicine to a patient in response to an earlier request, after he has become comatose and irreversibly ill. The Living Will is a statement of permission and desire for this kind of death.

3. Direct, involuntary euthanasia: mercy killing, performed on the patient's behalf without his present or past request; the individual is killed to end his suffering. Some examples are administration of fatal drug dosage to a terminally ill child or adult, shooting a person trapped inextricably in a blazing fire, and stopping the respirator on someone who is brain damaged.

4. Indirect, involuntary euthanasia: where nothing is done to prolong life and nothing is done to release the person from his condition, other than whatever is necessary to make him comfortable. This is current medical practice in many situations.

The religious-ethical defense of indirect, involuntary euthanasia is more generally accepted by ministers and priests of Protestant, Catholic, Jewish, Buddhist, Moslem, and Hindu beliefs than is recognized by the medical profession.

The Judeo-Christian heritage places great value on the wholeness of a person, which encompasses his spiritual, mental, and physical oneness as a human being of worth and dignity. When terminal illness cancels out all but the shell or body, the continuation of life through machines and drugs may be a gross violation of him as a person, and the aged or terminally ill may indeed have less fear of death than the suffering and the drawn-out process of dying (Fox 1976).

Weber (1973) makes a moral distinction between allowing patients with terminal illness to die and directly killing them; he maintains that there is a difference between direct killing and abandoning attempts to prolong life, that both are not euthanasia. He states that the terminally ill are best served by giving up attempts to extend their lives and concentrating on their needs as dying persons. However, such care cannot include activities that are lethal in intent. Proper care of the dying must include treatment of patients as whole persons; the human person is violated when either body or personality is violated. Respect for the human person implies a moral obligation to preserve health and prolong life. Weber suggests that respect for the dying may demand that we be able to stop trying to cure and try to help patients practice the art of dying — to die in a style consistent with life. This effort must be made before the person is near death; it is based on the perception that the overall good of the person may be served by allowing his illness or injury to take its course.

The ethical position which affirms the sanctity of life states that all lives are of equal value; each person's life is sacred. There is no need to prove one's right to life and no justification for taking another's life for any reason. Weber (1973) perceives that the quality-of-life ethic allows only some lives to be valuable and worthy of respect. That is a violation of the person; although the goal is to improve the manner of human living, who determines who should be killed and whose life is not of appropriate quality?

The sanctity-of-life adherents are also concerned about the quality of life, and they believe that the quality of all lives suffers unless each person's life is considered inviolable because of its very existence. A dying person's relationship to those about him symbolizes the relation of all men to one another. From this point of view, to practice direct euthanasia — even at the request of the patient — is to weaken the claim of all to the right to have others' respect, and to be inviolable when weakened.

However, not to fight death to the last ditch is compatible with respect for life, and the good of the patient is not necessarily the same as the desire of the patient. All acts have a moral quality, regardless of their intent or purpose; it is always evil to kill a man even for reasons of mercy.

Control of the human person is implied both in direct mercy killing and in prolonging life as long as possible, rather than allowing the person to die naturally when he is terminally ill. However, problems of possible abuse arise here also. Many people object to indirect euthanasia because of the possibility of abuse; they fear that the voluntary principle will be extended to force professionals to withhold care from handicapped or aged persons when they could indeed recover. Who would enforce the laws and monitor the enforcement of *voluntary* euthanasia is also a concern.

> *[However, even] those who vigorously oppose euthanasia are frequently equally opposed to prolonging the vital functions in an obviously "dead" body. Technological progress has made it possible to maintain for a considerable time the appearance of life in a moribund or actually dead patient. The respirations can be kept going; the heart function can be supported. . . . Such measures hardly seem warranted in the case of a chronically ill person in whom stoppage of the heart or breathing is merely the final outward manifestation of death. (Elliott 1974, p. 88)*

Elliott does not regard it as killing when the medical profession refrains from treatment that serves no curative or rehabilitative purpose for the patient. Resuscitation is not appropriate when it would only renew the patient's suffering. He does not believe that the terminally ill patient is necessarily freed from discomfort by large doses of narcotics. Many terminal patients die in a tangle of glass jars, pipettes, tubes with needles in veins, mouth, nostrils, bladder, and sometimes surrounded by bars and pulleys. The family can scarcely reach the dying patient through all this paraphernalia, and at the time when the patient may need it most, the support of family and friends is severely curtailed; the closest thing to him is a monitoring machine. This ordeal of technology hastens the death of the personality, which is composed of conscious decision, integrity, and self-possession. To be at home, to have quiet and restful light, comfortable temperature, books, tasteful food and drink served at reasonable times — this is the final boon a family can give their loved one. Sometimes that is impossible, but often it can be managed with the help of friends, a visiting nurse, a home health aide, or a private-duty nurse. Private-duty nursing is expensive, but less so than useless or repetitive x-rays, laboratory procedures, and the other extras reflected on the hospital bill. Also, in his own home the patient is not an object; he is not manipulated. He can remain the prime mover of events surrounding his care.

The public is now much more aware of the practices of institutional care and they are less and less tolerant of the technology. It is well known that poor or apparently unimportant patients are more likely than others to become research subjects. However, even the well-to-do person may be kept alive after he is personally dead in any meaningful sense of personhood. Better-educated people who are more sensitive to their rights frequently try to avoid institutionalization as long as possible. Elliott finds little ambiguity in the definition of extraordinary support. He would include artificial respirators to promote breathing; heart massage, the use of a pacemaker, or other machines for stimulation of the heart muscle; the use of a kidney machine to replace worn-out kidneys; transplant of vital organs; prolonged medication to create favorable blood pressure; and prolonged intravenous feedings (1974, p. 96). When such treatment would not be considered extraordinary remains a question that tends to be answered in economic terms. It is reported that the cost of keeping a hopelessly injured patient alive for a year is about $30,000 (Elliott 1974, p. 105). The decerebrate patient who lies in bed for a year, comatose, with heart and lungs maintaining function because of machines, is occupying a bed that could be used by perhaps 26 other patients during that year who might recover to live fully human lives.

The literature supports Fletcher's (1973A, 1973B) comments that passive euthanasia is common practice, and not abhorrent to either practitioners or families when the aim is to allow death to come gently. Supportive measures are not used to prolong the dying process when there is irreversible brain damage and intractable pain. Medications are given to eliminate pain, even if they shorten the process of dying; letting the patient go, while rejecting any measure that adds to discomfort, is not unusual.

Fox (1976) says that too often society has emphasized the importance of mere existence, so that everything possible was done to extend a life — often at great suffering, indignity, grief, financial burden, and emotional strain for patients, families, and caregivers. Currently, even those who are not comfortable with the concept of elective death do not perceive the need for a rule of vigorous treatment in all situations. However, the discussion is now being pushed by philosophers and others past the concept of refraining from life-saving treatment to the necessity for some principles or guidelines for actual lethal intervention. There is some gut-level feeling that letting an individual die is in some way different from killing him, or even from providing him with the means of death; that actually doing harm to others is worse than merely allowing it to happen. This is reversed in the consideration of good, rather than harm; it is better actually to do good than merely to allow it to occur. This leads to the question of whether death is a good or an evil. If death itself is natural, whether it is good or evil will depend on the character of the life that is cut short. Therefore, if continuation of life is a perceived evil to an individual, then providing him with death can be considered a moral action and active intervention to do so can be viewed as more moral than merely refraining from actions to prevent death. Fletcher puts the question clearly enough, and the rationale for the answers of those who would advance the view that treatment providing direct voluntary and involuntary euthanasia is principled treatment.

What, then is the real issue? In a few words, it is whether we can morally justify taking it into our own hands to hasten death for ourselves (suicide) or for others (mercy killing) out of reasons of compassion. The answer to this in my view is clearly, "Yes," on both sides of it. Indeed, to justify either one, suicide or mercy killing, is to justify the other. *The heart of the matter analytically is the question of whether the end justifies the means. . . . however, to hold that the end justifies the means does not entail the absurd notion that any means can be justified by any end. The priority of the end is paired with the principle of "proportionate good;" any disvalue in the means must be outweighed by the value gained in the end. . . . the really searching question of conscience is, therefore, whether we are right in believing that* the well-being of persons *is the highest good. If so, then it follows that either suicide or mercy killing could be the right thing to do in some exigent and tragic circumstances . . . (Fletcher 1973A)*

The guidelines on caring for the dying issued in 1976 by The Swiss Academy of Medicine identify medical, ethical, and legal considerations in the practice of euthanasia (in the Hastings Center Report, June 1977). They suggest that "it is medically justified to abandon a therapy or limit oneself to alleviating suffering if in deferring death one prolongs suffering beyond what is bearable and if . . . the affliction has taken an irreversible turn with a prognostication of death." However, it is clear that passive rather than actual euthanasia is considered: "According to Swiss Penal Code active euthanasia is a punishable, intentional homicide. Active euthanasia remains punishable *even when done at the request of the patient*" (italics ours) (Swiss Academy of Medicine 1977).

There is an extensive and erudite literature on the subject of the right of the competent adult to refuse treatment; on the desirability of the prolongation, or cessation of extreme care measures in the presence of irreversible conditions, or extreme cost to society; and on the philosophical and pragmatic differences between active and passive euthanasia (Rabkin et al. 1976; Hanink 1975; Cassem 1975; Fletcher 1967). There is very little in the professional journals about the implications of active euthanasia. The differentiation is made, and the possible abuses of active lethal intervention may be pointed out, but the clinical literature does not really address the problems. Ethicists and philosophers build logical and tidy arguments either in support of or against active euthanasia, but persons with clinical responsibility are more likely to make the assumption that active euthanasia is not in question, and go on to discuss who should make decisions about passive euthanasia. This is probably not unrelated to the legal implications of active euthanasia or to the statement adopted by the American Medical Association that "the intentional termination of the life of one human being by another — mercy killing — is contrary to that for which the medical profession stands and is contrary to the policy of the American Medical Association" (Rachels 1975). As pharmacologists, physicians, and nurses become more sophisticated in the use of pain-relieving and behavior-modification techniques, the question of active lethal intervention may become less urgent because compassionate reasons may dwindle in number and the discussion around who should make the decision not to initiate (or to discontinue) life-prolonging activities may be sufficient to generate adequate guidelines. It may be enough merely to let the patient die. It is suggested that this decision is "subject to moral appraisal in the same way that a decision to kill him would be subject to moral appraisal; it may be assessed as wise or unwise, compassionate or sadistic, right or wrong" (Rachels 1975). Therefore, while physicians may have to distinguish between the two activities as a matter of law, they should not give the distinction "any added authority and weight by writing it into official statements of medical ethics" (Rachel 1975). Morison (1971) identifies three modes of treatment open to the physician attending the dying patient: the use of all possible means to keep him alive; cessation of extraordinary means, but continuation of ordinary therapy; and active intervention to hasten the termination of life. There is much discussion about the movement from the first to the second of these steps but some agreement that the step may be taken. The questions are usually ones of when and how. However, medical opinion appears to be against ever taking the third step, although philosophical literature, poignant comment from victims (e.g., Alsop 1973; Morgan 1971), and the suicide rate all point to the need for consideration by clinicians that active euthanasia may sometimes be the decision most in the interest of the patient.

A primary difficulty, of course, is that if lethal intervention becomes legal, administration of the agent, whatever it is, will probably be the responsibility of the caregiver. The current official medical position is clear; active euthanasia is not considered, although there may be discussion of guidelines for the provision of passive euthanasia. Nurses, however, may be more willing to hear the arguments. In the study by Brown et al. (1971), nurses were more likely than physicians to hear requests for passive *and* active euthanasia; they were more uncomfortable when physicians did not practice negative euthanasia than when they did. They were also supportive of active euthanasia; however, it is worth noting that this finding is age-related — older nurses are not so likely to support this as younger ones. A majority of them reported they would practice passive euthanasia with a signed statement from the patient requesting it.

Nurses were also more likely than physicians to support the use of a professional panel to help with difficult decisions on the subject, rather than depending on an individual decision-maker. The changes in society since 1971 support the notion that a replication of the study would identify changes in the direction of more, rather than less, support of euthanasia by nurses.

Beauchamp (1976) reports that nurses still do not see themselves as autonomous decision-making agents in skilled judgmental areas of care or in response to patients and families. However, as expanded and primary-care roles are developed in hospital, clinic, and home care, nurses will have to reexamine their functions with respect to management of life and death. The nurse is responsible for her decisions and their consequences, including decisions to give or not give life-preserving service. She must therefore be aware of the legal, ethical, and medical perspectives of death and euthanasia.

As the domain of nursing takes shape under the aggressive leadership of women (and men) who need no longer consider nursing activities to be second-best to and dictated by medical activities, nurses will be faced with difficult decisions. The findings of Brown et al. (1971) indicate that nurses already hear more requests for euthanasia than is reported by physicians. Frequently they may be the only constant resource for families. They must be articulate and skilled in communicating with families and patients about death and its various aspects.

The nurse–practitioner must confront situations involving passive euthanasia; failing to feed patients, or to stimulate them, or give them cardiopulmonary resuscitation, or allowing infection to take hold. Even in choosing not to act, she makes a decision. With increased responsibility, authority, and status will come increased personal risk. The courts have to date been inconsistent in their treatment of mercy killings, although on the whole they have been lenient. It remains to be seen whether the nurse practitioner fares differently from the medical practitioner in the courts. If she acts in good faith, with the best interest of the patient at heart, it seems unlikely that she will be the object of judicial retribution (Beauchamp 1976), but sexism is not unknown in courts of law and the majority of nurses are female. In any case, nurses have a professional commit-ment to optimum human interaction, to go beyond curing, and to consider the dignity of the persons for whom they care (Epstein 1976).

Murray (personal communication 1978) points out that the nurse's role is surely not to distribute death as she would distribute medications. Rather, she should intervene to help patients experience the final part of life as a period in which they can give as well as receive. Certainly no one can teach about suffering, dying, and death as well as the person who is facing and pondering his own ap-proaching death. Ideally nurses can be involved with patients so that patients' lives remain meaningful because of the relationship, so that through the last days love, hope, peace, and the retention of humanity are possible. The dying patient has social significance, but staff must risk involvement. The nurse's role is to *care* for the patient and his family, to maintain their comfort physically and emotion-ally, to share humanity during the last contact with humanity, and to speak for life.

There can be no quarrel with this perception of nursing. The very real ques-tion still concerns the *means*. Does "speaking for life" in any given situation dic-tate that life is prolonged to the extent that this is possible or that in common humanity a suffering or an irreversibly comatose patient is allowed to die?

Public Policy

There is a burgeoning legislative activity around refusal of treatment and eutha-nasia, and by the end of 1977 eight states* had passed and enacted Natural Death Acts.

In his analysis of the legislative proposals on refusal of treatment and eutha-nasia, Robert Veatch, of the Research Group on Death and Dying at the Hastings Center, identifies and analyzes bills that apparently legalize active killing, bills that would clarify the rights of competent patients, and bills that clarify decision-making for incompetent patients (Veatch 1977). He states that since 1969 over 85 bills have been proposed. It is obvious that the legal constraints on profes-sional decisions are only a matter of time. Bills that apparently legalize active euthanasia do not distinguish clearly in their texts between mercy killing and omission of treatment; although none of them refers explicitly to active killing, the implication is that *if* the bills are passed, the act of killing will be legal in certain specified conditions. Veatch (1977) points out that the bill introduced into the British Parliament in 1969 defines euthanasia as "the painless induce-ment of death," and would make it lawful for physicians to "administer eu-thanasia."

Physicians may prescribe, but nurses implement treatments; they are also those persons most likely to be giving care to terminally ill patients. The ethical and legal components of euthanasia are ambiguous, and public policy is fluid.

---

*California, Idaho, Arkansas, New Mexico, Nevada, Oregon, Texas, and North Carolina.

For those persons who would never in any circumstances administer a lethal drug or discontinue a treatment, there is no ethical dilemma. For those who may consider that there are situations in which these activities are compassionate, and in the best interests of patients, the possibility of euthanasia is inextricably intertwined with the rights of patients both to receive the best possible treatment and to refuse any given treatment.

References

Alsop S: Stay of execution. SR/World (18 December 1973), pp. 20–23

American Nurses' Association: Code for Nurses with Interpretive Statements. Kansas City, Mo., ANA, 1976

Annas GJ: Rights of the terminally ill patient. J Nurs Admin 1 (2):40, 1974

Beauchamp J: Euthanasia and the nurse practitioner. Nurs Dig 4 (5):83, 1976

Blaylock JN: Characteristics of nurses and of medical-surgical patients to whom they react positively and negatively: a synopsis of findings. Nurs Res Conf 8:113, 1972

Bloom SW: The Doctor and His Patient. New York, Free Press, 1963

Brockway GM: The physician's appeal to first-hand experience. Hastings Cent Rep 6 (2):9, 1976

Brown JS, Rawlinson ME: Sex differences in sick role rejection and in work performance following cardiac surgery. J Health Soc Behav 18:276, 1977

Brown N, Thompson D, Balger R, Laws EH: How do nurses feel about euthanasia and abortion? Am J Nurs 71 (7):1413, 1971

Cassell EJ: Illness and disease. Hastings Cent Rep 6:27, 1976

Cassem N: Ever say die? Linacre Quart 42:86, 1975

Castles MR: Game theory as a conceptual framework for nursing practice. In Barnard M, Hymovich D (eds), Family Health Care. New York, McGraw-Hill, 1973

——: Professional codes and personal values: The implications of incongruence. In Reilly D (ed), Teaching in the Affective Domain. New York, Charles B. Slack, 1978, pp. 9–16

Coe RM: Sociology of Medicine. New York, McGraw-Hill, 1970

Crane D: Dying and its dilemmas as a field of research. In Brim O, Freeman H, Levine S, Scotch N (eds), The Dying Person. New York, Russell Sage Foundation, 1970, pp. 303–325

Culliton B: The Haemmerli affair: Is passive euthanasia murder? Science 190: 1271, 1975

Drummond E: Communication and comfort for the dying patient. Nurs Clin North Am 2 (1):55, 1970

Dyck A: An alternative to the ethic of euthanasia. In Williams R (ed), To Live and to Die. New York, Springer-Verlag, 1973, pp. 98–112

Elliott N: The Gods of Life. New York, Macmillan, 1974

Epstein C: Active and passive euthanasia: Nursing implications. Nurs Dig 4 (4): 54, 1976

Flaherty MJ: The nurse and orders not to resuscitate. Hastings Cent Rep 7 (4): 27, 1977

Fletcher G: Prolonging life. Washington Law Rev 42:999, 1967

Fletcher J: Ethics and euthanasia. In Williams R (ed), To Live and to Die. New York, Springer-Verlag, 1973A, pp. 113-122

———: Ethics and euthanasia. Am J Nurs 73 (4):670, 1973B

———: The Ethics of Genetic Control. Garden City, N.Y., Anchor, 1974

Fox N: A good birth—a good life—why not a good death? Nurs Dig 4 (2):24, 1976

Georgopoulous BS: The hospital as an organization. In Georgopoulous B (ed), Organization Research on Health Institutions. Ann Arbor, Institute for Social Research, University of Michigan, 1972, pp. 1-46

Greene WA: The physician and his dying patient. In Troup S, Greene WA (eds), The Patient, Death and the Family. New York, Scribners', 1974, pp. 85-94

Hanink J: Some light on "double effect." Analysis 35 (5):147, 1975

Hendin D: Death as a Fact of Life. New York, Warner Paperback Library, 1973, pp. 60-82

Heritage Dictionary, s.v. "Euthanasia." Boston, Houghton Mifflin, 1977

Illich I: Medical Nemesis. New York, Pantheon, 1976

Jameton A: The nurse: when roles and rules conflict. Hastings Cent Rep 7 (4):22, 1977

Kübler-Ross E: On Death and Dying. New York, Macmillan, 1969

Lach S, Lamerton R: The Hour of Our Death. London, Geoffrey Chapman, 1974

Lasagna L: Life, Death and the Doctor. New York, Knopf, 1968

Levin P, Berne E: Games nurses play. Am J Nurs 72 (2):483, 1972

Lieberman M: The physician's duty to disclose risks of treatment. Bull NY Acad Med 50 (8):943, 1974

Mauksch HO: Patient care as a perspective for hospital organization research. In Georgopoulous B (ed), Organization Research on Health Institutions. Ann Arbor, Institute for Social Research, University of Michigan, 1972, pp. 159-171

Morgan LG: On drinking the hemlock. Hastings Cent Rep 1 (3):4, 1971

Morison RS: Death: Process or event? Science 173:694, 1971

———: Dying. Sci Am 229 (3):55, 1973

Murray R: Personal communication, 1978

Neville R: Ethical and philosophical issues of behavior control. Paper presented at the 139th Annual Meeting of the American Association for the Advancement of Science, December 27, 1972. New York, Institute of Society, Ethics, and the Life Sciences, Reading no. 804

Pappworth MH: Human Guinea Pigs. Beacon, Boston, 1967

Parsons T: The Social System. New York, Free Press, 1951, chap. 10

Parsons T, Fox R: Illness, therapy and the modern urban American family. J Soc Iss 13:31, 1952

Quint J: Personalizing institutional care of the dying. Arch Found Thanatol 2 (2):60, 1970

Rabkin MT, Gillerman G, Rice NR: Orders not to resuscitate. N Engl J Med 295:364, 1976

Rachels J: Active and passive euthanasia. N Engl J Med 292:78, 1975

———: Active and passive euthanasia. Nurs Dig 4 (4):52, 1976

Robinson L: Psychological Aspects of the Care of Hospitalized Patients. Philadelphia, Davis, 1968

Robinson M: The pediatrician and the dying child. Arch Found Thanatol 2 (1):13, 1970

Scott WR: Professionals in hospitals: technology and the organization of work. In Georgopoulous B (ed), Organizational Research on Health Institutions. Ann Arbor, Institute for Social Research, University of Michigan, 1972, pp. 139-156

Shubik M (ed): Game Theory and Related Approaches to Social Behavior. New York, John Wiley and Sons, 1964

Steinfels M: Ethics, education and nursing practice. Hastings Cent Rep (August 1977), 4:20-21

Swiss Academy of Medicine: Swiss guidelines on care of the dying. Hastings Cent Rep 7 (3):30, 1977

Ufema J: Dare to care for the dying. Am J Nurs 76 (1):88, 1976

Veatch R: Analysis of Legislative Proposals on Euthanasia and Treatment Refusal. Institute of Society, Ethics and the Life Sciences. Hastings-on-Hudson, N.Y., 1977

Weber L: Ethics and euthanasia: another view. Am J Nurs 73 (7):1228, 1973

Wilson RN: Patient-practitioner relationships. In Freeman HE, Levine S, Reeder LG (eds), Handbook of Medical Sociology. Englewood Cliffs, N.J., Prentice-Hall, 1963, pp. 273-275

Chapter 6

Nurses' Perceptions

In this study, nurses were randomly selected from a roster of all nursing-service personnel involved in patient-care activities.* The roster included nursing assistants, orderlies, licensed practical nurses, staff nurses, team leaders, and head nurses. Supervisors and nursing administrators were excluded, with the exception of those evening and night supervisors who were the only registered nurses on duty on the division during those shifts. The roster nurses were stratified by shifts, in order to examine whether there were differences in perception between night and day nurses, but since most of the subjects rotated shifts, this analysis was not carried out.

Two kinds of institutions were visited: institutions in which cure was the primary goal and institutions in which care was the primary goal. In two of the institutions visited both goals were observed; that is, the acute-care institution had a long-term care annex. Although institutions were randomly selected from the Guides Issue of Hospitals and nurses were randomly selected from personnel rosters, the findings are not interpreted as though random techniques were utilized; the subjects are all volunteers, and the institutions are all located in one state, within driving distance for the senior author. The study was exploratory, and the design was compromised by the requirements of the various institutional review boards. However, the responses of this sample of nursing

---

*It was our intent to interview those members of the nursing staff who were actually giving direct patient care at some time during their working days; therefore, it was expected that the sample would be heavily loaded with nurse assistants and licensed practical nurses and this was, in fact, the case. Selection of the nurses was carried out as here described (see also Appendix A).

185

caregivers provide a realistic assessment of the difficulties and rewards inherent in institutional care of patients who will not recover. The nurses interviewed were on the whole humane and caring individuals; they wanted to provide the best care to their patients. If they were also defensive it is only to be expected. Nurses are blamed for much that they do not perceive they have the power to change. They endure long hours in stressful settings and provide support which is usually not recognized or rewarded by either physicans or patients, although they look to these groups for *their* support. The nurses who agreed to be interviewed were without exception interested in improving the quality of the care received by patients. They wanted to do what was best; they frequently indicated that they did not really know what was best for any given patient or that if they could identify the patient need and the appropriate nursing intervention, they did not have the authority or time for implementation.

For study purposes nursing personnel were categorized as follows:

> *The professional nurse* is employed by the department of nursing service, has a baccalaureate degree in nursing and a state license to practice nursing, and is involved in patient care.

> *The technical nurse* is employed by the department of nursing service; has a diploma in nursing or an associate arts degree in nursing, as well as a state license to practice nursing; and is involved in patient care.

> *The licensed practical nurse* is employed by the department of nursing service, has completed a licensed practical nurse program or passed an equivalency examination, has a state license to practice nursing, and is involved in patient care.

> *The nursing assistant* is employed by the department of nursing service, has completed the institution's in-service training program, and is involved in patient care.

As status in nursing is in inverse relationship to the amount of time spent handling the body of the patient and in direct relationship to years of education, it is not surprising that a random selection of nursing personnel giving direct care to patients should elicit only four nurses with baccalaureate degrees; one diploma nurse and 26 associate-degree nurses completed the sample of 31 registered nurses. Nurse assistants were most heavily represented (35) and licensed practical nurses least heavily represented (17). Comparisons were made when appropriate of similarities and differences between registered nurses and other nursing personnel (Appendix A). The interviews which follow are not identified here as to the status of the subject. All subjects responded to the same questions, and all subjects were caring for terminal patients in an institutional setting at the time of interview.

Attitudes of physicians and nurses reflect general social attitudes (Kneisl 1968). While they are treating seriously ill or dying patients they must handle their own feelings as well as those of their patients. Their education has emphasized the necessity of remaining cool, calm, and clear of judgment because although families and patients might misinterpret such behavior as uncaring and unconcerned, showing concern may cause them to lose confidence. Showing any signs of feeling may be considered to indicate lack of control; instructors teach that a measure of hardness and insensibility may be essential to practice. In addition, education still emphasizes that professionals cannot expect too much from obviously less knowledgeable lay persons. Reasons to share information with them or listen to their feelings are not identified.

Almost in spite of their education, doctors and nurses do care about people. In spite of the anecdotal and experiential data identifying discourtesy and depersonalizing behaviors in nurses, most of them are concerned for their patients. As one nurse suggested, after the interview was concluded:

> R: Of course we care! How can you nurse if you don't care about people? You may be tired, or sick, or under stress or angry, or just not like certain patients, but you have to care. There are easier ways to make a living if you don't!

Whether, or how, caring should be manifested is an unanswered question for many.

> I: You said something I'd like to explore a little bit, that sometimes you cry. You indicated in the context of your statement that you felt this was not a good thing to do. Do you think you should not cry?
>
> R: Well, I don't know. You know, nurses are supposed to be so strong, but . . .
>
> I: Are tears a sign of weakness?
>
> R: I guess people think they are. I always feel so foolish, because I want to say something to the family, and yet sometimes I can't even look at them because I can't even talk. We had a 28-year-old girl who I did a nursing assessment on, on a Thursday night, and she'd never really talked to anybody, but she really opened up, and I talked to her for about an hour and a half, and the next morning she started bleeding and they took her to the operating room and she died that night. And I was trying to tell her husband some of the things she talked to me about. I couldn't even . . . I talked to him for a little while, but I started crying and I couldn't talk. I'm about to cry now, thinking about it.
>
> I: Don't you think that was probably helpful to him, to know that somebody else cared about her that much?
>
> R: Yes, it might have been, I don't know. He didn't say a whole lot, because he was about to cry himself, but . . . you'd think that after awhile you'd get hardened, that you'd build up some kind of a shield, but I seem to be weaker now in that sense . . . not weaker, but more prone to get emotionally involved with the patient than I was when

a student. Well, not when I was a student, because that was really bad, but right after I got out I was, you know, really . . . I had good control. But since coming to this hospital it seems just the word cancer implies death to me, and I hate to think about anybody having to die, and being in pain before they die.

If the professional behavior of this nurse is not appropriate, it is obviously not for lack of caring.

NURSES' PERCEPTIONS OF PATIENTS

How Should Dying Patients Behave?

In spite of the school of thought that prescribes dignified, peaceful death, nurses in this study generally were less reluctant than their patients to accept idiosyncratic behavior in patients. This group felt that patients should behave in whatever ways made them feel safe and comfortable, and that there should be no effort to move patients into certain prescribed behaviors. However, almost half of the nurses expected cooperative behavior from patients. Registered nurses were more likely than other nursing personnel to allow individualized behavior, and some of their responses to the question "How should dying patients behave?" include the following.

R: Well, I expect when they're told, I expect them to cry and be upset. And a lot of times we don't see the doctor tell them, so we're not quite sure when they were told, or if they were really given any specific . . . And usually . . . they're depressed and I don't hear much from them. They don't say too much, and when you talk to them — this is generally — they seem to be pretty short, and they'd rather be by themselves, turn over and face the wall, and stay out of groups — isolate themselves. And then when they — I would say generally when they've been here three or four times . . . you know, you see them very negative, or different behavior patterns. A lot of it is just the individual personality, besides just the illness. . . .

I: You told me how people do behave, how they're likely to behave. How do you think they should behave?

R: Well, I guess that's how they should behave. I guess that's how I would behave, I mean. I would be very bitter at first, if I were told, and I would be very mad, because it was me, and I guess, not someone else.

I: So there isn't any one way that everybody should go? Should everyone die with dignity, or peacefully or any of these things that sometimes we say?

R: Perhaps they didn't live with dignity, or didn't live peacefully. How could they die that way? You have to meet each situation on an individual basis. I find it very difficult to get the idea that you can set up established norms, other than trying to get a good total patient picture. I think this is the only way you can help . . .

I: So the norm really is for nursing?

R: To individually evaluate, because each patient is an individual.

I: And there is no norm for each patient?

R: To me there isn't, no.

R: I'm not sure how they should. I don't see anything wrong with withdrawal. I think it's a normal reaction, that if you're trying to separate yourself from something which you don't want to continue with, you just start blocking out what is happening and you withdraw from that particular situation, this being life.

I: What they're withdrawing from, is life?

R: I think so.

I: If you had a patient who yelled and screamed and shouted, "I don't want to go," right up till the last minute, would that be all right?

R: Well, it would be all right. I don't know how I'd handle it, I haven't had that experience.

I: But if there is somebody who wants to fight every step of the way at the top of his voice, is that appropriate behavior in the institution?

R: For him it would be appropriate. He wouldn't be ready.

I: You think when they get ready they withdraw?

R: I think they're prepared then.

R: Well, I don't know if there's any certain way they ought to behave. I mean everybody's different and everybody's got to be different.

I: And that's all right with you?

R: Yes.

Although registered nurses generally would not identify a norm for patient behavior and espoused the right of individuals to behave in whatever way they could, they did not believe that dying patients should be allowed to experience pain and anxiety. The staff should facilitate a peaceful passage without undue interference with the process when it is inevitable.

R: If they have to be given medicine to help them, to relieve their anxiety, they should have it. If there's anything to give them medically to make their death easier . . . within the normal range of medication and nursing procedures that we do for the patient, I think dying people are entitled to a . . . [*long pause*]

I: It sounds like you think a quiet death is the best kind of death.

R: Yes, I do.

I: And you think it's the responsibility of nursing and medicine to help provide that quiet death?

R: Yes, I do.

R: Well, I feel that they ought to die with respect, and they ought to have, we ought to give them a certain amount of privacy. . . . I think patients should die the way that they feel . . . the way they feel best, and we ought not to interfere with it the way we interfere at times.

When nurses did identify expected patient behaviors, it was likely to be the norm of acceptance — of the peaceful and dignified dying, at home and/or in a position of faith, which is described in the literature.

R: If a patient is going to die, I don't see why he should have to die in the hospital. Why not die at home? That's an added burden here in the hospital — to die. Just go home, just be in your own surroundings, die with people that you know.

I: On whom is it a burden to die in the hospital?

R: Well, it's not the nurses. It's mostly the patients. It's really a burden on the patient. I mean how would you like to . . . I mean, I can't even stand going to the doctor's office just knowing if I have to stay there. I've never been in the hospital, but knowing I'd have to stay there, knowing I'm going to die there, that'd really frighten me.

I: So you think perhaps they would be happier at home, if it could be arranged that the care could be given there?

R: Yes.

I: Do you think most families would accept this?

R: Some families. Some families would. I wouldn't say the majority. . . . But if it was up to the patient, I'd say he wanted to die at home.

R: Well, I think he ought to be prepared.

I: How, how are you prepared?

R: Well, just be a gentleman or a lady . . . as you have all your life.

R: How should they behave? Well, when I come to die I hope that I can go out graciously myself. Now I may not, but that's . . .

I: Graciously. How would you behave if you were gracious?

R: Frightened. But underneath [sic] the medication, I hope there'd be a good nurse along to give it to me. I had an experience the other night, you see. A gentleman began to cry and I talked with him for a while, and he quieted down. So I hope that some nurse will be good enough to talk to me sometime.

I: You would like to go graciously . . . that is quietly?

R: Yes.

I: And with someone to talk to?

R: Yes. Someone to take the time to hold my hand, like I did.

Several nurses identified the nursing responsibility to keep patients clean and cheerful.

R: I don't think that they should be laying there with a pad under them in a wet bed. To me, that's not only not cleanliness, but its undignified . . .

I: Clean, dry, and comfortable is part of dignity?

R: Absolutely.

I: I'm still not sure I understand what you mean by "with dignity" — what that would involve besides the physical thing.

R: Well, of course, to me cleanliness and comfort and dignity all kind of go hand in hand.

Patients are required to be brave.

R: Well in an adult way. . . . I'd like to be able to greet it happily, you know. Be able to, all the way to the very end keep a small bit of humor, and meet it respectably.

I: Stiff upper lip?

R: That sort of thing. Yes, I would, personally.

I: You think this is appropriate behavior for everybody when they die?

R: I think so.

R: I think the main thing . . . he sees himself, he sees his own self-worth and that he is worthy enough of a person that there is something there worth saving and having go on . . .

I: You're telling me what he thinks or feels. Tell me what he should do.

R: I think that what he does is that he doesn't become completely involved in himself, he still retains the ability to look out and appreciate other people. What they're doing for him, know that they still have problems that he's already been through.

R: I don't believe I have a set pattern, the way I think people should react, except what I mentioned, that it seems to me they should

accept it. I don't think they have to be reading their Bible every
day. I don't think they have to sit and worry about "I was angry
to that woman when I was a child, and I wonder where she is and
if I can apologize."

I: I hear you indicating that you think there should be a certain acceptance of the situation when there is no other . . .

R: Yes. I know this would make our job easier. I would hope it would
make the patient's job easier. But this is my feeling. But I would
like to believe that I'm tolerant of those who cannot take this, right
away.

Some subjects responded to the question with statements of desirable
patient-nurse interactions, how the nurse should be and how the patient should
be. Staff should provide information and share patients' fears; patients should
allow staff to do so, and cooperate.

R: Well, I don't know. I think a person should know that they're going
to die. . . . I would want to know that I probably wouldn't be here
much longer. I think that a patient has this right, especially if they
are clear at all in their mind, and I think that the family and doctors
should talk to them about it, and not put it off. . . . I think someone
should be told that he is going to die.

I: So you think a person should die informed?

R: I do.

I: You've been telling me how the people around him ought to behave,
that is, they ought to tell him. How should he behave?

R: . . . he shouldn't just give up. He should keep on hoping. . . . miracles
have happened, and he should try and be cheerful.

R: I don't think they should be a model patient.

I: What do you mean by "a model patient?"

R: You go in and you say "Good morning, Mr. Jones." They say "Oh,
good morning, Miss Smith," and are cheerful. Because there's got to
be some sorrow involved . . .

I: So they don't have to be cheerful?

R: No, not all the time, I'd say at least fifty percent of the time.

I: How else should a patient be?

R: Cooperative.

I: Cooperative with what?

R: With what the nurses want, the doctors want.

I: Why?

R: If they cooperate it could prolong their life that much longer . . . and if he's got any fear, I think that he should confide that to the nurse. She won't have all the answers but there's no use keeping things like that to themselves, because it only burdens them more . . . if he could talk to the nurse . . . she could act as a sort of mediator.

R: I don't know. I think if it was me I'd be terrified. I don't really know how they should behave; 'course we'd all like for them to behave as if absolutely nothing was wrong, they were going to get well and go home. Because then we wouldn't have the pain of the burden.

I: . . . but you're not telling me they should do that?

R: No, no.

R: This is what I think should be: If they are accepting to the point of cooperating with what has to be done, and if they at least try to enjoy what there is to enjoy, and live for the moment, and try not to be so depressed that they're fighting everything anyone tries to do for them, in that it holds them down and holds them back, and that you cannot tell how ill they are because their depression interferes and gets in the way. And if they try to have enough faith to be uplifted without being so hopeful that they're not willing to accept what the usual is, which is inevitable death in a terminal disease. And of course I realize it isn't always like this; I'm not sure, of course, how I would be, and everybody tries to judge by themselves.

Some strong religious statements were elicited from this group of nurses.

R: . . . to answer that, it makes me have a little self-examination, because I should be in this group too, right? And I believe that we are creatures made in the image of God. And that we are built for eternity, that we are here just for a few years. And so I think that we should be peaceful and we should have a grace about us and we should exhibit dying grace — to be peaceful — and are willing to see our Saviour.

R: I think if you're a religious person, and you know everything's right with God, I think you can accept it. I think that's the way things should be — when I came to this hospital . . . I had quit my other job and didn't have a job any place else, and I didn't . . . I'd looked at several hospitals and nobody needed any nurses, which is strange, but I actually prayed about it, where I should end up and . . . there was an opening here, and I got on here. And I felt like God sort of wanted me to do something for the patients here, people who didn't have any hope left. But since I've been working here, I don't feel I've done what I came to do. I feel that so many times I'm just speechless. And a lot of times I cry, you know, I just come out of the room and cry. And that upsets me, because I don't feel I'm giving them enough support. But I think if a patient can have a . . . I mean, if a patient knows, you know, that there's a life after death, and that God has a reason for taking him, the patient can accept that, then I think he can accept dying much easier. So the ideal thing would be for everybody who's going to die should, you know, have a strong faith in God, and then I think they can handle anything.

Some nurses could not identify behavioral norms for patients; however, when they were asked, "How would you like to die?," they could identify personal norms for dying. These were likely to agree with the accepting, dignified, peaceful statements in the literature. *All* subjects would like to be informed, and most nurses would like to be "good" patients. However, whereas a personal, "preferred" norm may be identified, it was made clear that even "bad" patients should get support and care from nurses, who should tolerate "bad" behavior.

> *R:* I'm gonna be nice when I die, but if the patient wants to be bad, I think that's all right.
>
> *I:* When the patient is bad, what do you mean by that?
>
> *R:* Be angry, or something like that. If they want to be that way, it's all right with me.
>
> *R:* Well, they probably can't help doing this [being angry or complaining] if they're worried, and they should get TLC.
>
> *I:* So the behaviors that are difficult . . . you perceive as being something the patient can't help, and you would respond with TLC?
>
> *R:* Yes.

Many of the nurses perceived, realistically enough, that how patients should behave must be condition-dependent.

> *R:* Well . . . that's a very broad, difficult question. I guess first of all it would depend on probably the pain that they're in at the time, maybe, what they're dying from, and what kind of physical shape they're in. . . . I think that the length of time they had been in the hospital would have some bearing on how they felt at any particular time. I'm thinking that a person who has been bedridden for three or six months would be more depressed than one who hasn't been in bed that long.

How Do Dying Patients Behave?

It was not easy to elicit behavioral statements in response to the question "How do dying patients behave?" Nurses responded with terms like "acceptance" and "personality change" and could not always describe observed behaviors that led to these inferences. However, the statements are in agreement concerning two factors: patients behave individually, different from each other and different from their own previous behavior, and they are afraid; as one veteran nurse put it: "Mostly I see fear."

> *R:* It varies depending on the patients and their preparation. Some with complete acceptance, some with total apprehension regarding the whole thing. Generally I think they are somewhat apprehensive and want someone with them during this period of time.

> *R:* I think once a patient reaches a certain stage they realize — they know they have not much time left, and usually, I'd say nine-tenths of the time there's a personality change with these patients. . . . How their personality is going to change depends on that individual. And you just have to kind of feel your way around.

> *I:* What behavior do they manifest which leads you to remark that they had personality changes? How do their behaviors change?

> *R:* Well, some of them become very . . . oh, what shall I say — they just don't want to have anything to do with anybody, they want to be totally left alone to their inner feelings.

> *I:* What do they say or do that makes you think they want to be left alone?

> *R:* Well, they'll struggle if you try a certain nursing procedure on them. . . . Some patients become very combative. They realize they're dying and they say "Why, why are you trying to help me? Why don't you just let me go?" It really becomes kind of a problem to know exactly how to handle them when they reach this stage.

> *R:* I think they die being lonesome and not able to communicate their real fears. Maybe they can't really accept them. I don't know.

> *I:* Do you think if we'd behave differently in nursing that they would talk to us?

> *R:* A lot of them over here are scared and they're afraid of dying.

> *I:* I don't know how somebody behaves when he's afraid. What do they do?

> *R:* She acts afraid because she's afraid to be left alone in the room. She wants somebody there with her to reassure her all the time. If her family's not there, then she's constantly calling for little things. She's scared to be left alone. She's just scared to be there by herself.

> *R:* It's just a withdrawal right towards the end. It's very obvious, and you can tell that death is coming, because they are withdrawing, they're not . . . they have no will to continue, and their vital signs and everything are corresponding, almost, to this.

> *I:* What do patients do that makes you say that they are withdrawing?

R: They sometimes ignored your presence, they don't talk to you when you're talking to them. They don't talk to their family much. You ask them to do something and they just give no response at all, no negative response, just no response. No actions towards your maintaining their physical care. They lie very, very still, they don't turn. They don't want to eat, they don't want to drink.

The need to help patients continue to hope is identified, although even with hope withdrawal is expected.

I: Why do you think it [Bible reading] helps them?

R: I don't know. They sort of . . . It's something that gives them hope.

I: What do they say or do that makes you think that they have this support?

R: Well, they talk about maybe verses in the Bible, or just how they feel about reading it. They say themselves that that helps, that's what they have left.

I: What other things are they likely to do?

R: Some patients become sort of withdrawn, sort of, you know, just quiet. Like maybe they've just given up and they don't want to think about it, but just know they're going to die and just going to suffer it out. . . .

I: You mean withdraw from interaction with other people, or . . .?

R: Right.

Some subjects will withhold information in order to keep patients hoping.

R: Many times a patient will say, "What's this all for, what are you people trying to do? — Why don't you just let me die?"

I: What do you say when a patient says this?

R: I say, well, first of all I tell them that they're not dying . . .

I: Even if they are?

R: Yeah. —I try and relieve this feeling of being scared. Because I think this complicates the matter in getting better or getting well. Because if someone's afraid to do something, afraid to exert any effort, then they almost, like you say, lose the will to go ahead.

I: So you think if you told them the truth, that they were in fact dying, they would lose the will to undergo treatment that would perhaps keep them alive . . .?

R: For a longer period of time. . . .

I: If you were going to die in six weeks, wouldn't you want to know it?

R: If I was a bedridden patient and only had approximately six weeks to
    live, no, I don't think I'd want to know.

I: You wouldn't want to know?

R: No. If I was a patient that was able to be up, ambulatory and able
    to move around, and was given a date of six weeks or two months,
    knowing that I would die in that time, yes, I might say I would like
    to know, then, but not being a bedridden patient, because that would
    be the only thing on your mind, you know, the whole time that you
    were just lying in bed.

R: I think those that do that [gripe] feel insecure, they want reassur-
    ance.

I: Do you reassure them?

R: The best I can.

I: What do you tell them?

R: That I . . . you know, just make things as comfortable for them, and
    I tell them that just look on the bright side of things, you know.
    And I try to keep 'em smiling, cheerful.

In summary, most of the nurses, regardless of level of education and years
of experience, believed that dying patients were very individual in their behaviors, although they were more likely than not to be fearful and very dependent.
"They want to hang on." They require ("demand"; "need") someone in the
room with them a good part of the time. It is interesting to note that several
professional nurses spontaneously indicated that the presence of the nursing
assistant might be of equal or greater support to the patient than the presence
of the registered nurse, who might be perceived by the patient as too busy or
too "professional" to be able to spend the time.

Do Patients Know They Are Dying?

Not all of the nurses believed that patients should be informed of their prognosis, although most of them felt that this was appropriate if it was done compassionately, that the patient was at the same time reassured that he would not
be abandoned, and that everything possible would be done to postpone death
and to ensure physical comfort in his dying. However, the nurses believed that
most patients know the prognosis without being told, although some might
deny it.

When asked why they think patients know, nurses described the many
cues they are given: physiological cues ("They sense the body changes") and
personnel or family cues ("They are moved closer to the station; we make
rounds more frequently" and "Their people don't visit"). Under these circumstances, an alert patient would have to exercise a very strong denial mechanism
not to know.

Also, patients sometimes verbalize their knowledge. They ask questions; they speak of everything in the past tense. And most frequently there is a change in their behavior—toward withdrawal and hostility ("They resent your taking care of them").

What Do Dying Patients Need Most from Nursing?

However the nursing behavior which meets the need is described, dying patients need stability and reassurance. In response to the question "What do dying patients need most from nurses?" promptness, understanding of many things, and availability are mentioned. It is clear from the replies that the goal of the nursing actions is to reassure the patient that he will not be deserted.

I: What do you think they need most from nurses?

R: Understanding and . . . just have a nurse to check on them every few minutes. Ask them how they feel, if there's anything they can do for them.

I: When you say they need understanding from the nurse, what does that mean? Understanding of what?

R: That a nurse is willing to stand and listen to what the patient has to say or answer any questions for them. Just be willing to stand and listen to what they have to say.

I: Understanding that they need that?

R: Right.

R: I think that my presence is probably one of the most important things they need. They ask not to be left alone. And if they don't have family with them, then it's the nurse who must fill this role. So, being in the room. If I'm doing anything, that's O.K. If I'm not doing anything, if I'm just sitting there, I think that's meeting their need.

R: Attention. These patients are reaching out for life, they're reaching out for somebody to listen to them, to care for them. . . . many of them might like to talk about the world, what the news is. They want to be kept in touch with life. No one's experienced death to tell them about it of course, so they just want to hang on to what is, what they understand.

I: Do you think the dying patient needs you to be a link between him and the rest of the world?

R: Definitely.

R: I think the nurse has to understand that the patient is dying, and that the patient's moods are changing, they're changing fast, that they're lying there getting weaker each day. Just compassion and under-standing.

R: I think reassurance, just being their friend and letting them feel like somebody's there to help them through this time. I think that's what I can do best for them. I mean, of course, outside of medication to keep them comfortable.

I: When you talk about reassurance I'm not quite sure what you mean, because you can't reassure them that they're going to get well.

R: No.

I: Apparently you reassure them that there's going to be somebody there with them?

R: Right . . . patients that, you know, a lot of times they're afraid, and they don't like to be left alone for any length of time.

Most of the nurses assumed a basis of good physical care — this is primary. When that care is provided — and in the provision of that care — the need of the patient for reassurance is met. It is also clear from the above responses that nurses do understand that patients who are dying need not to be deserted — not to be left alone. (It is not ignorance of the need that sometimes keeps nurses from these patients.) Further, such patients must be approached with an attitude of compassion: "They need your love, you know," although this seems difficult to operationalize.

R: I think he needs love.

I: Tell me about that.

R: I think, any patient . . . you'll have me crying . . .

I: Are you distressed? Do you want to stop?

R: No, you're not distressing me. We've had five deaths in the family recently. I mean, this is why I've been like this. But I think any patient that's this ill, if their family isn't there or can't be with them, they need the reassurance that there is someone who cares. And I think this is where the nurse can do her best at that point.

R: Love. Understanding.

I: How do you manifest love and understanding to him? . . .

R: I think they can tell by your manner, I really do. Your manner and your mannerisms and the tone of your voice also.

R: Tender loving care.

I: How do you make your care tender and loving?

R: Let them know you care about them, let them know you're in-terested.

Several of the nurses made it clear that needs were as likely to be as idiosyncratic as behaviors, but the presence of an accepting somebody is always
necessary. Touch was perceived as important: "Going in there and holding his
hand," "Move them from one position to another—push a pillow here or a
pillow there so that they are comfortable." One nurse summarizes neatly: emotional support, freedom from pain, and cleanliness are required, and she sees
them as equally important.

> *R:* I think that he needs all three things. I think that he needs emotional
> support. I think religion has a lot to do with some patients, it helps
> them a lot. I think being kept pain-free. Being kept neat and clean
> and this is also good for the family and loved ones around them to see
> that they're taken care of. I don't think, can't think of anything more
> than that.

What Do You Do for Dying Patients?

The question "What do you do for dying patients?" was answered compre-
hensively; both instrumental and expressive activities were identified by almost
all subjects. When the responses were examined by level of education, registered
nurses were more likely than licensed practical nurses or nursing assistants to
report expressive tasks. This appears realistic, in view of the usual hierarchy of
nursing assignments in which the physical tasks that have obvious instrumental functions (baths, bed-making, toileting) are usually the responsibility of
lower-echelon personnel. Responses frequently provided some version of "What
the doctor orders" and tended to identify goals rather than activities.

Patient comfort is a major item of concern to all nurses, although there are
some obvious differences in perception of what leads to comfort. Reassurance
is a function of instrumental activity; the expressive component of care may be
provided when the patient understands he will be clean and comfortable, and
that someone will be there when he calls.

> *R:* For the dying patient? The main thing that needs to be done is to
> make this person as comfortable . . . if the person is bedridden, make
> him as comfortable as possible. I know sometimes it becomes a chore
> to turn these patients every hour from side to side to prevent decu-
> biti. You need to physically care for them, but not only that, you
> need to take time to sit at the bedside if you have to let something
> else go, just talk to them, give them mental encouragement, even
> though there may be nothing, you know . . . I think . . . some real
> personal attention, just talking to the patient can do a lot more than
> one realizes.

> *R:* I think comfort is the most important thing. To make sure that they
> are resting and if they have any wants or needs that I can provide,
> then I do so.

I: What kind of needs can you meet?

R: Physical needs, mostly . . . Just nursing care . . . comfort, if they need a back rub, or want something to eat . . . very basic needs is about all I can do. If they ask me to call somebody for them I can get someone who can call for them, their social worker . . .

I: You don't feel comfortable trying to meet emotional or psychological needs?

R: I think that the most important thing I can do is to be with them.

R: Well, I do what the doctor orders, and I do everything I can to build up the patient's morale and make him as comfortable as possible.

R: Well, it just goes back to the basics again, to keep them as clean and comfortable and quiet, hold their hand maybe if you have time, even if they don't seem to be aware of it. That's the way I would like it to be anyway, if I couldn't have my family with me — a lot of people don't have.

Most of the nurses were realistic — time would not be spent if time and staff were not available, and frequently they were not.

R: Not enough, I'm sure. If they want to talk, we talk to them. If, of course . . . we don't have a lot of time. I mean we don't have time to spend in hours in the rooms with them, which is bad that we don't have enough time for our patients. But we try to keep them comfortable. We try to keep their spirits up.

What is done with and for patients is individual — conditional on nursing assessment of patient needs.

R: I try to spend as much time as I feel the patient needs from me. I don't think you can take all terminal patients and lump them into a big lump and say, "You do this for the cancer patients." You can't do that because everybody's an individual and everybody has to be treated differently. But I think you feel the patient out, and if they need more of your time you've just got to find time to give it to them. They need a lot of consolation — they need a lot of reassurance . . .

R: I think it depends on the patient. Some patients want to talk, you know, and I feel like if they want to talk, then we should listen to them, that we should be near them. And when a patient is dying, we always try not to leave them alone, we try to stay with them . . . Some instances the patients' families are involved, and you have to give them, the families, support that they might need if their relative is dying. So each individual is different — it depends on what the patients' needs are, in general.

I: You say you sometimes have to give the family support. How do you
       do that?

R: You have patients that may be dying and if it is a long, drawn-out
       procedure, and the family wants to stay with them, you just don't
       go in, check the patient, and not say anything to them. You try
       to stop and see if maybe they want to talk. Maybe they've been
       sitting there for hours. You offer them a cup of coffee or see if they
       want a glass of water, and I think all of this is important to the
       patient.

I: You extend your interaction, your nursing interaction to the family?

R: That's right.

Some nurses were offended at the thought that dying affects nursing care,
and pointed out that care is the same regardless of whether the patient is
terminal.

R: I don't do any differently than I do for any other patient. I treat all
       the patients the same, or I try to, pretty much so. My patient care is
       no different for the terminal patient versus the nonterminal. It's
       exactly the same.

R: I try to treat this patient the same way I'm treating the patient in the
       next bed . . . not making a point of this one being more ill . . .

The importance of the presence of a supportive family is incorporated into
the nursing assessments.

R: . . . try and make them as comfortable as you can. Try and help the
       family, and I tell the family about—even though a patient is un-
       conscious, the hearing is the last sense normally to go, and that they
       shouldn't stand in the room and talk, I mean, and whisper. That they
       should talk to the patient and tell them who they are and that they're
       here to see them and that they care and . . . make the patient feel
       wanted up until the very end. I think working with the family really
       is probably one of the biggest . . . the family is the one is going
       to be there 24 hours when the patient's dying, and if they can give
       them good support. . . . And they're really the ones that the patient
       [wants] .

As can be seen from responses, personal values affect professional behavior
in the context of what one actually does for the dying patient.

I: What do you do for the dying patient?

R: I think a lot of it depends on your attitudes toward death. If you
       haven't resolved for yourself as an individual how you feel about

dying and death, you can give very external, very superficial . . . care to the patient. You can do all the externals, but you can't really relate to the person.

I: So you encourage them to live . . .

R: Rather than to just die. Maybe that's the wrong approach. If they know they're going to die, there should be a way to support them, but I don't have the finesse, I guess, to really do that . . . Well, I mean . . . if I know somebody's going—I'm just trying to think. It's hard for one to generalize, you know, I just have to . . .

I: I know; if it's easier to just give specific examples of your behavior, that's O.K.

R: But with this particular man, when he said he didn't feel like . . . I made it a point to go in and talk to him more, and the family, together, you know. And I commented on how she [his wife] was really devoted to spending a lot of time, you know, with him, and how much I'm sure it must have meant to him. And comment on different things, like this, or one other patient that we had got interested in a hobby at the last. He was making some leather purses of some sort, you know. I tried . . . why tell him there's no use in starting that, he probably can't finish it? I didn't say anything like that . . . I just encouraged him [to live a little every day].

What Is the Most Important Thing You Do for Dying Patients?

As suggested by responses cited earlier, the nurses were unanimous about the importance of reassuring the patient that he will not be left alone. Again, physical comfort and a sympathetic ear were stressed—all toward providing reassurance best expressed by a willingness to spend time at the patient's bedside.

In this sample of nurses there was much spontaneous expression of feeling against the use of heroic measures, although they are reluctant to give them up altogether.

R: Well, again I feel like it's—the most important thing is that the patient is comfortable and peaceful as possible. But I'm not sure this is always done at the moment. Depending on what their medical needs are, many times this takes priority, it seems like trying to meet whatever crisis is causing the death, you know, so many times that takes priority over seeing that the patient is comfortable and peaceful. . . . [But] I think we really can't [abandon crisis intervention] because we've had these other experiences. If you don't ever have an experience like that, then you could say definitely you know, if you know your patients are going to die, it would be better to let them alone. But you can't always say that.

Families are not forgotten; indeed, their needs may take precedence, particularly when patients are comatose. Families are also encouraged to support patients, and nurses perceive their most important task to be the facilitation of that support.

R: He [the husband] was all right as long as she was breathing, although he knew that this was the end, but still when it happened it was just really awful. So I stayed with him more because I felt like I could help him more, because I'd been there, . . . before, not just one who walked on the scene when it was all over.

R: You know, it's funny, because when you're the patient lying there, and the family comes in and they all whisper and everything, and you feel like "My gosh" . . . this is the way I would feel, and sometimes the patients express it to you. Like, "I'm lying here in this bed, and I'm really odd to them. And I don't know how to react, and they don't know how to react to me" — and you sort of play a game, like you want to avoid the word "cancer" completely in any sort of conversation, and everything is the weather . . . So I try to talk to the family and you know, keep the patient comfortable.

I: Do you think the patient would rather talk about something besides the weather? That he would like to talk about the fact he has cancer, and he's afraid of upsetting the family? I'm not sure I understand.

R: I think that the reason why a patient doesn't say anything about it is that he doesn't want to upset the family.

I: Do you think it would be supportive to him if he could say something about it?

R: When he needed to. I would give him the opportunity to talk, but I wouldn't try to drag things out of him, how they feel about it you know.

However, although nurses emphasize the value of family support, some believe it is important that patients continue to interact with the staff, even patients who are withdrawn and uncooperative. Nurses should encourage any patient to talk, and be there to listen. This is especially true for the dying patient, but the patient has a responsibility to help himself as much as he can.

R: In terms of importance I'd have to say talking. . . . Just having somebody to talk to.

I: You think that would take some of the pressure off?

R: Yeah, I really do.

I: Even if the patient is withdrawn and uncooperative, you think it takes pressure off for you to be there and . . .

R: Right, I do, because not only with the dying patient, but with the other patients too, they become attached to the [nurses], and look forward to seeing them.

R: Well, listening to them would be right at the top of the list I think . . . I will listen as long as they want to talk.

I: Do you listen to all your patients that way?

R: Many of them. Most of them.

I: Not just the dying patient?

R: Always the dying patient though.

R: Being a friend.

I: Can you explain that just a little?

R: Well, just being there, trying to give them the right amount of understanding when they need it, trying not to get so involved that you can't stand it, and also trying not to give them so much understanding that they just fold up completely, but trying to be honest and not giving them the impression that something is true that you don't know is. . . . Sometimes it seems necessary to talk to someone very frankly and tell them that they're interfering with their treatment, and try to sort of like give them some discipline.

I: You think discipline is something that can't go by the board just because the patient is dying?

R: No, I don't think it can.

R: Well, I think if I had to answer one word I think I'd say listen. I don't mean just hear. I mean really listen, to the patient, because I think that's what they want. I think they want someone to listen to them and not just brush 'em off.

R: Hmm . . . I think the most important thing would be to listen to whatever the person has to say, and in some form try to keep them happy but yet you still don't lie to them and say maybe you'll be all right tomorrow you know, when you know this person is dying. And I think you should listen to everything they have to say.

Do You Spend Time with Dying Patients? Doing What?

Although the patients responded that the nurses saw them frequently, the nurses were more likely to hedge. They spent as much time as they could, but the amount depended on how much time they had to spend. In spite of the belief that the most important thing they do for dying patients is be available, and listen — a most time-consuming activity — other duties with other patients would take precedence. They knew it was important, they tried to do it, but it was what could be done when the rest of the work was accomplished.

When the respondents who reported spending a lot of time with patients were questioned about how they spent that time, 45 percent of them cited carrying out instrumental tasks related to physical care. Some (20 percent) reported expressively oriented physical activity, and 29 percent mentioned verbal interaction. A realistic few (6 percent) indicated that what they did was directly related to the condition of the patient.

Those nurses who report they do not spend much time with dying patients — as well as a good number of the nurses who reported that they do — identify the work load as the reason they do not. They are willing to go in, they have no wish to avoid it, it would be good for the patient, but there isn't time.

On the whole, the nurses' perception that they spend as much time with terminal patients as they do with any other patient is not in agreement with the findings of other studies. As they, themselves, tended to bring up the caveat — if there is enough time — it is likely that their actual behavior was more in accordance with previous study findings than they realized. Informal and unstructured observations by the investigators suggest that nurses responded immediately to a patient's light, but were not likely to seek out such patients. However, the observations also suggest that both patient and nurse perceptions of nursing work load were accurate. The nurses were indeed extremely busy about many legitimate duties.

Do You Talk with Patients About the Fact That They Are Dying? What Do You Say? If Not, Why Not?

There was a great variety in all responses to the question "Do you talk with patients about the fact that they are dying?" — particularly when the further questions "If you do, what do you say?" and "If not, why not?" were added.

Those who replied with a straight-forward "No!" sometimes do not do so because it might distress the patient.

> R: I just feel that I would probably upset them more than I would help them, you know, because there isn't too much that you can say.

> R: No. I feel that that's just one of the most cold-hearted things anyone could do to go up to a patient and say, "You're dying," . . . I wouldn't do that. . . . in all the times I've worked here I've never heard anyone say that.

> R: No. Especially with younger people, no. . . .

> I: But what if he says to you, this 18-year-old person, "Oh, nurse, I'm so depressed. I've got a disease, and it's killing me, and I'm not going to live to be nineteen," then what do you say?

> R: I'd try to get out of that question as soon as possible.

> I: But see, there's a need here. The patient obviously needs to have

somebody with him, and if you're going to be with him, you're going to have to listen to him talk about the fact that he's dying. How do you respond?

R: That would depend, I think, on his disease . . .

I: He's got leukemia, and he knows it, and he's telling you.

R: But it would depend on him. Maybe he's . . . he really knows he's going to die, and he's really got that settled in his mind, you know. He's really accepted it. I don't know what I'd say.

I: Do you think it would be useful to patients to talk about the fact that they're dying?

R: . . . if they do believe they're going to die, they just might give up.

I: So you think it's probably better for the patient not to talk?

R: I think so, yes.

When they were pushed, nurses thought maybe they would submit to the conversation — be willing to try, if the patient needed to talk — but could not be sure this would be a good thing. Others perceived that they were simply not able to cope with such a conversation.

R: Not unless they bring it up. I'll listen to it for a while, but that's one area I haven't coped with yet. If they ask a blunt question, "Am I dying?" I shy away from that.

I: So you don't talk about it but more because of your own feelings than because you think it wouldn't be good for them?

R: That's right.

Some nurses adhered to behaviors reflecting a strong curative focus: (1) we never really *know* they're dying, there's always hope; (2) we've done all we can for them, now let's keep it light and cheerful; and (3) it's not my place to tell them anyhow.

R: . . . we don't know, and even the doctors don't know. Because we have a man that came here in '65, same year I did, and they gave him six months to live. He is still living, and he is much better, and working. So even the doctors don't know this . . .

R: No.

I: Why not?

R: Because there's always hope.

I: So you don't discuss with your patients the fact that they probably don't have too much longer?

R: No, no.

I: If a patient said to you, "Am I dying?", what would you tell him?

R: Our hopes for you are greater than what you have in your thoughts right now.

I: And if he wanted to go on and talk about it, how would you handle it?

R: Well, if he felt like he wanted to go ahead and talk about it . . . I would continue the conversation along those lines, and still give them hope.

I: O.K. You always hang on to that fact, that there's always hope?

R: Yes.

R: I'll say, "None of us know how long we have." You don't really kid with them, but you try to keep them a little lighter.

Patients are given cues not to ask by all the nurses — e.g., "Well, you've got a hundred years left!" The nursing assistants particularly were likely to refer the patient to the doctor for information, which seems only appropriate, since they have no authority to provide information. In any case, it is not a conversation most of them wish to sustain.

I: How do you get away then after you say this [refer them to the physician]? How do you leave the patient?

R: You mean, do I sneak out on the floor or do I walk out?

I: I mean, what's the next thing to be said?

R: Usually I just walk out after that. Haven't had any problems, they usually don't press it any farther.

I: You don't encourage them?

R: No, that's for sure.

One registered nurse, who admits her tendency "not to hear" the patient who talks about dying, discussed the difficulties of dealing with this within the time limits and the customary work assignments set. She identified a problem in communication between the nursing units; for instance, it is not a priority for the admitting nurse to inform the floor that a patient is talking about, or seems to wish to talk about, his death. There is no formal means of communicating this kind of thing in the way that exists for communicating information about medications or procedures.

Some who did not talk with patients would like to be able to do so — and would like some help in learning how. Others are comfortable with "orders" not to let patients know.

R: No.

I: Why not?

R: Because I don't feel as though I'm qualified or trained. . . . I feel as though I would be worried that I would maybe say something; instead of helping that patient I would hurt them.

I: So you feel you would like to have more information really, about how one can respond.

R: Yes . . . I feel as though I would be worried that I would . . . cause any more anxiety than the patient has already.

R: Oh no.

I: Why not?

R: Well, that's one of the orders not to.

I: Your orders?

R: I mean, we, we were just asked, you know, not to let them know that they were going to die.

Several methods of discouraging patients from initiating conversation about death can be identified. They can be put into a social role: "They get to be your friends"; there is not enough time "to talk with them about this; it does take time"; the subject is not addressed — "you talk around it" or the nurse just does not talk. However, even those nurses who generally did not discuss the subject with patients did, when harried by the interviewer, identify once more the importance of being available — primarily to *listen*.

Many of the nurses responded to the question in the affirmative, but usually it was a qualified yes. A tactful agreement, a change of activity, and inculcating enjoyment of the present were stressed.

I: You do say, "Let's enjoy what you have left." You would make that statement, or "You've got a little time left."

R: Yes, in a roundabout way I'd say something similar to that to them. I have in the past. Maybe not those exact terms, but . . .

I: Why do you object to the blunt statement? If a patient says, "Am I dying?" why do you then . . .

R: It's just not a good nursing ethic to do that, to say — to agree with them. Because . . . I think once a patient has decided that there's nothing left, and they don't care anymore, it becomes a very, very difficult situation . . .

I: For the nurse?

R: For the nurse, as well as the patient, psychologically. They've decided that this is it, they don't care, there's nothing else left for them in life. They are going to become such a horrible person not only to the nursing staff, but to themselves, it's not good for either one.

I: You think the patient should fight right up until the end. Is that what I hear you saying?

R: Yes, I really do.

R: If they want to talk about it.

I: What do you say to them?

R: Well, you, if they say they're dying and you might say, "Of course you are. We all die. But maybe it's not going to happen right now" or "Don't think that way." or . . . it depends on the patient . . . if they're the kind of person that is very frightened, well I wouldn't talk about it, you know.

I: Even if he brought it up?

R: . . . it takes a very strong person, I believe, to understand that he's dying and talk about it, and to want to talk about it.

I: Most of us would just as soon turn the other way and not think about it?

R: A lot of people aren't realistic, and they hang on as long as possible and hope that they won't. Of course if you know it's going to happen, there isn't much you can do but you can talk about it.

Nurses who reported talking about death reported various degress of comfort with the conversation. They were not comfortable at all, were somewhat comfortable (but finding it not easy), or are willing to listen to patients but are not able to sustain a long discussion.

I: So you just let them talk. Are you comfortable letting them talk?

R: Not too comfortable.

I: Why not?

R: Because I'm afraid they're going to ask me a question I'll feel I need to answer and I can't.

I: Are you comfortable with the conversation when it goes on like that?

R: Generally speaking. Less comfortable if the patient just wants a pat yes or no answer, if they just want reassurance that they're not dying.

R: No . . . but most of them whenever they realize they are dying, they just have to talk to somebody, they don't really care whether you talk back, they just want to unload, to get it off their chest. . . .

I: But you do listen. You don't say something cheerful and then walk away.

R: No.

Two of the licensed practical nurses with a definite religious orientation responded in a way that made the investigator uncomfortable, but which might be appropriate for the majority of their patients.

R: Only if they bring it up themselves and then I say very little, only I'll ask them if they're ready. Quite often I'll ask them if they're ready. Their opinion of "ready" might be different from my opinion of "ready." I never explain that word. I just ask them if they're ready. If they are, fine. And I tell them they have nothing to worry about, just to go to sleep.

I: And if they say they're not?

R: I ask them if they know what they can do to get ready.

I: You're not uncomfortable with this conversation?

R: No, I'm not. I have seen people die who . . . at the last minute ask for a minister. When it's almost too late they'll ask for a minister. But you have to wait until they ask before you send them that kind of help. Those grieve me. I worry about them because they're the ones that are scared.

I: You think people with religion are not scared?

R: Not as scared.

R: I ask them if they're prepared to go, and if they are interested, I try to help them, I'll tell the nurse to get the chaplain. If not, I won't bother. . . . I feel like that I've been some help, to the dying patient . . . because of my religion a lot of times, because of my faith, let's put it that way.

A few of the nurses gave an unqualified yes to the question. They perceived the discussion to be therapeutic to the patient, and are able to sustain it for that reason.

R: Yes, I do. They really need someone who will listen to 'em and if they want to talk about dying and they know they're dying and they want to talk to you about it, I think you should talk to 'em. And not say, "Oh, come on. We've all got to go sometime." If they want to talk about dying I think you should try to calmly talk to 'em about it.

I: Do you?

R: Yes, I do.

I: What kinds of things do you say?

R: Depends on what they say. Depends on what questions they ask. If they ask "Well, well now, you know, you've talked to the doctor, you know, how much longer have I got?" Well what can I say, other than I really don't know and that's the truth. How can I say? Because I don't determine. Your doctor doesn't determine. No man determines when you're going to die, not even you. So I honestly can say that I do not know.

I: And then do they usually go on to say something else?

R: Well . . . yes. I've had 'em ask me things like "Does everybody become unconscious?" . . . or "Do a lot of patients here have convulsions before they die?" or "Does everybody go into a coma first?" . . . or "What's the first sign that a patient is dying?" I've had them ask all kinds of things like this.

I: How do you answer them?

R: I try to answer them truthfully as far as possible . . . you go right back to being truthful. "I don't know. And that's the truth. I can't tell you." Because I can't. Maybe that patient's going to fool the doctor. Maybe the doctor says a couple of days. And a year later that patient may be . . . Well, maybe not a miraculous cure but that patient may be a lot better because I've seen that happen.

Be as honest as you can without destroying hope seems to be the unwritten rule among this group of nurses.

What Do You Like Most about Caring for Dying Patients?

The most frequent immediate response to "What do you like most about caring for dying patients?" was that there was nothing to like: "I don't care for it much at all, really."

R: What do I *like* most about it? I don't like it at all.

R: I hate death. I don't like to take care of people that die. I don't think anybody does. But it's all a part of your job, I think you just do the things that you think are important to them and the things that would be best for them, but then no one likes to take care of the dying person.

I: So you can't identify any one thing that you like most about it?

R: No, because I hate death.

R: Nothing, I really don't like it.

R: Well, I don't particularly like it, because it is depressing to me, but somebody has to take care of the patient when he is dying.

These respondents, however, all go on to point out that such care must be given, and must be good care. Nobody thought care of the dying would not be a nursing responsibility; they might not like it, but they were there to see that good physical care and emotional support were provided to all their patients.

When they were strongly encouraged to think of something they liked about it, the "feeling of being needed" was primary; however, "it doesn't have to be a terminal patient to get the same sort of satisfaction from helping another human being." If a patient one knows becomes terminal, and asks for services from a particular nurse, she would volunteer because the personal relationship is so much more important in terminal care. There was a tendency to describe what could be done for terminal patients, and this group of nurses did perceive them as different, although they would give the same physical care to the non-dying patient, and have the same professional attitudes about not facilitating dependence and about helping people to cope. It is interesting that although nobody cared to define nursing, almost everyone could recognize a good nurse.

A personal-growth component was also identified as what the nurse liked most about terminal care.

> R: It teaches me a lot about, oh, I'd say human nature. It just amazes me . . . these people who are dying . . . how they accept it. I haven't seen anyone here, or I can't remember anyone just screaming and saying, "I don't want to die, I don't want to die." They just seem to accept it. . . .
>
> I: . . . [Is it] fair to say that this is what you like most about the inter-action, is the fact that you do carry something away sometimes?
>
> R: Right. Because I can't say that . . . that would be about the only part of it that I liked. It's really hard for me.
>
> R: . . . when I see them facing it with courage and with hope and feeling that somehow life has been worth it all and whatever else that comes will be worth it too, I think this increases my own feelings of worth, my own feelings of hope.

One nurse said, "It makes me stop and think." Another perceived aging members of her own family in the patients. The feeling that one can help, that one is wanted and needed as a friend — particularly when the family and the community drop away — is also identified as a positive factor.*

> R: Mainly the cooperation of the patient and of the family. You feel like you're really wanted and doing something when you feel you're accepted by the patient and the family, too.
>
> I: A feeling of being wanted?
>
> R: Right.
>
> R: Oh . . . I really don't know. It just makes me feel good that I'm doing

---

*Only a very small minority maintained that terminal patients are no different from other patients.

something, you know. They're just not all alone, 'cause someday I'll be like that too.

I: Does it make you feel good you're doing something in a different way than doing something for a nonterminal patient makes you feel?

R: Yes, because a non-terminal patient can have . . . I mean, he can go out and take a trip and just really enjoy himself, but a terminal patient will be close to the hospital.

R: You get to know them as a person, you really do. If you care, if you really love nursing you get to know each of them as an individual, you get to know their needs. Things like they feel maybe they lack . . .

I: So getting to know the patient as an individual is what you like most about caring for a terminal patient?

R: Yes. Because every one's different . . . no two patients are alike. Their illness may be similar, but how they develop, how they progress as a person in the progress of their illness is an altogether different thing with every patient.

R: I think it's very rewarding work to be able to help someone in need. This is what nursing is all about . . . with . . . terminal patients, you really get to know them and really . . . do nursing care.

It became clear as the study progressed that nurses are just as likely to undergo reminiscence as are patients; the replies were concrete and anecdotal, and usually incorporated memories of one patient who had made an impression. These patients were likely to have been encountered early in the nursing career.

What Do You Like Least about Caring for Dying Patients?

There were a few nursing assistants who did not care to admit to a stranger that there was anything they did not like about caring for patients — including dying patients.

Some nurses identified the fact that "death occurs" as what they liked least. When this concept was examined with them, their helplessness — "nothing can be done," being reminded of their own deaths, and the feeling that the patient still may have things to do — emerged as components. Nurses expressed themselves poignantly, and at length. They could not always say why they felt as they did, and occasionally they would perceive the condition of the patient as affecting their feelings, but the general feeling was: "You know, it's a lot to lose when you lose your life." Clearly, it is a difficult task to observe such a loss.

R: The death. The death itself.

I: Why?

R: I guess I'm just soft-hearted, I don't know. It just . . . and I think I'm too easily inclined to get attached to a dying patient, especially, and I guess it's because at the time I work closer with a dying patient than a patient that's up and about. I guess that's the only reason. It's just . . .

I: So the death itself distresses you?

R: Right.

I: What if the patient is very old and in much pain?

R: Well then I can accept that, because I feel that they're better off, they're more comfortable and all, they're out of their pain and misery. I can accept it real well, but still it's just something that kinda touches you when one does die.

I: It really bothers you?

R: Yes it does.

I: Whether you knew the patient well or not?

R: Yes.

I: Have you talked to yourself about why?

R: Yes.

I: Can you share it?

R: Well my dad is a physician and he once, when I was small, took me hunting . . . my dad was telling me that I had covered them [the dead animals] up with a blanket and was sitting beside them, crying. And it's been that sort of thing ever since.

I: Do you still want to sit and cry?

R: No, not quite that bad any more. You know, it's a lot to lose when you lose your life, whether you're a dog or a cat or a human being. It's a very precious thing.

I: The only one we have?

R: That's right. When someone loses it, I feel bad about it, I really do.

R: The concept of death itself.

I: The concept of death itself. Can you expand on that a little?

R: You know that they're going to die. I think a lot of times when I see terminal patients, especially cancer patients, there's a lot of suffering that goes with it, sometimes death doesn't come easy. And I think it's just the hardship that goes along with the family, and the actual death itself, I guess.

I: I hear you saying two different things. You're distressed with the suffering, which is a different thing from distressed with the concept of death.

R: I guess I have contradicted myself there.

I: Well, feel free. But could you try to explain?

R: Well, I think it's hard to see a person die . . . It is for me. I don't think it's a pleasant thing, even though I think after a person's died he's maybe perhaps, better off than people who are suffering. I think just the time before the death would be better . . .

I: Would be better . . .?

R: Would be better than what I meant by death itself. I think the time immediate to death.

I: So that the dying rather than the death really distresses you?

R: That's right.
_____

R: When they're dying.

I: Can you explain that a little?

R: After you get attached to them you just don't want to see them die. It's just like one of your family. I just don't like to be around.

The characteristics of the required care are perceived by some as the least palatable part of terminal care. Such care is defined as frequently tiring and tedious; again, nurses are not comfortable with heroic medical measures when these procedures must be opposed to supportive care.

R: I think again the thing I least like are those times when . . . I know that a patient is apprehensive and when we are spending more time trying to do medical measures to try to prolong their life or . . . emergency type things that are necessary and the patient is alert and very anxious and there isn't time really to calm them and reassure them. And I think that's the hardest part.
_____

R: [It's] very difficult when you've got maybe two terminal patients on one end. You know, you've got a lot of work, because you've got all those patients plus those two, and so . . . it's just like you try [the nurses] . . . you get tired of that work on that end, they get tired of taking care of them, and they start . . . "That cranky Miss So-and-So," or something, and it's sort of a relief when a patient's discharged or sent to another hospital or something . . .

I: Or dies?

R: I don't think anyone would ever admit . . . or dies . . . but you know, I would have to be honest and say . . .
_____

R: Well, the fact that they're really sick and they need a lot of little things that aren't always too pleasant done with them, you know they have smelly discharges and things like that that aren't always too pleasant but I don't mind it really.

The concepts of defeat, of failure, are specifically identified.

> *I:*   Can you identify the thing you like least about caring for terminal patients?

> *R:*   I think possibly just the simple fact you've done all you can do, you can't do any more for them physically. It's maybe that the defeat has finally won over, though really it's not defeat at this point, but this is sort of a feeling you get after a period of time, a lack of real accomplishment . . .

Although supporting families — both for their own sakes and so they can continue to support patients — had been earlier identified as a nursing function, dealing with families was the least liked part of terminal care for many nurses.

> *R:*   Trying to watch after the family because there is a lot of emotion involved and you never know when something might happen to them because of this.

Having to tell the family the patient is dead was particularly difficult, and communication with family members is a problem.

How Do You Feel When a Patient You Have Taken Care of Dies?

In response to the question "How do you feel when a patient you have taken care of dies?" the nurses did not identify a professional norm; feelings seem to be of the same kind and intensity any person would have. Nurses may believe they should control or at least not manifest feelings, but they do not appear to believe they should not have them. "Crying" is seen as "not right" in terms of its effects on others, rather than as an essentially not-right thing in itself. Apparently it is all right to care, but you should not let the family or your colleagues, or, most importantly, the patient, become aware of it. Nurses warn against caring too much; some report that they do not, for instance, ever work in pediatric divisions because they cannot see children die without caring too much. They did not report feeling fear, and only one subject reported a feeling of awe. Loss — and sometimes relief — were identified. However, the death of a youthful patient generates anger in a youthful nurse: "You hate to see a young man go."

Feelings depended on the age and condition of the patient, and particularly on the presence of pain. Whether the patient was well known was a strong factor, and nurses were also quite concerned with the question of whether they had done everything they could. If they perceived the care had been good, they were more comfortable with the death.

R: Usually relieved, kind of, because quite a few times here it's pretty painful. So I'm usually kind of relieved that they've stopped having their misery.

I: And you're comfortable with that feeling of relief?

R: Yes.

R: Oh, that's difficult, depending on what your relationship was with the patient. If you had a very honest, open relationship with the patient, and perhaps you shared some feelings or shared some thoughts, I suppose you might feel saddened, but certainly, you know, conscious that things would go on as best they could. You would certainly be saddened by the death, but if you were able to accept your own feelings about it and the patient's, you would have fulfilled some immediate goals. It depends on the circumstances.

R: It sort of depends on the situation. Sometimes I don't think we did enough, and then it really bothers me, because I think we could have done something more to make it easier on them. I don't mean to save their life. I wish I had done this, or our plan of care should have been over a longer period of time. . . . And some of them I think we've done all that's humanly possible to help them.

R: Again, it would depend on the condition the patient was in before he died. If I felt that the patient had suffered tremendously I would be relieved to come to work and find that he'd expired. If it was a young person, that really didn't seem to be terrifically ill or incapacitated, I would be shocked to find that they had expired. I can't say any one feeling.

I: It depends on the individual patient?

R: Yes. I have one thing to add that might be useful. You asked the question, how do I react when a patient dies, did you not? I said that it would depend on the patient again but there is, there are some times when I personally am just relieved that I'm not going to have to take care of them anymore. Especially when the patient has been unconscious for a considerable amount of time and has had a zero prognosis for a long time, he's been a burden upon the staff. What I feel is he didn't have a flicker of life left in him, yet he was in pain and he was a burden to the people that took care of him and a burden to his family and to himself. And, sometimes I have a feeling of relief that is self-centered, it's not patient-centered.

I: Would you state that feeling to your colleagues here?

R: Yes.

I: Would you be comfortable [doing so]?

R: Yes, I would.

Loss and sorrow — "it hurts you" — are felt, and sometimes anger and frustration if the death is unexpected or preventable.

R: Lost.

I: Lost. Can you be a bit more specific, explain?

R: Like somebody has really died, that you'll never be seeing them again, they'll never be coming back, you'll never be sharing anything with them anymore. Just emptiness, you wonder what they're doing now, if they made it to heaven, if they haven't . . . they surely had to. It couldn't be hell. I mean, they have hell on earth.

R: Let's say mixed feelings, sometimes. Oh, sometimes, well it sounds very cruel, I'm almost glad because it's an end to the pain. In fact many times I am . . . if it's a . . . patient you felt something could have been done, then you become very frustrated and a little angry, at oh, at things in general . . . if it's unexpected, preventable, I'm angry. Not so much angry, I feel frustrated, like if something should have . . . something I could have done, or somebody could have done.

Only very few persons indicate that they are not affected by the death of those in their care. This seems to be related to the fact that death is an expected end, or that responsibility ceases with death, rather than with any lack of humane concern.

R: It doesn't bother me. I know they're out of their pains, miseries. When they die a natural death, I don't question it.

I: Do you have your patients around for quite awhile before they die here?

R: Some. And we get those in that die shortly after they're admitted.

I: The ones who stay longer, is it harder to see them go?

R: No ma'am.

I: The same either way?

R: Death doesn't bother me.

R: Just, they only come and go.

I: It doesn't distress you, then?

R: Oh no, no; of course I hate to hear or see anybody go but that's for somebody else to look in. I just take care of them when they're here, and if they're gone, well they're just gone.

Again, interaction with families is an important component to the nurses' feelings. Nurses may become distressed when families break down, because this triggers an unwelcome breaking down of the nurses' defenses. It is also interesting to see that subjects could and did move very quickly from how *they* feel to how families must feel. Many of the nurses who were willing to discuss patient behavior and nursing intervention were obviously not so comfortable in the discussion of personal feelings.

> R: I think it's a loss . . . if it's someone we have known for a long time and really struggled with through a complete process, I think probably I identify more readily with the family than a lot of persons do because I'm a pretty sentimental person. And, I don't know, I had a teacher tell me when I was a first-year student that the nurse that can't shed a tear with the family is not worth her weight in salt to begin with.
>
> I: You were fortunate in your teacher.
>
> R: And I don't think the family resent this. I think the family needs to feel and wants to feel that their family meant something to you as a person.
>
> R: If the family isn't here I'll put it this way, if the family isn't here, nobody's around, it doesn't bother me a bit when somebody dies. But if the family's here and they go to pieces and everything, then that bothers me.
>
> I: So it's the family rather than the patient that's likely to be a source of concern? What do you mean by really bothers me?
>
> R: Well, it kind of, I guess it kind of hurts me, 'cause I know that they're really tore up, you know, I don't know whether they're . . . they're hurt 'cause they lost a loved one, but the way I look at it the one that died isn't hurting anymore, he's not suffering anymore. But I know from going through it with my own family that you don't see it that way whenever some of your family dies.

Nurses were realistic in their perception that "you can't die with them," and developed strategies for noninvolvement, so that they could continue to function. There were some fairly explicit descriptions of protective devices, which included anticipatory grieving, intellectualization, and anger (not included in the excerpts from interviews included below), and a simple resolve not to become involved.

> R: Generally, I think that before they die, I start accepting the fact that they are, and after they have passed away, then I feel like I'm usually ready for it. I don't think there's anybody up here who has

totally surprised me, caught me totally off guard, unprepared, myself, to handle it. . . .

I: Do you think a sudden death would be more traumatic for you, so that you would perhaps react in a different way?

R: Um-hum.

I: If you weren't prepared, if you hadn't gone through this preparation?

R: Right. Working in a unit where accidents come in, I don't think I could handle it.

R: You can't get attached to the patients. So you can't have any real sorrowful feelings, I don't know just how you would say it. You feel sorry for the patient that has died but it can't interfere with the rest of your work and your other patients.

I: O.K. You have other responsibilities.

R: Right.

I: I hear what you're saying, but let me ask you why you think you can't become attached to your patients.

R: Because if you become attached to every patient, it's going to pain so to where you can't take it when they die. So working in a hospital like this, you just got to get a set attitude that you can't let it bother you.

R: I've already learned this lesson before I got here. I got terribly attached to a couple of women who were in the hospital about a year with cancer, and they were such good patients, such wonderful people, that I became involved and I learned then not to do it anymore.

I: Why?

R: Well, it's just not healthy for either one of us. Especially when they die. [Subject is crying.]

I: It hurts a lot when they die.

R: Yes, I was, even the last few days of taking care of them when you can see them slipping away, one patient especially, I was trying to take care of her one morning and I began to cry and the supervisor took me out of the room and would never let me back in there again. And then the other patient that I became fond of, expired while I was myself a patient in the hospital and I was bedfast and couldn't go and see her but they came and told me when she was gone. And I learned from those two experiences not to let my wall get broken down.

Would It Be Useful to Have a Structured
Discussion of Your Feelings?

There is no doubt that working with dying patients can be a threatening and even destructive experience, and some system of support for caregivers is necessary. There is some evidence to suggest that those who are most comfortable in this work operate within the network of a religious community, supported by the common beliefs and functions of their group.

Historically, the best care has been provided within a religious framework, and it may be that the ability to remain in equilibrium in the presence of death is related to shared beliefs in a deity. When the bodies are broken and wasted, and minds no longer respond, what gives meaning to the routines of care? There is no shared past to remember or to give meaning to the present, as there perhaps was when care was provided by families. The excitement of saving life is lacking, and there is no thought of repairing the broken body, retrieving the lost mind, and returning the person to full productivity. The belief that there is still something inviolate and of worth in the dying organism certainly gives some significance to the frequently unpleasant tasks.

In spite of the language used in discussions of patients' rights, dying is seldom dignified. The physical necessities of feeding and elimination, the presence of mucous and ulcers, the tendency of the weak to dislike having to depend on those who are stronger, the necessity to be grateful, and always, for both actors, the fear of the unknown, all preclude an easy dignity. In a relationship in which the tasks of one adult include the removal of feces from the person of another adult, there is bound to be some resentment on both sides. For both to retain dignity, they must retain some feeling of self-worth.

Nurses, as well as patients, are only human — with all the strengths and weaknesses implied by that statement. In order for them to stay in situations in which they may be frightened, tired, and disgusted, they must have some network of support. Religious communities devoted to the care of the sick and dying are not so common as they used to be, and in any case there are those who are not religious but who wish to do such work. Because a sense of community appears to be an important factor, it may be necessary further to develop the feeling of membership in the professional community. Nurses may need to affirm the ugly feelings of fear, resentment, guilt, and relief that are usually not reported, and continue to receive from colleagues a strong and consistent affirmation of the meaning of life and of their own worth. The process of dying does not automatically confer strength, courage, or a good disposition on either patients or nurses. Still, dying patients must be supported and cared for by nurses who must, in their turn, receive support and care. Is that support sought from or given by nursing colleagues? Do we trust colleagues who are also supervisors?

When nurses in this study were asked about their feelings, they tended to reminisce about patients, to discuss problems of care, to discuss the death scene, and had to be coaxed into discussion of their own feelings. When they were asked "Would it be useful to you to have a structured discussion of your feelings?" some nurses reported that it was (or would be) useful.

R: Yes, we talk about our feelings, as well as the patient.

I: That's useful to you?

R: Yes. I think it is because, I mean, you feel like, "Well, gee, I'm not the only one who feels like this." You know, "There's other people." Or you think, "Well, I don't know. It sounds like she must be getting a little too involved emotionally, so I'm going to watch it, I don't want this to happen to me."

R: I think it would because other nurses would . . . help you over your feelings or help you to understand that, "Well, he is a burden but he is a patient, you know, he is a human being." We have to understand this and we have to take care of that person!

The discussion may be quite informal, and may not include too much about personal feelings. Review of the death of a patient in small groups of trusted colleagues might be helpful, but not everyone can be trusted with feelings. Many nurses reported discussing their feelings with their families, rather than with colleagues.

R: I don't think it would really help me to take any better care.

I: But would it help you to deal with your own feelings better?

R: Possibly. No, actually when you talk to other people on the ward that you're working with, about, well when they're on duty with you when the patient dies or it's into the next day that some comment is made, then everyone will offer some comment.

I: So you do have this to some extent?

R: Yes. Yes . . . We do get it said I think.

R: We, well, I don't know, we don't usually much discuss missing the patient, although we do sometimes, but we do talk about the patients.

I: You reminisce about the patient, but you don't discuss your feelings, particularly.

R: Well, at the moment maybe, if the patient's been particularly close and everyone's upset and maybe people are crying, or something like that, you may somewhat reassure each other, but otherwise, if a patient died during the night and you come on during the day, then I think we usually release our feelings maybe by talking about the events that happened, and how the patient went, and how the family took it. But . . .

I: What happened rather than how you feel?

R: Yes, I think probably more or less.

I: Do you think it would be useful to you to talk in this "how I feel" way with your colleagues? You know, in some kind of structured situation?

R: It might be somewhat, but I think there's an understanding maybe that we all feel the same way . . .

I: Do you all feel the same way?

R: Well, yes, I think maybe we do . . . with certain patients I think we do, sometimes we have meetings; a doctor will talk with us sometimes if a patient we've been very close to is . . . looking very bad, and he feels they won't be here [more than] a week or a few weeks, he'll talk to us to kind of prepare us, and then I think we talk about it beforehand, during report that we know that the patient is getting near the end, and I think in this way we prepare each other, probably.

I: Are you ever relieved when a patient dies?

R: Yes, I think probably we are.

I: Are you guilty about that relief? Or do you see that as a respectable way to feel?

R: Well, I think sometimes that relief is just as far as work goes. We are relieved because the big burden of the extra care and the tension that you always feel when you know that — it's an emotional strain to take care of a patient under these circumstances. And I always think there's some relief that things are going to be back to normal. But again, it's a mixed feeling. It's a relief, and I don't think I personally feel any guilt for that, and there also is a sense of loss.

R: I don't think so.

I: Would you be comfortable in that kind of a situation, if others felt that need? . . .

R: I think I'd be uncomfortable at first, because I don't know too many of these people well. I think if I . . . well, with a couple of the people I know, I'd feel comfortable talking about death . . .

I: Your feelings toward death . . . ?

R: Yes.

I: But you would need to know the people?

R: Yes.

R: I think it would be very helpful, but I think it's a long time in coming. I think most people find this kind of situation very uncomfortable to work in. It's very difficult to get your personnel together and to talk out, because people are shy and they don't want to talk about it. They're afraid of what you'll think of what they say. I'm talking about staff personnel . . . and I think a lot of us in that situation, we're reluctant to admit things to each other.

R: Oh, I don't know whether it would or not. I usually go home and talk to my husband or I think you can talk it out with them at home, at lunch, or something like that and talk about it.

[The following was recorded after a discussion about informal nursing-station remarks that may sound flippant or disrespectful.]

I: You think it's just a way of coping with the situation?

R: That's what I think. And then, of course, different people say different things according to what their personality is.

I: Do you think it would be useful to you if you could discuss all these things with your colleagues?

R: Probably. I think it's useful to talk about anything.

I: Are you comfortable with this discussion about death?

R: Pretty much. Yes . . . I think more people ought to think and talk about death more than they do, because most of us have a tendency to, when the thought crosses our mind about our death or someone that we care for, we have a tendency to shut it off and not think about it. And I think it would be good because if we thought of it more we would be more prepared to accept it and handle it. We might be more prepared psychologically, and also for whatever there might be to prepare for spiritually. We might be more prepared. This should, at least, give us more understanding and more acceptance . . . to face death.

Some of the nurses who did not talk about their feelings believed it would be helpful to do so. Others felt that such discussion would be useless, or even threatening.

I: Do you ever share these feelings with colleagues?

R: Rarely.

I: Do they share theirs with you? Do you talk much about death and dying?

R: No.

I: Think it would help much if you did?

R: I guess it hasn't been till recently that many people did talk about it, you know or even start, so I think that maybe everybody has a tendency to shy away from it.

I: Everybody sure does. So you kind of shy away from it, do you think?

R: Yes, I think so . . . I think everybody does.

I: But you would not object to talking about it, if it became part of your professional duty to discuss it?

R: No. I think it would be very good, but as I say nobody [talks much about it].

I: You wouldn't look forward to it, would you?

R: Probably not.

R: No, I really don't, I mean it's just something that's just you. It's just really hard to explain your feelings whenever somebody dies — it varies with different patients.

R: No [I don't discuss feelings].

I: Do you think that would be useful to you?

R: I don't think so. Because they [other nurses] might not feel the same way about them as I do.

I: How do you feel about death?

R: I think it's as natural as being born, that's what I think, and when the time comes I think we should be allowed to do it.

I: Would it be useful to you do you think to have a more structured way of expressing your feelings when somebody dies, a conference?

R: It may, and then again it may not, because as I said, this is something that in our profession that you expect any time; even though people are up walking around, it doesn't necessarily mean that they will be here tomorrow.

I: So you think it's something that takes some getting used to?

R: You never get used to it, I don't think.

I: But you don't think it would help you that much to have some kind of conference when people die, about how you feel? You think it is just something that is part of — what? of your responsibility?

R: It is just something that talking with Mr., Mrs., or Miss is not going to alter the situation.

I: So it wouldn't do that much for you?

R: It wouldn't do anything.

However, it should be noted that even those persons who did not wish to admit their emotions, or who felt "they already know how I feel" had a story to tell the interviewer about some patient who had died, and about their feelings at that event.

SUPPORT FOR CAREGIVERS

Strauss and Glaser (1970) have said that the person who is able to confront his dying comes to terms with death in two separate processes. The first consists of facing the annihilation of self. The second involves facing dying as a physical, and perhaps mental, suffering and deterioration. Most frequently patients come to terms with dying and death by themselves or with the help of a few close loved ones. However, nurses may also be drawn into the process when the patient initiates talk about death, and they will usually try to listen, assent, and be supportive and compassionate. Sometimes they cry with patients and families. Some nurses, unable to act in this role, will abruptly leave the patient's room, ignore his statement and change the subject, or express a cliché about how well he is doing. Unless a patient shows composure about his dying, staff often lose *their* composure; even with composed patients, they may be unable to contain their fear and grief.

When the patient's conversation is only obliquely about death — for example, when it consists of reminiscences about the past — and is not unpleasant or repetitious, he has a better chance of inducing staff to participate in the closing of his life. Aside from the fear and grief inseparable from the care of the dying, a further barrier to adequate staff support of the patient or family is the staff's conception of time, and preoccupation with a work schedule. Additionally, often the number of professional staff on the unit is inadequate to care even minimally for the numbers of patients on a ward, especially when many patients are ill. Thus, in addition to the stresses imposed by their own fears, and their concern for patients, staff must deal with the guilt they feel because they have not spent more time and effort with dying patients.

Institutional rewards are mainly given for curative care; the few rewards reserved for persons working with dying patients are likely to be given to those nurses who are stoics, who hide their feelings. However, each dying patient is a reminder to the nurse of her own potential illness and death, draining her energy. She cannot support the patient and the family unless she is herself supported on the job — by colleagues, supervisors, or chaplain or psychologist consultants; as she works with the patient and the family and grieves with them over the death of the patient, eventually she can give no longer if she is not emotionally given *to*. She burns out. Regardless of her original psychological resources, her energy must be replenished if she is to continue giving. The refilling, the gratification, the rewards come partly from material goods (salary, fringe benefits, working environment) but more from the kindness, patience, approval, support, respect, affection, validation of ideas, encouragement and even challenge presented by medical and nursing colleagues and supervisors. To be openly empathic and communicative leaves nurses and physicians very vulnerable to loss, sadness, grief, and a sense of futility and failure.

Sonstegard et al. (1976) report three methods, in combination, to be helpful in providing adequate support to nurses working with dying patients: (1) the nursing hierarchy is available to the nurse on a 24-hour basis to explore feelings; (2) regularly scheduled group meetings exist for staff peers, in which everybody shares concerns, joys, and plans for their patients and their own concerns, problems, and needs; and (3) each nurse is assigned a specific time for a meeting with the unit head nurse to discuss her feelings (the head nurse in turn must have time to discuss her needs with another health-team member). Sonstegard et al. maintain that if intensive, repeated involvement is expected from the professional nurse, licensed practical nurse, or nursing assistant working with dying patients, then the nursing staff must be guaranteed that they will not be alone in that function. Nursing personnel are living, needing persons, not just automatons who go through the rituals of care of the dying without themselves being affected. They must take the initiative to meet their own needs in and out of work, and reach out to one another.

It is impossible to avoid involvement with patients as nurses perform care procedures; feelings of involvement should not be borne alone, but rather shared with the group because, indirectly, each one is involved.

Nurses who care for dying patients in one Southern hospital may voluntarily attend group sessions that are held weekly. The purpose of these sessions is to help nurses express the feelings engendered by their work with the dying and to analyze personal feelings and behavior, especially avoidance of the dying patient, feelings of repulsion at his appearance, or anger at his dying as a representation of staff's failure.

The group helps the nurses to set small goals with the patients and to see how they are helping patients in small ways, to recognize that sitting with a patient is as important as physical care, to realize that not every patient expects cheery news each day (Living With the Dying, 1974).

One of the major differences in care of the dying and care of those who will recover is the necessity for nurses to deal with patients' feelings regarding dying and death. Nurses who are able to help patients verbalize such feelings may help patients, but are themselves victims of anxiety and stress (Vachon et al. 1978). Vachon has set forth some realistic guidelines for maintaining coping mechanisms in staff working in palliative care units.

1. *Individual staff members should be encouraged to gain personal insight so as to understand and acknowledge their own limits. It should be acknowledged that one's limits vary over time and extra support or time off may have to be provided when staff members are under a high degree of stress. However, the needs of patients do deserve priority and if certain staff members constantly require considerable support they might be encouraged to seek employment elsewhere.*

2. *A healthy balance must be maintained between work and an outside life. While this type of work demands considerable personal involvement and cannot realistically be a 40-hour a week job, there must be times when staff are totally off-call and left to pursue their own life-affirming activities.*

3. *The individual must be careful when his or her "need to be needed" becomes too great and he or she attempts to be everything to everyone. This work is probably best accomplished by a team. Although*

> *many in the field are strong individualists, a team approach to much of the work is crucial.*
> 4. *The individual must maintain a support system at work and outside the work setting. Hospice units must make some provision for ongoing staff support through the use of visitation, psychiatric consultants for the staff, weekly staff support meetings or other models which seem appropriate to a given unit. In addition individuals should be encouraged to seek relationships outside the work setting for additional support. All too often staff members working in hospice settings become a closed social network, isolating themselves from friendships with others outside the field.*
> 5. *For those working in isolation it may be wise to seriously consider on-going contact with an outside consultant and/or therapist who can offer guidance as needed and provide much needed support as well. (Vachon 1978)*

Observers are in agreement (for example, see Elder 1976; Vachon et al. 1976; Vachon 1978; Reland 1077) that nurses—and physicians—need to be themselves supported if they are to be able to care for and give emotional support to dying patients and their families. What is less clear is how such support is to be provided. The proposed activities (group interactions, outside consultants, education of staff to the need to work through their feelings, etc.) require two components presently in short supply: *trust* among colleagues (both within discipline, in other disciplines, and in supervisors) and *time* to interact, to be educated. Staff time is expensive, and institutions may not be as willing to absorb the cost of the support system as they are to absorb the cost of the more tangible equipment required by curative procedures.

The nurses in our study expressed a need for some support; however, many of them indicated they would be more comfortable obtaining it from significant others away from the work setting (and frequently did so). There is some question whether the members of such a hierarchial structure as the presently constituted "health team" can be comfortable exposing their vulnerabilities to each other. However, a series of independent formal support systems (e.g., for physicians, for nursing supervisor, for team leaders, for staff nurses, for licensed practical nurses, and for nursing assistants) is ludicrous—although this arrangement may exist on an informal level with physicians sharing their concerns with other physicians and nurses doing so with other nurses.

There is some evidence (Kotulan 1977, reporting on the National Institute for Occupational Safety and Health) that stress is inversely related to power; persons without power to make changes experience more stress. Those persons with the least power to make changes in the health-care system are those who are most exposed to the pain and suffering of the dying patient. It is not surprising that our study's nurses identify a nursing norm to keep cool, to bounce back, and to be careful of involvement, nor that nurses are reported to encourage denial in patients.

Certainly it is not difficult to point out the problems in both education and practice. Professionals are taught how to become expert in the management of technological instruments and tools, and do not emphasize sensitivity and commitment to internal resources and strength (Kübler-Ross 1975). The literature, exemplified by Kübler-Ross's report, indicates that caregivers are not taught or encouraged to recognize that caring behavior is as much a part of the helping process as working with drugs, instruments, and tools. Kübler-Ross (1975) suggests the need to abandon in the health sciences the focus on diseased organs and efficient technology, and instead to emphasize the person, his special needs, his humanness. However, it is only fair to point out that his person, his special needs, and even his humanness are inextricably part of his disease, and the impersonal and efficient tools of the technology frequently cure the diseased organ. In an effort to develop skills in the therapeutic use of self, caregivers must not lose sight of the therapeutic use of those fine and delicate tools that do so much for patients. What is required for quality care is a focus on the patient, rather than on the equipment or the requirements of the institution. The therapeutic use of the self is not necessarily in conflict with the therapeutic use of the technology; care addressed to the diseased organ can be combined with care addressed to the person.

Nursing curricula include the means of providing comfort, understanding, and emotional support, as well as physical care. However, reactions to dying and death are influenced by the culture and by past experience with the dying. Unless nurses can analyze and resolve their feelings, the functions which were taught cannot be practiced effectively. This analysis and resolution is not an easy task, and it cannot be accomplished without support from supervisors and peers. If the provision of comfort, understanding, and emotional support to patients is as important a part of nursing as carrying out medical orders, equal time must be allocated to the effort. This means time for caregivers to deal with feelings associated with dying and death, as well as time for expressive interactions with patients. Few of the personnel who are in immediate and enduring contact with dying patients and their families now exercise the power to demand the time to nurse (as they define nursing) or to have their own needs met in order that they can continue to meet patients' needs.

References

Anon.: Living with the dying. Newsweek 84:89, 1974

Beland IL: The burnout syndrome in nurses, part I. News and Views 31 (4):3, 1977

Elder R: Dying and society. In Caughill R (ed), The Dying Patient: A Supportive Approach. Boston, Little, Brown, 1976

Kneisl C: Thoughtful care of the dying. Am J Nurs 68 (3):550, 1968

Kotulan R: These jobs can drive you crazy. Detroit Free Press, 18 September 1977, pp. 1A, 2A

Kübler-Ross E: Death: The Final Stages of Growth. Englewood Cliffs, N.J., Prentice-Hall, 1975

Sonstegard L, Hansen N, Zillman L, Johnston M: The grieving nurse. Am J Nurs 76 (9):1490, 1976

Strauss A, Glaser B: Patterns of dying. In Brim O, Freeman H, Levine S, Scotch N (eds), The Dying Patient. New York, Russell Sage Foundation, 1970, pp. 129-155

Vachon MLS: Motivation and the stress experienced by staff working with the terminally ill. Death Education (Winter 1978)

Vachon MLS, Lyall WAL, Freeman SJJ: Measurement and management of stress in health professionals working with advanced cancer patients. Death Education (Spring 1978)

Vachon MLS, Lyall WAL, Rogers J: The nurse in thanatology: What she can learn from the women's liberation movement. In Earle AM, Argondizzo NT, Kutscher AH (eds), The Nurse as Caregiver for the Terminal Patient and his Family. New York, Columbia University Press, 1976

Chapter 7

Strategies of Care

The difficulties of caring for the dying are related to the lack of cultural norms for guiding the relationships between patients, families, and staff. Assumptions about what must, should, or could be done are ambiguous since care has been shifted from the home to the hospital. Communication between caregivers and patients is difficult; death, like sex, politics, religion, and finances, is seen as a private topic into which caregivers are unwilling to intrude. Also, caregivers are likely to be unfamiliar with death; many have not personally known a dying person prior to their education.

Care of the dying is likely to involve the intimate bodily care of one person by another person, and there is an obvious correlation between prestige and the provision of such care. The more intimate and long-lasting the usual interaction with the patient, the less likelihood that the provider of care will be in a position of prestige and power. If there are strategies of nursing care which are specific to dying patients, licensed practical nurses and nursing assistants are the people who will probably be implementing the strategies. It is unrealistic to think of nursing care as being provided only by registered nurses. Indeed, even within that single category three levels of basic education exist, so that patients are not the only ones confused by the question of who is able to carry out which nursing functions. Nursing as it is defined by educators and curriculum experts is somewhat tenuous and amorphous; there are few legal constraints prohibiting almost anyone from carrying out the *independent* functions of nurses. Patients frequently report they do not know who is a nurse and who is not. If the status of the nurse is not made obvious by what she does, then those activities are not solely in the domain of nursing. However, when the dying patient is moved away from the ICU, and begins to wait, it is nursing personnel who help to beguile that wait.

Two questions arise here: whether there are salient factors differentiating the care of the dying from the care of those who will recover, and whether there are salient factors differentiating the care given by nursing personnel who are differentiated by levels of education. The second question is not addressed in this book. Nurses are identified as their patients are likely to identify them: those persons employed by institutions to give nursing care. No effort will be made to assign the few strategies recommended here to any level of nursing.

How does nursing care of the dying patient differ from care of those who will recover? The dying will generally require a great deal of physical care, but physical care is basic to all nursing, regardless of the diagnosis or prognosis. The nursing goal always includes help with those bodily activities the patient would carry out alone if he were able, without demeaning him in any way, and without nurturing unnecessary dependence. This is the care which is now given mainly by persons who are not registered nurses, and is perceived by patients as what nurses do. Physical care correctly given is reassuring and supportive, but this is true for all patients, and not just for dying patients.

The difference might lie in the extent of the responsibility to do as little harm as possible. No patient should become a victim merely because he is a patient, but the dying are perhaps more vulnerable, and more in need of reassurance which is impossible to give. Most probably, however, the salient factors are not to be found in either the needs of the patients or in the tasks and responsibilities of the staff, but rather in their attitudes and behaviors. Therapeutic modalities are affected by the nurses' ability to tolerate uncertainty — they know that patients will not get well, but they do not know when and how they will die — and by their ability to tolerate their own helplessness and lack of control. Nurses are also affected by a sense of confidence in professional skills, as well as by conceptions of self. Toleration and self-confidence will necessarily affect the amount of time nurses are willing to spend with patients, their willingness to allow the patient to talk about his or her death, and their willingness to ignore the organizational constraints on the provision of information.

We are not dealing in this section with the meaning of death, whatever that may be to any individual; we are dealing pragmatically and empirically with the fact that someone must care for the dying. There is some agreement in the literature that dying persons need certain things from the people around them: the regular presence of some significant other, honesty, and room to talk, to grieve, to die. Empirically, the people around them are nurses. Dying patients also need care other than that which is oriented to their dying. They must be bathed, turned, fed, and medicated — in a word, nursed. However, nursing the dying apparently does differ from nursing the living, although the tasks may be the same. Certain patient needs can be identified, and some of these are considered here.

PSYCHOLOGICAL CARE

If the patient *denies* his condition, the denial should be accepted as necessary for him. As he begins to feel secure with staff he may be encouraged to face reality; staff should not probe or force him to talk about his condition.

If he is *angry*, it will help him if staff will listen to him talk about when he became ill, who was involved, and the details about the present situation. Blame for his feelings, defense of the medical team or treatment, return arguments, or statements about how well off he is should be avoided. Staff should remain open and calm, and if necessary, repeatedly listen to the same story (Cassini 1974).

If he is *bargaining*, he should be encouraged to talk about the good deeds he will do if he is allowed to live. Staff should not contradict his plans, but rather promote a sense of hope: they may help him to achieve his desired goals if that is possible, and help him modify them if necessary.

The *depressed* person may be helped by staying with him in spite of his tears, listening to his sorrow, sitting with him in silence, and avoiding cheery conversation (Cassini 1974). The depression accompanying terminal illness can be reduced by helping the patient realize that family members and professional staff feel more useful and at ease when they can help to take care of him. People measure their worth by their ability to help others, especially in a loving relationship. To be the constant recipient of care, attention, and kindness, as happens to the patient, is intolerable for some people. But if the helping efforts of family, friends, and staff can be interpreted as an expression of love to the patient (as it permits the patient to be helpful to them), then he may feel less useless and dependent. Staff and family may review with him the many times he has been helpful to others, and point out he now deserves to be helped. To be lovingly cared for can be comforting. To be taken care of routinely, as an obligation, can be demeaning (Koenig 1973).

The dying patient who is in *suspicious awareness, mutual pretense,* or *open awareness* presents a special challenge. Often he appears very cooperative, cheerful, friendly, and well-adjusted. Although it might be expected if the patient, the family, and the nurse are all aware of the terminal illness that open communication would be easy, this is not necessarily true. The aware patient may be so gentle, well-educated, or soft-spoken that he remains very much in control of the conversation, and no one cares to mention anything that might distress him. He may, because of personality characteristics, be liked very well, but staff may be unable to bring themselves to spend much time with him. When they do come, they may talk at a superficial level to avoid showing feelings of sadness. They may engage in physical care primarily to make up for lack of communication, and rationalize that the family, which appears to be devoted to the patient, is adequately meeting the patient's emotional needs. Staff should recognize such feelings and behavior, and consider the amount of energy it may be costing the patient to retain constant composure, to be a "good patient," in order to protect himself from avoidance by the nurses (Kübler-Ross 1969).

The patient may have *worked through his grief* and have no need to talk. His primary concerns may be his comfort, easing pain, and the little pleasures the day may bring. He may be involved in making final arrangements in business, in setting old wrongs right, and in making his farewells. It may be that such behavior merely represents a deeper level of denial, as how far acceptance can go is relative. Some cover for deep denial may be desirable, given the difficulty in accepting one's own nonbeing. If some degree of repose is achieved, it is unlikely that the patient will say much about dying, or if he does, it will be to one or two people with whom he feels closest or most comfortable (Reeves 1974).

PHYSICAL CARE

During a cursory survey of texts devoted to nursing measures for patients with medical or surgical disorders it was noted that many of these books do not index "dying" — rather, they index medical diseases or subtitle dying under the heading of "death," as though dying patients were no longer considered to be living. Few pages (perhaps five to ten in an entire text) are concerned with nursing measures for dying patients (Harmer and Henderson 1958; Kozier 1972; Matheny et al. 1972; Brunner et al. 1970; Fuerst and Weitzel 1974).

The more recent references are likely to discuss psychosocial needs and psychological reactions of patients, with some attention also given to staff attitudes. However, nursing measures are fully described under the headings of the medical or surgical conditions — for instance, cancer of the breast, colostomy, laryngectomy, etc. There is no effort here to present a comprehensive section of nursing interventions in the care of physical needs of the dying patient. The many excellent texts (see previous paragraph and see also, for example, Beland and Passos 1975; Brunner et al. 1970; Murray and Zentner 1979; Matheny et al. 1972; Carini and Owens 1974) and journal articles written on the care of patients with medical or surgical pathology provide adequate information concerning nursing treatment of physical problems. Some few care measures that are *especially* relevant to the physical care of the dying patient are mentioned here; the reader is referred to the above-mentioned texts for comprehensive descriptions of physical nursing activities related to medical conditions.

Four developmental tasks have been described for the dying: to manage reactions to symptoms of the terminal state and pathophysiology; to prepare for impending separation from loved ones; to react to the prospect of going into an unknown state; and to adjust perceptions of how life actually was lived in relation to a desired life (Birrin 1964). Most dying persons know that death is near and will say so to those able to listen. Often discomfort and suffering are great earlier in the illness and in the early stages of dying, but dying is often relatively easy right at the last — regardless of how great the earlier suffering. A brief interval of peace may come before death, and apparently most people do not suffer pain or agony at the end, as many persons who have remained conscious to the end testify to the persons sitting with them (Worcester 1961).

Physical changes during the last hours before death include mottled skin and cyanotic lips and nailbeds (resulting from hypoxia); a thready, weak, or absent pulse; hypotension; and either a subnormal or elevated temperature. Shortness of breath and Cheyne-Stokes respirations, which occur when death is imminent, occasionally cause a patient to become panic-stricken, but most deaths are a quiet "slipping away" with only a few seconds of struggle or restlessness at the time of death (Walker 1973).

The mental condition of the individual near death varies from deep coma to full alertness, and the patient may appear comatose when he is really able to be aroused. Even a comatose patient may just before death recover consciousness and be able to speak a few sentences. Regardless of the apparent state of consciousness, he may be able to hear. Usually in the process of dying, consciousness and the ability to communicate thoughts are gradually lost, but the person may be able to signify assent or dissent by slight movements of the head, hand, or eyes. An acute observer may notice that often an individual's mind is active until the end, although he may appear stuporous.

The process of dying is a progressive rather than simultaneous failure of vital functions, usually from the lower part of the body upward. Sensation, reflexes, and motion are lost in the legs before they are lost in the arms. Sphincters relax, peristalsis ceases, and the stomach distends with contents ingested prior to loss of the ability to swallow. With relaxation of the sphincters incontinence of urine and stool occur. The folly of giving oral medicines or nutrients is evident; they will be regurgitated or quickly eliminated. Later, there is an equal chance that the fluids given by mouth will run down the trachea. Worcester (1961, p. 36) takes from earlier physicians the classic picture of the individual who is very near death:

> The eyes glazed and half closed, jaw dropped and mouth open, cold and flaccid lip; cold, clammy sweats on head and neck; respirations hurried and shallow or slow and stertorous with rattle; pulse irregular, unequal, weak, and immeasurably fast; prostrate on back, arms tossing in disorder, hands waved languidly before the face or grasping through empty air, or fumbling with bedclothes.

Physical care of the dying person includes providing relief from pain, and the help necessary to permit good nutrition, hygiene, elimination, and rest. Meticulous physical care provides emotional and physical rest for the patient, and should be paced slowly enough and with intervals to lessen fatigue.

Specific Areas

MOUTH CARE

As long as the patient can swallow, water should be offered with increasing frequency but in lessening amounts. When even a few drops cause choking, a water-soaked gauze can be placed between the lips for the patient to suck on. Except for respiration, sucking is the body's last instinctive action, and thirst the last craving.

The patient's mouth often is open, the tongue edematous, dry from lack of saliva, immobile so that it pushes against the roof of the mouth. Chips of ice wrapped in gauze, placed well back between the gums and cheek, or a light film of vaseline applied to the tongue help relieve the discomfort of the excessively dry mouth when the patient can no longer swallow. The ice in gauze is preferable because its moisture evaporates without causing choking. If there is too much fluid in the mouth from regurgitation, gauze wicking placed between the cheek and gums, extending between the lips, affords relief from choking. In both of these situations, the patient should be turned to one side to allow gravity drainage from the mouth and to prevent the tongue from blocking the airway. Additionally, the upper part of the body should remain as straightened as possible, and the neck should not be flexed on the body (Worcester 1961).

The mouth can be a significant source of discomfort or pain in people dying from oral cancer, cancer of other body parts, or chronic diseases, and often becomes dry and sore. Moniliasis or other infections, taste disturbances, halitosis, drooling, and disturbances of chewing, swallowing, and speech are often present. Further, the drugs that the patient receives may also cause side-effects or toxicity symptoms in the mouth. Inability to eat or talk may be perceived as deprivation, a precursor to loss of relationships. Emotional reactions of others to the condition of the patient's mouth may be a source of embarrassment and shame.

The mouth of the patient requires the care he would give it if he could — so that it remains comfortable, usable, and as attractive as possible to the patient and others. The lips, oral cavity, and teeth should be kept in as optimum a condition as possible.

As total bodily deterioration progresses, the mouth increasingly becomes the most convenient, and later the only, mode of communication as hands lose coordination and the person loses will and strength for writing. The mouth remains the last area for gratification and satisfaction with which the patient is able to indulge himself or can be indulged — through eating desired foods, talking to loved ones, and requesting desired satisfactions (Kutscher 1972).

Mouth care should be done by the patient as long as he can do so. As he becomes weaker, his mouth often hangs open, saliva drools, and ulcerations and halitosis develop. He may be unable to swallow or expectorate mucus, so that aspiration by suction or a gauze wick helps remove secretions. Use of a soft toothbrush or cotton-tipped applicator to clean teeth, gums, tongue, and the inside of the cheeks, as well as swabbing the mouth tissues with mouthwash, glycerin, or ointment help to keep tissues moist and sweet smelling (Beland and Passos 1975).

NOSE CARE
Nose care is often neglected but is essential for comfort and nasal respiration. Mucus crusts should be removed with tissues, gauzes, or cotton-tipped applicators moistened with normal saline. Water-soluble jelly can be used for lubrication of the nares (Fuerst and Weitzel 1974).

EYE CARE
Proper care of the eyes adds to comfort, vision, and appearance. Cotton balls

or gauze, moistened with normal saline, can be used to cleanse the eyes, removing crusts from eyelids or mucus secretions from the corners. If eyes are dry, they stay open; several drops of cottonseed oil instilled in the conjunctival sac will prevent friction and ulcerated cornea.

MAINTAINING NUTRITION AND HYDRATION

This task is a special problem because dysphagia, anorexia, nausea, and vomiting are symptoms common to most terminal illnesses. The diet should be modified as necessary for as long as possible. If the dying person desires a meal of bread, butter, jelly, and beer, and can retain it, he should have it. Concern about providing "the basic four" for the terminally ill person should not deprive him of the joy of eating something he really wants, even if the combination of foods appear strange. Gastric-tube feedings and intravenous fluids are given as the person's condition deteriorates, and the special measures of care for each of these procedures (described in medical–surgical nursing texts) should be followed.

In terminal illness, nutrition *is* difficult to maintain. During chemo- or radiation therapy, the resultant nausea and vomiting causes the patient to eat little, and become dehydrated and malnourished. Anemia frequently results, and efforts should be directed to prevent and correct it. In the patient with cancer, anorexia may result later from liver or gastrointestinal metastasis or bowel obstruction. As death nears, normal activities of the gastrointestinal tract decrease; although nourishment remains important, offering large quantities of food is contraindicated as this may lead to distention and further discomfort.

Taking antiemetic drugs before meals may help. The patient should be allowed to eat and drink whatever he likes and can tolerate so that he can remain as active and strong as possible. Exercise, assistance with walking, and eating in a dining room rather than in bed may improve his appetite. Wherever it is taken, food should be the correct temperature, tastily prepared, attractively served, and chosen by the patient. Often sweet foods or liquids are tolerated less well than tangy or sharp foods. If it is necessary to assist with the meals, the patient should be fed in an unhurried manner.

Mouth ulceration often results from treatment; anesthetic mouthwash may help as well as avoiding citrus fruits and highly seasoned foods. In the presence of this condition, bland foods are usually tolerated best, although they may not be the choice of the patient.

As the person becomes weaker, nasal tube or gastrostomy feedings or hyperalimentation may be ordered by the physician to maintain nutrition and intravenous fluids to maintain hydration (Beland and Passos 1975; Fuerst and Weitzel 1974).

MAINTAINING ELIMINATION

The patient often alternately has constipation, impaction, and diarrhea. Bulk foods, fluids, stool softeners, and enemas, or an antidiarrheal medication will be given as indicated. Urinary retention or oliguria may be present, especially in the presence of dehydration.

It is necessary to keep an accurate record of intake and urinary output as well as of bowel movements. Urinary output may be scanty because of inadequate intake or renal deterioration; or urinary frequency with small output may occur. A bladder-control program may be initiated. Later an indwelling catheter may be necessary, although this should be considered a last resort. Giving the patient fluids and placing him on the bedpan every two hours frequently regulates urinary output and prevents a wet bed. Constipation can be prevented by fluids, some type of exercise program (even in bed), regular meals, daily prune juice, and a glycerin suppository routine. When the patient ingests little, only a small amount of fecal material will be eliminated. Constipation and impaction may occur, which at first may be misdiagnosed because of the diarrheal leakage. If the patient does not have a bowel movement at least every three or four days, he should be digitally examined for impaction. Enemas are fatiguing and should be used as a last resort.

Often the dying patient has urinary and fecal incontinence because of loss of muscle tone. When this occurs the perineal area must be kept meticulously clean. The patient should be cleaned promptly and in a matter-of-fact way, removing soiled and wet linens to reduce odors and maintain hygiene. The patient who is conscious feels like an infant — dependent, a burden, embarrassed, and even devastated — when he cannot maintain controls. No caregiver should ever add further to these feelings with harsh words, a punitive attitude, or by being negligent in care.

CARE OF THE SKIN

Care of the skin must be more than routine in the effort to prevent decubitus ulcers. The skin and bedlinens must be kept dry, clean, and unwrinkled. Pressure points should be massaged frequently with lotion or mineral oil to keep the skin moist and soft and to maintain circulation. Backrubs promote comfort and circulation and allow time to talk with the patient. Daily isometric exercises maintain circulation and muscle tone, if the patient is able to do them. If possible he should get out of bed and walk. If the patient is too weak for either of these attempts, passive range-of-motion exercises maintain circulation, joint movement and muscle tone, and relieve pressure on various body areas. The use of an alternating pressure mattress, lamb's wool, silicone pads, water beds, and rotating beds are all measures to help prevent decubiti (Beland and Passos 1975).

Early decubitus care involves exposure to air and light — heat lamp with a low-watt bulb (40) placed 18 to 24 inches from the patient for 20 minutes — and keeping the area dry and clean. If the breakdown is extensive, debridement is done and the decubitus is packed with iodoform gauze that permits healing and granulation. The ulcer may be packed with sugar and covered with gauze, as local irritation by the sugar stimulates wound repair processes; granulation tissue forms and the acid pH of sugar increases vasodilation as well as being bacteriocidal (Beland and Passos 1975).

PERIPHERAL CIRCULATION

As death approaches, the temperature usually rises above normal. Simultaneously, peripheral circulation fails so that the skin feels cold. There may be diaphoresis, with cooling of the body. Bed linens and gowns should be changed frequently. Using light-weight bedlinen and supporting it on a bed cradle (so that the linen's weight does not rest on the patient) adds to his comfort. If he is picking at his bedlinen, it may be because he is too warm.

Alcohol or tepid water sponges provide relief. Although in the past patients complained of being too hot, this complaint may not be as common in today's air-conditioned, cold rooms. A light sheet is the only needed covering. A well-ventilated room with moving air, such as an electric fan, promotes comfort and cooler sensations for the patient.

POSITIONING

The patient must be kept in proper alignment but does not have to remain in the dorsal recumbent position. A text on medical–surgical nursing or fundamentals of nursing may be consulted for information on how to properly position a patient on his back, his side, or his abdomen. Pillows or towel rolls will be needed to support the dying patient, as he will be too weak to remain in the position in which he is placed. Misalignment, which causes fatigue and discomfort, must be avoided. If the patient has respiratory distress, the orthopneic position aids respiratory movements. Turning the head to the side or placing the person on the side helps to prevent airway obstruction. If the dying patient feels more comfortable with pillows under his knees or arms, or additional pillows under the head, these can be placed to avoid pressure. This is not the time to be concerned about thrombophlebitis, or a head thrust forward; comfort should be the primary concern.

The most comfortable position may be lying on the back, with head slightly elevated and supported with one or two pillows, a pillow rolled and placed beneath the knees to support the legs in a slightly flexed position. Any position will be uncomfortable if it is maintained too long; frequent small changes are essential (Price 1959, p. 779).

ENVIRONMENTAL CONSIDERATIONS

Many texts advise placing the dying patient in a private room, or pulling the bed curtains around him if he must remain in a multibed room. This may, however, add to the sense of loneliness and isolation, although when he is near death such arrangements do allow privacy for the patient and his family. In any case, he should not be left alone for long periods.

The room should look cheerful, be well-lighted and ventilated, but free from drafts. Vision gradually fails as death nears; the patient sees better if the room is not darkened. Odors in the room are often a problem because of sloughing tissue or infection. Scrupulous attention to patient cleanliness will, with good ventilation, help overcome odors. Drops of oil of geranium, oil of eucalyptus, and oil of orange are effective room deodorants. One or two drops of neutroleum alpha is lasting and pleasant when applied to the dressing or bedclothing. Powdered charcoal on the dressing or potassium permanganate solution 1:2000 as a wound irrigation often helps. Activated zinc peroxide is effective in cleansing and deodorizing the wound. Since odor-producing organisms require an alkaline medium, the use of buttermilk or yogurt on dressings is helpful because their acidity prevents odor-forming bacteria from growing. Commercially prepared products can be disseminated from a bottle with a wick, or by means of an electric deodorizer to absorb odors. Deodorizer sprays may cause nausea (Brunner 1970; Beland and Passos 1975).

MANAGING COMPLICATIONS

As with any patients, the terminal patient must be observed for complications. Metastasis is always possible in patients with malignant tumors.

If bone metastasis is present, the patient is likely to develop hypercalcemia because bone destruction causes an increased load of calcium in the blood, which eventually the kidneys can no longer excrete. Symptoms include nausea, vomiting, polyuria, dehydration, personality changes, lethargy, muscle weakness, fatigability, and (finally) coma. Treatment involves restoring electrolyte balance through hydration with up to 4 liters per 24 hours of high-sodium fluid if the cardiac condition permits.

Metastatic tumors to the spine cause severe neck and back pain, muscle weakness, numbness, and loss of sphincter control, and (finally) quadriplegia or paraplegia. If pressure on the cord is relieved when sensory loss is just beginning, the paralysis is usually reversible.

Bone metastasis and demineralization cause spontaneous fractures, especially of the hip. Patients and staff must guard against fractures as much as possible by avoiding sudden twists and great pressure or weight against the body; patients are cautioned to avoid lifting, pushing, or climbing. The major complication to be anticipated near the end is hemorrhage, owing to erosion of blood vessels by the tumor, secondary necrosis, or sloughing of tissue following irradiation (Brunner et al. 1970). Suctioning to maintain an airway and use of direct-pressure dressings are the main nonheroic measures.

Pain

The control of pain is an essential component of the care of the terminally ill patient, and *who* should manage the techniques of pain relief is being considered in the literature. Whether pain management will be vested primarily in patients or in staff may depend on the organization of task activities and of sentiment in the institution. Strauss et al. (1974, p. 566) have pointed out that "the staff is not genuinely accountable for much of its interaction with or behavior toward patients in pain." The balancing of priorities when both patient and staff must choose among options of endurance and relief in terms of the consequences of the decision is not easy. Staff may not agree among themselves, and may not agree with the patient. When there is discrepancy in choices (for instance, staff's withholding narcotics — in the commitment to longer life or patient safety — from a patient who would prefer relief from pain and a shorter life), misunderstanding and mutual antagonism ensues (Strauss et al. 1974). Staff concern about addiction may appear unwarranted to terminal patients in severe pain.

There is some evidence that pain is really intractable in only a very few cases. The use of synergistic drugs, of relaxation techniques, and the time-honored but frequently neglected nursing measures of positioning, backrub, creation of a quiet environment, and letting the patient decide what will best alleviate pain and promote comfort will most likely control pain. Staff discomfort with the drug dosage in pain relievers such as the Bromptom Cocktail (Mount et al. 1978),* and the belief that techniques of relaxation are not scientific in origin create problems with the use of such measures. There is no overt objection to the older nursing measures described above; however, they are time-consuming and not particularly exciting—or they are difficult to do, and have fallen into disuse.

Pain is not simply the result of physical illness or disease but is also determined by anxiety level, knowledge, death expectation, fear of disfigurement, cultural norms, and past experience with pain. The gate-control theory of pain suggests that the amount of pain transmitted from peripheral fibers to the brain is determined by sensory input from the body as well as by brain activities that exert a descending influence on the gate system. When the amount of pain to the brain exceeds a critical level, pain is perceived and relief measures are required.

Cancer pain is best understood with the gate-control theory. Lesions of different kinds of tissues may produce pain that varies in intensity and duration. Pain is influenced by psychological and social factors, as described above (Melzack et al. 1978).

Pain has many meanings and can be a catchall term for many different feelings. It may represent a challenge, an enemy, loss, weakness, punishment, fear of the unknown, of losing control over behavior, of losing independence, and of becoming depressed, quarrelsome, and unlovable. It may be the result of or represent unpleasant feelings concerning life situations or relationships. Chronic pain represents endlessness and meaninglessness. Pain may also bring grief and anguish. Pain interferes with all aspects of life, including love and sex. Some patients may see a value in pain, considering that it encourages self-testing, self-awareness, spiritual growth, and appreciation of other sufferers (Copp 1974).

Medication alone is not enough to provide optimum comfort; the quality of nurse–patient relationships may exert a greater influence on relief than medication. Talking about feelings has a cathartic effect for both patient and staff; while not all patients can talk about their feelings directly, most can do so indirectly.

---

*The Bromptom Cocktail is an oral narcotic (usually morphine) given with a phenothiazine. The morphine blocks sensory input to the brain at many levels. Morphine and phenothiazine decrease anxiety and the emotional and evaluative aspects of pain; the mixture reduces the expectation of pain and the related fear.

The Bromptom mixture achieves these results after milder analgesics are no longer effective because the pain is too severe. The syrup is perhaps better than the tablets because it is easier to swallow if the patient is dysphagic, and the dose is easier to adjust to need. The mixture may be used for many months without dose escalation (Mount et al. 1978).

However, although pain, anger, and depression about approaching death can be devastating, they are also a private matter. Staff do not have the right to force their way into private things; even in the midst of pain, the integrity of a person's right of privacy must be respected. The nurse can and should offer help, presence, and availability to the patient, but the feelings of the patient must be recognized verbally and generally, so that it becomes *his* choice how much of the self to reveal and how to respond (Wygant 1967).

Frankl (1971) suggests that persons in pain can be helped to find meaning in the experience, find a way to react, and understand or be conscious of the conditions of the pain. However, for meaning to be found in suffering, the person must be allowed to suffer and helped to see suffering as enabling rather than degrading. Staff must recognize courage in suffering and help the patient to express his hurt; neither staff nor patient can deny the suffering. The temptation to administer pain-relieving medication is overwhelming; staff may succumb before the patient is ready to do so. The choice of whether to endure and seek meaning in the pain or to seek relief should always lie with the patient — as should the modality of pain expression or pain relief.

As suggested earlier, the quality and the intensity of the pain, as well as the characteristics of the response are influenced by the unique past history of the individual, by the meaning he gives to his expectations about pain, by his mental and emotional status at the time, and by the pain-producing stimulus. The pain threshold is approximately the same for everyone; perception of the pain and reaction to it vary. Fear and anxiety almost always increase the felt pain.

Prodomal signs and symptoms of severe pain include restlessness, tremor, generalized uneasiness, anxiety, irritability, muscular aches, vertigo, nausea, vomiting, and diarrhea (Copp 1974). These signs and symptoms are associated with many illnesses without pain, but in order to initiate comfort measures, prevent the pain, or (at the least) decrease its severity, staff must be alert to the possibility that they are pain precursors.

Chronic pain leads to a vicious cycle of fearful anticipation, occurrence, anxiety, and depression; the pain is a constant reminder of the patient's condition.

Short-term pain is tolerable. Severe or continued moderate pain is depressing and demoralizing, as even when the individual is pain-free for several hours, he knows the pain will return. He becomes preoccupied or even obsessed with pain, unable to think of anything else for very long periods. Patience and tolerance are limited; little things seem too much to handle. Even the smallest amount of added discomfort — for instance, a painful examination — becomes too much to stand. As pain continues, tolerance to it decreases, and larger doses of narcotics are often asked for. Pain causes the patient to feel neglected and rejected; even when he is getting efficient, prompt, kind care, minor slights or delays are magnified (Cashatt 1972).

Although an individual's threshold does not actually change, perception and tolerance are affected by age. The older person reports less initial pain and greater relief from analgesics (Belleville et al. 1971).

Dimensions of staff's work with pain include not only diagnosis and management but also responding to the patient's expression about pain, minimizing or preventing the pain, helping the patient to endure pain, and controlling personal reactions to the way the patient is enduring his pain (Strauss et al. 1974).

In institutions, in almost all wards, there are expected pain trajectories — the staff has repeatedly experienced certain courses of illness and pain and is prepared to work with patients who manifest the usual pattern. When an unexpected pain trajectory appears — for example, when a patient insists that relief measures are not controlling pain — the ward may not be organized nor the staff psychologically prepared to handle the event. Patients who present an unexpected pain trajectory are often labeled uncooperative or difficult, and relations between such a patient and staff deteriorate. Most patients come to hospitals because of chronic illness; patients with chronic diseases are most likely to present an unexpected pain trajectory. Thus the patient who is in the hospital the longest, or repeatedly, is most likely also to suffer staff rejection. Some of the rejection and poor relationship results because the patient who has endured illness, pain, and medical care for some time is quite knowledgeable about routines and what relieves his pain. Staff may have less experience with his routines of relief. Often drugs are changed without his knowledge when the patient enters the hospital, and it is not unusual for drugs to be ordered that are ineffective, or to which the patient is allergic or responds idiosyncratically (Strauss et al. 1974).

These patients tend to mistrust staff, although they also realize they are at their mercy and must "court" them for care. The application of game-theory notions (see Chapter 5) by staff would make the patient a knowledgeable partner in his care, to be consulted about the best possible way to manage his pain. Because staff and patient often perceive different options in pain management — enduring pain and longer life versus avoiding more pain by shortening life or undergoing major neurosurgery — use of game theory can assist staff and the patient to talk about the perceived options and arrive at a consensus acceptable to both, but most especially acceptable to the patient. Discrepant priorities frequently result in mutual antagonism and rejection. Strauss et al. (1974) suggest that much of the negative aspect of the inefficient management of pain that can occur for chronically and terminally ill patients could be avoided if the individual nurse or staff member was held accountable for her actions and interactions, and not just for techniques and procedures.

RELIEF OF PAIN

McCaffery and Hart (1976) maintain that nurses' pain-relief activities fall into these categories: (1) administering pharmacologic agents; (2) administering placebos; (3) altering pain stimulus or source; (4) assisting the patient to use physical activity if he is able; (5) providing distraction; (6) suggesting psychotherapy; (7) discussing pain with the patient; (8) remaining with the patient; and (9) providing the comfort of touch.

Copp (1974) found that patients who are in pain want different things. Most stress that they want nursing and medical personnel who listen, teach, and talk, and who will be present as a source of strength and as a protection from feared invasion, intrusion, disaster, or death. A small number want contact with natural elements — sunlight, oxygen, earth, grass, plants, trees, flowers, an opportunity to walk in their environment, and an opportunity to touch their possessions as a source of strength. The comfort of the familiar is most important to hospitalized patients.

According to Copp's (1974) study, nurses and doctors can do the following to help patients in pain: (1) do *not* hurry, stay to talk to the patient; (2) be prompt with comfort measures; (3) try to be understanding; (4) have confidence that what they are doing or giving will work, so that the patient also has confidence; (5) see patients as individuals; and (6) get to the cause of the pain, do not merely give pain pills. Further, nurses should not tell the patient he does not really hurt; ignore the patient or consider him a neurotic; be too casual or flip; assume the pain medication is always effective; or become calloused. Finally, patients prefer having to interact with only one doctor and one nurse per shift.

There is some agreement among clinical investigators as to nursing measures used to alleviate pain, either with or in place of medical or surgical modalities. McCaffery and Hart (1976) suggest the importance of remaining with the patient — a measure cited throughout this book — and discussing pain with the patient and continued care after intervention.

Remaining with the patient when he is in pain may serve several purposes, one of which is to prevent or reduce social isolation. The nurse may remain quiet, so that the patient can initiate conversation if he wishes. Her presence conveys that others care; further, the patient with pain has greater anxiety, and the desire to be with another person increases as anxiety increases.

Touch can convey a wide variety of meanings and may be a helpful addition to remaining with the person in pain. Touch conveys that dependency is allowed during stressful periods, such as intense pain or high anxiety. The patient who is striving for independence may reject touch; yet, during pain he may reach out for the nurse's hand. A firm responsive touch is then appropriate. Touch may help control anxiety through relaxation measures such as a backrub or gentle stroking of a painful area; firm pressure to a painful area can also be effective.

Discussing pain with the patient may be done in several ways and geared to achieve different purposes: to obtain the patient's trust, and convey concern; to mobilize the patient's coping mechanisms; to reinforce and stabilize his coping abilities; and to change his attitude toward pain related stimuli. When the patient says he has pain, he should be asked to further describe his pain; the nurse should not disagree with the patient or convey that he is not in pain. By listening to the patient's description, the nurse and the patient decide on the best intervention, which might be repositioning instead of analgesia administration. Also, if the patient knows what to expect in the way of pain and how to help minimize it, he can cope better. When painful treatment is required, the patient can visualize ahead of time the ordeal and think about the realistic information given about the procedure; he is then less likely to be overwhelmed by the pain or anxiety, especially if he knows that the nurse will be there to support him through the situation. Some patients need more time to mentally prepare than others do.

Continued care after intervention for pain is often neglected. The patient needs to realize when the source of pain has been partially or completely altered so that he need not anticipate or experience any more pain. Thus his level of anxiety can decrease and he does not misinterpret other stimuli as painful. Also, the patient needs to assimilate his painful experience so that he can handle future episodes if they should occur. Verbal reenactment of pain, what happened, and of his emotions and feelings help him to resolve the stress of pain.

In many instances, how well the patient is able to handle his pain is partially dependent on what the nurse does. When the nurse is confronted with a patient who expects or feels pain, she can intervene to help him cope with his immediate experience and also influence future pain experiences.

Pain relief is desirable for humane and moral reasons as well as to improve the patient's psychological and physiological welfare. Total elimination of pain may not be possible, but usually distress can be relieved to a considerable degree. Narcotic analgesics are more effective when used with other comfort measures such as positioning, backrub, distraction, relaxation techniques, and with nonnarcotic drugs such as tranquilizers.

The treatment of intractable pain with analgesics and narcotics may have several aims:

1. To identify the cause, which may be the disease, constipation, position, etc.

2. To prevent pain with regular administration of analgesic.

3. To help erase pain memory; as the anxious anticipation and memory of it lessen, the amount of analgesic needed lessens.

4. To maintain an unclouded sensorium by carefully regulating analgesic dosage.

5. To help maintain a normal affect — neither depressed nor euphoric, so the patient can relate to the environment.

6. To have ease of administration with oral analgesic so the patient retains some independence and mobility; oral administration is preferred over the parenteral administration utilized when the patient is cachexic.

Because the fear of pain is likely to be intense, causes of what might otherwise be sensed merely as discomfort must be considered. These elements include lack of rest, which decreases the ability to tolerate pain; the weight of the bedclothing on the body; or edema from blocked lymphatic vessels, which may add to discomfort for cancer patients.

Gentle handling with every procedure, turning and/or positioning, the attitude that something can and will be done to relive the pain, and the sensible use of diversion may precede the use of medication as pain-relief strategies. When medication is required, the following factors must be considered: (1) severity; (2) whether pain is continuous or intermittent; (3) the patient's level of anxiety and perception of the pain, as well as his projected lifespan; and (4) whether the cause of the pain can be removed (Beland and Passos 1978).

In the treatment of terminally ill patients, withholding narcotics is merely cruel; there is no need to worry about addiction. However, less potent drugs should be used earlier in order that the patient will get more relief later from narcotics. Analgesic drugs should be given prior to painful procedures. It is well to remember that during the night, when there are fewer distractions, patients will need more of the prescribed medicine, or to have it combined with a tranquilizer to enhance its effect. Giving a small dose of the analgesic every two hours rather than a regular larger dose every four hours may be helpful. Part of the benefit of any drug is the patient's faith in it; the nurse's suggestion that it will work adds to the likelihood of relief.

Severe pain may be treated surgically; ulcerated areas are excised, obstruction relieved, or pain impulses are prevented from reaching the brain by cutting sensory nerves, nerve roots, or tracts in the spinal cord. Such surgery is a last-resort measure. Nurses must remember that interruption of the sensory nerve supply means that the patient also loses the sense of pressure and of heat — predisposing to other complications (Beland and Passos 1978).

There is clinical and research evidence to suggest that medication does not always relieve pain. However, when the patient enters into the decision-making about the pain therapy, suggests what measures he believes would be most helpful, and has the final choice about which one of several possible comfort measures should be used, he is more likely to obtain relief (Moss and Meyer 1966; Billars 1970).

Placebo research indicates that suggestion is effective in relieving pain, and staff conviction that a medication will bring relief results in greater patient comfort than when the medication is given with no suggestion that it will relieve pain (Billars 1970; Gliedman et al. 1957).

Undertreatment for pain with narcotic analgesics occurs frequently because physicians prescribe insufficient dosage, or intervals between administration are too long, or nurses give less of the medication than is ordered.

There is evidence that codeine, Demerol, or morphine are more effective if combined with another drug, such as aspirin or Tylenol (acetaminophen) or with a tranquilizer such as Thorazine (chlorpromazine). Doses of analgesics and intervals between administration should be determined by the patient's comfort level and overall response (McCaffery and Hart 1976), although certainly possible and actual side-effects, toxic and idiosyncratic reactions, and allergic responses must be considered.

Detailed information about major narcotic analgesics, their effects on patients, and their effective use is contained in the McCaffery and Hart (1976) reference, or in standard pharmacology texts. For example, Mount et al. (1978) report:

> *The standard mixture at St. Christopher's and St. Joseph's Hospices is: variable amount of morphine, 10 mg cocaine, 2.5 ml ethyl alcohol (98%), 5 ml flavoring syrup, and a variable amount of chloroform water, to make a total of 20 ml. Most chronic pain is controlled with 5 to 20 mg*

of morphine per dose. Usual sequential doses of morphine are 2.5, 5, 10, 15, 20, 30, 40, 60, 90, and 120 mg of morphine. This elixir is always given with a phenothiazine, which helps decrease anxiety, potentiates the narcotic, and as an antiemetic, reduces morphine-related nausea and vomiting. Prochlorperazine, 5 mg in 15 ml, causes little sedation. If the patient remains restless or agitated, chlorpromazine, 10 to 25 mg, may be given.

Administration Guidelines: *Morphine elixir in 20 ml dose with phenothiazine every 4 hours daily — sometimes q 3 hours. Night-time dose omitted if patient sleeps pain free.*

If pain is excruciating, start with a higher narcotic dose, then decrease the narcotic until the analgesia is without sedative effects. Dose alterations should be made q 48-72 hours during this period. Only one component at a time is varied — the morphine or the phenothiazine — because they are synergistic.

The initiation of narcotic therapy produces transient sedation for 48 to 72 hours, but pain can be controlled with only temporary sedation. Dispensing morphine and phenothiazine separately allows greater flexibility in adjusting the dosage. When the patient is free of pain, the drugs can be combined for ease of administration. The patient's condition is carefully monitored for 24 hours to determine whether augmentation of one or two specific doses at periods of peak activity is required. If parenteral medication becomes necessary, the equivalent dose of morphine is one-half of the previous oral dose. The adverse effects of all narcotics is considered; Sedation; nausea and vomiting (controlled with phenothiazine); constipation (prevented with stool softener); and tolerance-dependence (not so much of this exists in the presence of the pain of malignant disease; undertreatment of pain may actually cause craving and psychological dependence). Additional adverse effects include extrapyramidal effects and orthostatic hypotension. Other therapies to control symptoms are also used: these include radiotherapy, peripheral nerve or intrathecal block, neurosurgery, physical measures such as splinting and passive exercises, and the maintenance of a pleasant supportive environment. *

Regardless of the medication, patients often work out methods that reduce the intensity of the oncoming pain. They use a range of muscular activities varying from very strenuous work or play to complete inactivity. They use words: profane, prayerful, or nonsensical. They concentrate on specific exercises, phrases, or games. They time the taking of drugs (prescribed and nonprescribed). They apply heat or cold, use breathing exercises, try certain body positions, or use ritualistic behaviors such as rubbing, pounding, pacing, rocking,

---

*Mount B, Ajemian I, Scott J: Use of Brompton Mixture in treating the chronic pain of malignant disease. Garfield C (ed), Psychosocial Care of the Dying Patient. New York, McGraw-Hill, 1978, pp. 396–403

or biting. Sometimes they use rituals or distraction methods dating to their childhood. However, patients are often afraid to use familiar rituals to relieve pain in the hospital because the staff may laugh. While patients seem quite able to manipulate the environment to produce comfort and to cope with pain while they remain at home, they often seem at a loss to know how to cope in the unfamiliar hospital setting (Copp 1974).

Focusing is a common coping style, and may take the following forms:

1. *Counting of objects, holes in the acoustical ceiling, flowers in the drapery, tacks in the upholstery, or tiles in the floor, or doing mathematical problems, letter arrangements, or series. Counting is used to focus and distract from pain.*

2. *Seven major types of words are used to focus on in order to cope with pain: control words ("I won't scream"); supplication ("Let it be over soon"); intercession ("Help me, Jesus"); memorized words (prayers, rhymes); repetitive words (nonsense syllables); derisive words ("This is stupid"); evaluative words ("It's going to end soon"); and anxious words ("I can't stand this")*

3. *Deep thinking and visualization, including prayers, concentration exercises, focusing on lights or shadows, mentally reorganizing cupboards, or recalling specific routes of previous travels may be used to distract from pain.*

4. *Separation attempts, deliberate attempts to separate mind and body, to deny a part of the body; the patient may imagine the hurting part as dropping away, or try self-hypnosis.*

5. *Distraction strategies, which include smoking, reading, talking to others in pain, whistling, blowing, panting, pounding, or squeezing.*

6. *Having people around may decrease the pain unless the other person is a sick roommate. Often a specific person is sought during pain because of special personality qualities. (Copp 1974, pp. 492–495)*

RELAXATION TECHNIQUES

Relaxation techniques are a useful adjunct to medication and other pain-control therapies, or may in themselves serve as control therapies. Four elements are necessary for relaxation techniques: (1) a quiet, calm environment with few distractions such as background noise; (2) a mental device or stimulus that can be repeated silently or in a low, gentle tone; (3) a passive attitude; and (4) a comfortable position. Breathing is done through the nose, with conscious awareness of respirations. The relaxation practice should be continued for 20 minutes once or twice daily (Benson 1975).

Conscious relaxation is safe, simple, practical, not difficult to teach, and is always available to diminish pain, relax muscles, promote sleep, and promote a calm, alert frame of mind as well as a sense of control over pain. If the technique is to be well-utilized, the patient must be in the correct posture to minimize muscular stress. An explicit effort to put the mind at rest is made by focusing on a center of concentration outside the body. Deep breaths are accompanied by mental instruction to body parts to relax, beginning with the legs and feet and progressing upward. At the point of maximum discomfort, shallow, more rapid breathing is done only briefly to avoid hyperventilation. Light massage and continued rhythmic breathing can lessen pain (Stewart 1976).

Patients in pain identify a variety of nursing roles. These include:

1. *A controller, who relieves or denies relief.*
2. *A communicator, who tells, validates, or interprets.*
3. *An informant, who can or cannot be trusted with personal, private data.*
4. *A judge, who decides if reported pain is reasonable, timely, expected.*
5. *An avoider, who refuses to report that medication does not relieve, and acknowledges the patient's pain only to the intensity that she can tolerate.*
6. *An empathizer, who lets the patient have his own experience; authentic empathizers state their understanding of the patient's pain experience; pseudoempathizers describe their own experiences, detracting attention from the patient.*
7. *A barterer, who gives relief in return for good patient behavior. (Copp 1974, p. 495)*

In their discussion of the treatment of the terminally ill patient, Schmalz and Patterson (1978) state that after open discussion among the physician, the patient, and the family, a therapeutic approach geared to the patient's comfort can be instituted. They suggest the following comfort care guidelines.

1. *Comfort care should be initiated whenever patient and physician agree that all reasonable measures for control of the disease have failed.*
2. *The purpose of this care is to minimize discomfort without specific or direct attention to the underlying disease.*
3. *The plan should be flexible but specific in its detail and should be known to all concerned with its implementation. It should include roles for family members or others the patient wishes to be involved in the process, with no restrictions on the frequency of personal contacts except for those set by the patient.*
4. *All treatment and medication will be prescribed to minimize symptoms.*
   a. *Drugs, procedures, fluids, and so on not clearly needed to relieve symptoms will be omitted.*
   b. *Measures to relieve pain and discomfort are provided as requested by the patient with no concern for addiction or habituation. Other measures for relieving symptoms include measures such as oxygen that may help dyspnea as may morphine; salicylate may relieve the discomfort associated with fever, and nasogastric suction should be used only as needed for distension.*
   c. *Routines such as repeated physical examinations, measuring vital signs, and recording weight, intake, output should be discontinued.*

    d.   *Emergency measures should not be used to prevent death, although symptoms are always treated.*

5. *The plan should be reviewed at regular intervals and whenever the patient desires.*

6. *Alternatives in types of care and in settings that are needed in order to provide for changing patient needs should be available on a standby basis. Such alternatives allow the patient to move from home to hospital to hospice or nursing home as his requirements for care fluctuate. . . .*

If patient, family, and physicians agree on these guidelines, there are no ethical or legal issues to confront. With this acceptance of death, dying may become less of a defeat, and again will come to be recognized as an inevitable consequence of living. (Schmalz and Patterson 1978, pp. 20–21)

THERAPEUTIC COMMUNICATION

Communication *with* the patient is as essential to his well being as communication *about* him among caregivers; the nature of his progress to recovery (or death) depends on what he knows about his illness, the implications of the illness, and what verbal or nonverbal messages he receives from staff concerning his continuing importance to them. Inappropriate messages frequently impose dependency on patients, in spite of their best efforts to remain in adult control.

It has been suggested that the dependent status of patients has historical roots; that early hospitals were primarily conceived of as places in which to confine the sick in order to protect the well. This reasoning continues to be functional for a small number of highly contagious diseases. In addition, many patients are temporarily dependent because of their illness or injury. Much of the hospital routine imposed upon all patients, however, involves forcing them to be needlessly dependent upon the institution. Basic necessities such as food, "clothing," and shelter are prescribed and provided. The expression of initiative is limited or punished. Many patients find themselves cut off when they have the temerity to ask questions about themselves. Medications are administered by others. A routine is established and enforced. Social interaction with the outside world is restricted; personal privacy is invaded; the patient's body is given up to the ministrations of others; and the territory he occupies is subject to invasion by numerous strange people at any time of day or night. (Straus 1972, p. 218).

Patients report that the most important component of their care is that of having some control over their own treatment. However, hospital staff assign the patient roles that are to be played — to be a good patient, and to die on schedule at an expected time and in an expected manner. Although patients do not necessarily go through the stages discussed in the literature, most patients do go through denial a number of times. The behavior while dying reflects or parallels previous behavior when under stress. Nursing assessments include obtaining information as to how the person behaved in less stressful situations or during periods of failure. Previous patterns determine if he will surrender or fight, despair or deny. Talking with a dying person is a special task. Mere conversation differs from a professional exchange. In conversation, the talk is about things, dates, events, the surface of the world. In professional exchanges, the focus is on the feelings and the emotional tone of the patient minimizing facts sometimes. When using psychotherapeutic methods with the dying person, the therapist does not introduce the topic of death. The patient is allowed to bring up his feelings — and he will, because they are uppermost in his mind except when he is in a state of denial. When the patient is able to discuss his feelings, the therapist does not try to evade the feelings or the statements that are made. The focus may be on manifest or on latent levels — topics of fact (burial arrangements, etc.) or feelings (the wish for extension of life). The concern of the therapist is not with interpretation but with promoting comfort. The professional exchange may touch on other stressful periods of life, and earlier successes and happiness. The patient sets the pace. The therapist can safely and quickly become a significant figure to the dying person as the person's life will soon be over.

Schneidman suggests specific guidelines for psychotherapy with dying patients, as follows.

1. *The goal is emotional comfort. Tasks may include helping to tie up loose ends, giving the patient as much stability as is possible.*
2. *Rapid development of transference and countertransference is appropriate, as is the quick establishment of rapport, helping the patient to feel attached to the therapist, and the professional to feel and show interest and love.*
3. *The therapist must move with the moods of the dying person, his efforts at control, and denial, and include plain talk about ordinary things when this is indicated.*
4. *Intervention may take the form of listening, making suggestions, giving advice when asked, acting as a liaison with the family and other staff, arranging for social services, such as an ombudsman.*
5. *It is not necessary to do much interpretation; the patient need not die with any great degree of self-insight.*
6. *The patient may not be able to resolve past life crises, but can be helped to put his affairs in order.*
7. *The dying person sets the pace for the exchange.*
8. *Denial will be present, and should be accepted by the therapist; it is a part of the process of dying, and allows hope never to be entirely abandoned.*
9. *If necessary, the therapist should establish therapeutic relations with the closest survivors, to help them with their mourning.*
10. *In order to invest in the patient's welfare, the therapist, like other health professionals, needs a strong support system. (Schneidman 1978, pp. 201-208)*

It is interesting to note Hannan's (1974) description of her experience with patients with cancer. She reports that they seemed to respond better to her when she changed her verbalized focus with them. This nurse found that when she spent time talking with patients, in order to help them with grief and other feelings, at first patients seemed relieved from the catharsis. Later, however, they would say "I'll be all right," and try to avoid the nurse (and, indirectly, the disease) and the dependency the situation implies. When she switched her approach to interest in *learning* what patients go through rather than *helping* them, the patients were more open, expressive, talked longer, said more, and seemed to invite a relationship. Nurses tend to emphasize their role of helper, putting patients in a dependent relationship. This report suggests the use of game-theory notions (again, see Chapter 5) that allow the patient to function in a peer relationship with staff.

Informing

There is no doubt that among the aspects of the hospitalization experience that are perceived as very stressful by patients is lack of meaningful communication on the part of hospital staff. Such events include the individual's not being told his diagnosis, not knowing the reasons for or results of treatment, not having questions answered by staff, having doctors or nurses talk too fast or use words not understood, and presence of a staff that appeared to be always hurrying (Volicer and Bohannon 1975).

While many health professionals advocate telling the patient that he is terminally ill, Gottheil et al. (1974) contend that knowledge of approaching death may not always be warranted.

Knowledge of impending death is not always accompanied by acceptance, courage, or dignity — denial, fear, anger, or depression may be the patient's feelings. All patients do not progress through Kübler-Ross' (1969) five-stage model.

Some evidence suggests that knowledge of impending death and the associated depression may decrease life expectancy; the individual loses the hope that may be literally keeping him alive.

Traditionally, knowledge of impending death permits the person to put his affairs in order, if he has the energy and motivation. Knowledge may help the family and medical staff to communicate more openly, but it may be easier for the family and medical staff to remain silent, or make excuses, and bear the burden of deceit. The signs and symptoms that indicate decline of the patient are not necessarily questioned by the patient; some patients do not want to know and do not hear the truth when it is discussed. Informed patients are not always more cooperative, cheerful, calm, or easier to talk with. Often the patients prefer comfort, protection, hope, and compassion rather than the truth, followed by staff and family expectations of courage. The professional may want the patient to accept death and simultaneously retain hope and the will to live; the paradox may be impossible. Additionally, the "honesty" of the staff may convey to the patient that they have given up.

There are no guidelines about who should be told, by whom, and when.

Should the patient be told his specific statistical life expectancy, the medical facts of diagnosis and prognosis, or given general information about his condition and the treatment plan by the nurse and doctor? Gottheil et al. (1974) question whether knowledge of coming death is a human right; humanness would depend on a number of factors inherent in the sharing of knowledge. Along these lines, Saunders (1974) believes that everyone knows they are dying but may not ask direct questions about it or want direct answers. While staff should give no false reassurance, they should not assualt the patient with unwanted information either.

In communication with the dying, the patient should always take the lead, and staff should always be available and approachable. Honesty and truth are in the relationship rather than the words.

However, staff seldom even consider withholding information about their condition from patients who are not terminal, even if the information is stressful or shocking in nature.

Denial and distress may indeed occur in the patient who is informed of death too quickly or abruptly by someone who does not know him well, without taking the patient's readiness into consideration. After unexpected shocking news, denial functions as a buffer—enabling the patient to collect himself and with time and understanding mobilize less radical defenses (Kübler-Ross 1969).

As illustrated by interviews in Chapter 6, one of the reasons it is difficult for nurses to communicate with dying patients at all is their concern over saying something that will distress the patients. If kindness, sensitivity, and tact are utilized as they would be with other patients, dying patients will not crumble into despair at anything said by nurses. Patients are not so fragile, and nurses are more likely to convey sensitivity and warmth than they believe they are (Koenig 1973).

Information exchange among the patient, the family, the nurses, and the physicians must occur in order to provide continuity of care and reduce feelings of uncertainty and neglect. Open communication is mandatory for good care. Staff should inform the patient fully about his care routine and the expectations of the institution, and convey that they welcome his suggestions about how to carry out procedures or treatment measures so that he is most comfortable. He should be encouraged to be active in making decisions about his care as long as he is able. However, this demands honest information and flexibility and willingness of the staff in order that a patient may actually enter into his care planning. Giving information, teaching, or counseling does not mean that staff tell him absolutely everything known about his condition or prognosis. Lengthy explanations of pathophysiology are inappropriate and usually not understood, and staff cannot predict when he will die. What the patient needs is basic information clearly presented so that he can decide what is best for him to do: to begin or refuse a new therapy; to omit routine measures such as a bath; to take more of the prescribed analgesic; to use nursing measures such as positioning and backrub instead of medication to relieve discomfort; to sleep without sedation if he can; to eat something contraindicated on his diet. If strict routine is avoided, the patient will be willing to state preferences, give suggestions, and enter into decision-making. If he senses that plans can be changed to meet his needs, he will be more willing to follow a schedule when there is no choice, without losing self-esteem or sense of integrity. If at all possible, he should be assisted to maintain the roles of spouse, parent, or other significant roles as long as he desires, so that he can be commended for his role behavior as a person. He needs to be told that he is doing well in the personal sense, and can take pride in performing cooperatively with his own treatment and care. A comment such as "You are coping well in a difficult situation. I admire your strength in dealing with a hard problem." should be directed to the patient (and family) to encourage and support them (Koenig 1973).

For those nursing and medical personnel who proceed from the game-theory orientation rather than from the perception of patients in the classic Parsonian sick role (see earlier in this book), there is no doubt that patients must be informed of both diagnosis and prognosis. The only question is: How can an individual be informed in a way that is most protective of him? Hogshead provides the following guidelines.

1. *Keep it simple. Perhaps as a result of apprehension or uneasiness, there is a tendency to go into too many details and technicalities.*
2. *Ask yourself, "What does this diagnosis mean to this patient?" Many patients are simply unable to comprehend the nature of the diagnosis, in which case methods must be found to gradually educate them.*
3. *Meet on "cool ground" first. It is very unpleasant to walk in to meet people whom you have never met before, knowing you have to give them a piece of really bad news. It is always easier to handle if you have some earlier relationship to the patient or his family, and have some notion of their background and possible reactions to the news.*
4. *Don't deliver all the news at once. It is a good idea to try not to provide too much information at the first sitting. People have a marvelous way of letting you know how much they are able to handle. Like the newspaper that printed "all the news that's fit to print," I feel that the patient has the right to all information that he is prepared to handle. This may mean that the full disclosure has to be spread out over two or three sessions.*
5. *Wait for questions. A long pause will allow the question that tells you where to go next.*
6. *Do not argue with denial. A characteristic response in many patients is outright denial of the reality of the situation. No matter how illogical the denial, it is serving a purpose, and there is nothing to gain by battering down the denial with logic. This usually leads to loss of rapport with the patient. In general, the patient will "hear" the message when he is ready to accept it. It is sufficient that he has been told at least once in some form that condition "x" has been discovered.*
7. *Ask questions yourself. Ask the patient to tell you what you have told him, or ask him what it means. Oftentimes you will be surprised at the answer. Or, ask the patient what the doctors at such-and-such a hospital have told him.*

8. *Do not destroy all hope. There are a hundred ways of handling this, and it requires real tact and experience to be able to acquire the necessary skill. "Most people with this kind of injury don't walk again" is a useful kind of treatment.*

9. *Do not say anything that is not true. This would be the most cruel blow of all. (Hogshead 1978, p. 129)*

Hogshead suggests that, sadly enough, there may really not be a right way to deliver the bad news — only various levels of wrong.

Kavanaugh (1974) is in substantial agreement with these guidelines. He believes almost everyone should be told, and the only real questions are when, how, and who tells. He suggests information should be given immediately after the diagnosis is medically certain — but "padded in hope." There is no easy way, but it is perhaps better if there is no "act of telling — only a two-way conversation open enough to allow the patient to announce his dying if he chooses." There is no "proper" person to do the telling, although Kavanaugh suggests many persons may be more qualified than the physician to perform this task. The patient's need is for a confidant(e) who will instigate and allow honest talk. The ethical need is that each one know as much of the truth as he wishes to know, in a way he can accept.

Listening

Communication with the terminally ill patient is recognized as an essential but frequently neglected nursing intervention, but listening (rather than talking) is the activity most likely to meet the needs of the patients.

As interviews cited earlier show us, the patient should be allowed to take the lead in conversation, but it can be initiated with questions or comments about his family, the pictures or floral arrangements at his bedside, or his past work, interests, hobbies, and special talents. No topic should be avoided that the patient wishes to talk about, and nonverbal communications are important indices of concern (Cassini 1974).

If the patient introduces the subject of dying into the conversation, he wants to talk about it and hopes staff or family will listen. He is more likely to initiate such a conversation, and to confide in some people than others; whom he chooses may depend on how he feels about the person, but also on the person's ability to listen to conversation about dying without uttering pseudoreassuring clichés. Often the listener will be tested first with some obtuse statement; the patient will not indicate explicitly what is on his mind (Cassini 1974).

However, if the patient wishes to talk, he will give some kind of signal. Ambiguities, ambivalences, trailing sentences, discrepancies between verbal and nonverbal communication are all cues to a listening ear. If signals are picked up gently, he may talk. When he gives such signals and then does not talk, it may mean the listener failed to pick up on cues, or responded too strongly.

Questions should be responded to as simply, and as honestly and positively as possible; false reassurance avoided. The patient can be invited to talk about himself and his feelings through open-ended questions that are related to his initial remarks and concerns. If he talks about death, *listen.* The nurse is not really expected to have any answers or to expound any philosophy or beliefs. If she answers from a feeling of concern and interest, it will be difficult to say anything wrong. Attention should be focused on the patient; listening to him will convey that his concerns have meaning to staff, and in turn, he will feel a sense of esteem and hope. If he cannot or does not talk about his feelings, he can be helped to reduce tension and depression through other means — crying, physical activity, or sublimative activities such as in occupational therapy.

Although nurses are encouraged in their education and by the literature to talk with the dying person, or to encourage him to talk if he seems reticent, some patients do not talk about their concerns and give every evidence to a warm but persistent nurse that they do not want to talk about death. Such reticence may reflect a person who is shy under all circumstances; who is self-contained, and has accepted death; or who is trying to deny or exclude perceptions and thoughts from his mind. Getting a patient to talk as an end in itself may constitute an unnecessary intrusion into the person's right to privacy and dignity. Nursing the quiet patient necessitates acceptance of his silence. The nurse must be able to relax, be at ease, and sit silently. The individual may speak in erratic spurts, especially about a difficult subject; it is necessary to listen closely for small clues. Repeating or restating what is said in order to clarify his perception — and the listener's own — is useful. The nurse can convey that she is trying to understand what the patient is perceiving, thinking, and conveying; the use of touch conveys caring in a nonverbal manner, although this, too, should not be an indiscriminate intervention (Stackman 1973).

Evans (1971) provides support for the importance of the factors addressed in the professional literature when she describes the months her husband was dying. She speaks of the fears, anxieties, and questions which are so much a part of the family of the patient that it is hard for them to realize that the medical personnel do not realize what they are. She contends that medical personnel offer no information or support unless they are directly asked, and identifies the need for more empathic, involved caring by staff, more flexibility with rules, and constant attention to the expression of hope when facts are presented. The hospital experience and the indignities that accompany it are described. The family and patient need to be perceived as living people; the person with the terminal diagnosis is still living and should not be mourned too soon by the medical personnel or the family. The few genuinely caring doctors, nurses, and friends are recalled vividly and were essential for support during the crises to both the family and the patient (as was demonstrated in our interviews with patients). The line between denial and hope is slim; hope is essential. She describes how hope — the patient's wanting to live, and returning to the home setting, and being surrounded by loving family — kept her husband living for months longer than was predicted.

Nurses need to know what the doctor has told the patient in order to assess the patient's immediate reaction, what he actually remembers, and what he wants to be told. When nurses do not know what the patient was told or knows, they become defensive, do not wish to talk with the patient, and avoid him.

Too often the nurse must infer from the patient's behavior what he knows and wants to know in order to explore with him what his condition means to him. The patient may be suspicious about his condition but unwilling to confirm his suspicions unless he has pain, disability, obvious lesions, severe symptoms, a family history of the same illness, or specialized medical treatment. Sometimes the patient resists all efforts to talk about any aspect of his condition because of a natural reticence or a desire to proceed with tacit communication. For such a patient, the advantages of not being explicit are that his condition can be denied or seem less real; others cannot react to something that remains unspoken and anxiety is less high. Tacit communication can be successful in that the patient is grateful for being spared the emotional pain of discussing his fate or of losing face by being forced to react in a manner that conflicts with his self-concept. Trust and respect for the nurses are strengthened when the nurse understands the patient well enough without relying on verbal communication. Tacit communication preserves the "as if" quality of the patient's life without interfering with the relationship.

Sometimes the patient who doesn't say much verbally is honest within himself in the privacy of his own mind, although he appears to staff to be denying. He intuitively senses that once members of the medical staff present him with clear, undiluted prognostic details, therapeutic efforts may be considered to be meaningless because they are aimed at a lost cause. Even the patient who is most honest with himself nurtures some tiny seed of hope (Verwoerdt and Wilson 1967).

Patients like nurses to talk with them if the nurse is a good listener, if the patient is ready to talk, if he gets information he wants, or if he gets a message to his doctor. Patients do not like talking with nurses when they feel forced to talk regardless of whether they feel like it; if nurses use only nonreflective conversation, which is boring; when nurses encourage patients to talk about their troubles, all at one time, and then never reappear; or when nurses interrupt or cut off conversations when patients try to talk.

To be accountable for conversation, and to evaluate the effects, nurses must have continuity of contact with their patients (Benoliel 1970). Patients can benefit from purposeful conversation with a truly listening nurse in many ways. When they can talk about their feelings with such a nurse they are better able to cope with them. They can feel supported in dealing with their problems. The nurse who will raise questions and give honest feedback can serve as a sounding board for the patient faced with difficult decisions, problems, and concerns. She can support patients as they manifest self-pity, guilt, and hostility because families do not do more, or because staff are to be blamed for threatening behavior.

Nurses who have developed stereotypes about what constitutes a "good patient" do not serve as nonjudgmental, therapeutic listeners. If the patient talks about death, the nurse should answer with open-ended questions so that he continues talking. Talking to a quiet listener will help him to work through his feelings. Again, no answers are expected, and for the nurse to admit she does not have one is supportive. The patient will decide how much and what he wishes to discuss. He may wish to do a life review, to talk about phases of his life, or what has meaning for him. He needs assurance that his life — and therefore his death — has meaning; that he had a contribution to make, that he made an impact. Family can be involved in this conversation. If the patient expresses regret about his life, the nurse must listen without correction or judgment. His confession of misdeeds, whether real or imagined, allows him to express his feelings about his past and to right things in his own mind.

If it is not possible to talk with the patient when he first mentions his concerns or questions, he should be informed the nurse will return, and approximately when. On the return to his bedside, she should refer back to his earlier comments, indicating a willingness to talk about his ideas and feelings at this time.

Nurses become "significant others" to patients for different reasons: as a function of time spent with the patient; when there is no family available; and to some extent as a function of basic personality structure. Self-disclosure is easier for some than it is for others, and both nurse and patient must endure self-disclosure in meaningful discussion of death. It may be that before the "professional exchange" (Schneidman 1978) can occur, the parties to the exchange must each become significant to the other. Staff who are most comfortable in a less personal relationship may find it difficult to give good nursing care to the dying.

Weisman (1972) points out that even experienced psychotherapists find themselves withdrawing from the presence of imminent death, despite efforts to remain in contact. The threat of annihilation is too great, the sights and smells are too unpleasant, and the atmosphere of hopelessness and helplessness are too distressing. Nurses remain, to the best of their ability, and nursing measures are enhanced by Weisman's reminders for the therapist:

1. Accept the terminal patient according to what he would be like without the disease so that he is not seen as the disease or lesion.

2. Encourage him to talk about how the illness has changed him.

3. Ask about him, his possessions and the pursuits that seem to be meaningful still.

4. Preserve his self-esteem by the way you communicate.

5. Monitor your own feelings — denial, apathy, fear. Elicit key persons for their support.

6. Convey acceptance, clear communication, candor, compassion, and accessibility to make the patient feel safe in the relationship.

7. Do not insist on talking about death or underscore the gloom of illness; however, do not persist with empty optimism.

8. Include the patient in decisions about his illness and give him information.

9. Help the survivors to accept the inevitable death.

Whatever guidelines are accepted, lay and professional authors are agreed as to the major impact of honest and compassionate communication with the dying patient.

REASSURANCE

A relatively long time can pass between a person's first distinct awareness of the certainty of his own death and the point at which he actually enters a dying course. Buehler (1975), who studied patients with cancer, points out that after the initial shock of learning of the diagnosis of cancer, the patient begins reading social and physical cues regarding the illness that tell him whether he is improving, on a plateau, or deteriorating.

Two major classes of cues affected the patients interviewed in the Buehler study: hopeful cues and nondying trajectory cues. Hopeful cues — as well as the lack of dying-trajectory cues — that are presented explicitly or implicitly have a strong and positive impact on patient attitudes toward the disease and the prognosis. Most of the 124 patients in Buehler's study who were receiving radiation therapy at two medical centers did not perceive their futures as threatening. Rather, they vacillated between doubt and hope.

Sources of doubt included new and unexpected symptoms, any additional or unexpected stressor related to treatment, financial concerns, or the temporary absence of the doctor. When the source of stress was relieved, so were the doubts. Hopeful cues included direct statements by the medical personnel of "We can help you"; the patient being encouraged by the personnel to join the battle in fighting the cancer (to be in control and actively involved in treatment and aligned with the doctors and nurses against the disease); being treated at a leading medical center; and the hopeful attitudes of the staff.

Staff generally felt they should foster feelings of hope and cheer in the patients, ignore or combat patient depression, and maintain a positive attitude all of the time. They emphasized that treatment of cancer is more effective than ever, the importance of team approach to treatment and research, and the increased survival rates for specific diseases. In this staff, positive attitudes by staff and patient were emphasized because the hopeful patient is more cooperative and easier to care for, better tolerates stresses of treatment, is less depressing for staff to be around, and can serve as an inspiration to staff. Staff hopes seemed more derived from global statistical success rates than personal knowledge of patients they had treated; Buehler believed that this glowing generality might function as a buffer when they encounter patients who are deteriorating and dying.

Hopeful patients contribute to their own treatment by remaining optimistic, tolerating side-effects of treatment in a more accepting manner, making fewer emotional demands on staff (which enables staff to conserve energy that would be needed for cheering up the patients and each other), serving as models for other patients, and acting as a source of hope for staff.

Staff saw their function as providing improvement for patients rather than the managing of dying. They did not give cues that could be interpreted as indications of ensuing death. Responsibility for managing dying after the radiation therapy course was shifted from the staff at the medical center back to the local physician or to the center's oncology unit.

Four conditions which existed in this study and which influenced the hopeful attitudes of the patients were:

1. Patients were in active treatment, which temporarily forestalls longer-range concern about the future.

2. Patients were surrounded by staff with a strongly manifested hope ideology.

3. Patients believed the medical center had superior treatment capabilities.

4. Patients had a built-in rationalization for symptoms associated with their disease: symptoms were the consequences of the treatment.

Ashby (1975) suggests that the refusal to die or to accept the partial death of helplessness is the motivation or factor that keeps patients alive when all the odds are medically against their living. Patients who remain confident and determined in spite of severe illness or hazardous surgery often live for many more years than predicted by the doctors. On the other hand, patients who give up the will to live or who cannot imagine themselves as continuing to live will die, without clear medical cause. Usually the underlying feeling is hopelessness, helplessness, or extreme submission. Experiments in a wide variety of animals in the laboratory as well as numerous case histories indicate that a perception of helplessness can induce depression, shock, inability to function, and death.

What can be done to prevent loss of will to live? Understanding and comfort from friends and relatives are most important. Teaching people to recognize early signs of hopelessness and despair in themselves could help. The relationship that the nurse establishes with the patient can become highly significant because the nurse can help the patient to realize that he is welcome in the world, giving him something to live for.

Persons fearful or angry about their imminent deaths are more likely to survive longer than predicted by their doctors than are persons who are less frightened or more resigned to death. Long-term survivors are frequently angry about their situation and become more angry and resentful as the death nears. These patients are cooperative with staff, friends, and relatives. Short-term survivors tend to reach out or wish for death and become depressed near death (Braden 1975).

However, even with the evidence that individual survival is not so predictable as the statistical rate, staff are seldom in a position to reassure the patient that he *will not die.* They are always in a position to assure him that death *may* not come to him as soon as might be expected. The real area of staff reassurance, however, lies not in the prediction of the event or the time of death, but in a very real ability to support the patient through the dying process. The fears of the dying have been well identified by many investigators. Cassini (1974) lists being left alone to die, abandoned; having unbearable pain; being disfigured; losing independence; and losing sanity. While staff cannot assure the patient that his family will remain constant, they can offer themselves as surrogates. This will involve some emotional involvement by the professional with the dying patient; it is necessary for reassurance to the patient that he will not be abandoned. However, feeling interest in and compassion for the patient does not mean that other tasks are neglected. These tasks are also accomplished efficiently, carefully, thoroughly, and effectively — but the patient may be helped by knowing that the person caring for him is capable of emotion as well as efficiency.

As there is now some evidence that very little pain is intractable, patients can be reassured that they will not suffer physical pain. Other physical symptoms (e.g., nausea, vomiting, dyspnea, dysphagia) are not so well controlled, particularly in patients with cancer who are receiving chemotherapy or radiation. However, attentive staff can tend and support patients through the worst of these symptoms, keeping the final hope of remission alive. Disfigurement is not in the control of nursing staff; the appropriate reassurance in this instance is staff perception that physical disfigurement does not detract from the *person*, and that staff will not avoid the patient because he is disfigured. Fears of loss of independence and loss of sanity can be addressed by staff attitudes: that staff do not demean, do not judge, and do not abandon. As these fears of the dying patient are examined, it becomes obvious that the major nursing reassurance is that the patient will not be abandoned or avoided, and that disfigurement, dependence, and confusion will not drive the staff away. It is perhaps the only reassurance which is wholly within the power of nurses to give, as pain medication and other medical treatments depend on physician directives and nurses cannot control family behavior (although they may "persuade"), and in the course of disease the patient may indeed become dependent, confused, and disfigured. Nursing staff, however, can promise to stay with the patient in spite of these events, and continue with the nursing care.

There is one further reassurance that staff may or may not be willing to provide: the information that there is some empirical evidence that death, when it comes, brings happiness (Woodward 1976, p. 41).

Various researchers are reporting experiences with dying patients which indicate life after death. Patients who appear dead on arrival at the emergency room or in an intensive-care unit but who are resuscitated sometimes later describe the experience and what they recall when their bodies were apparently lifeless.

> *The patient feels himself rushing through a long, dark tunnel while noise rings in his ears. Suddenly he finds himself outside his own body, looking down with curious detachment at a medical team's efforts to resuscitate him. He hears what is said, notes what is happening, but cannot communicate with anyone. Soon his attention is drawn to other presences in the room — spirits of dead relatives or friends — who communicate with him nonverbally. Gradually he is drawn to a vague "being of light." This*

being invites him to evaluate his life and shows him highlights of his past in panoramic vision. The patient longs to stay with the being of light but is reluctantly drawn back into his physical body and recovers. (Woodward 1976, p. 41)

Psychiatrists are beginning to study these near-death experiences rather than dismissing them as hallucinations or delusions because an increasing number of patients are being resuscitated and reporting similar experiences afterwards. However, whether patients' religious or philosophical beliefs about life after death bring comfort during the time of dying is, again, not in the control of nurses. What nurses can provide in the way of reassurance is nonjudgmental attitudes, whatever the behavior of the patient, and the promise that good physical care and emotional support as possible will be provided until the end.

THERAPEUTIC PRESENCE

Kavanaugh (1974, p. 10) says that the "continued presence of a special someone who dares to walk the edge with us . . . [a] concerned confidante can help the patient remain in touch with reality." Although this section is concerned with the therapeutic effects of the mere presence of the nurse, it is a mistake to believe that nurses can or should assume the responsibility for the role identified by Kavanaugh. Nurses have many patients, and care activities other than "continued presence" must be done for dying patients. To be a special someone and only a continued presence does not utilize the skills of nursing. When the patient has no other confidante, nurses may serve in that role, but it is not the primary nursing responsibility. It is important to delineate limits here, and to do so without apology. Nurses *must* care for bodily needs, and should do this in such a way that patient self-esteem is supported. But they should not feel guilty if they are unable to "walk along the edge." They may not have the time, the skill, or the strength to do so, and certainly not the love for each dying patient that this role requires.

However, with equal certainty, it is part of the nursing responsibility to remain with dying patients when they are needed, and to add to the care they give some offering of themselves. When some portion of the self is part of the nursing care package, the presence of the nurse becomes therapeutic. The comfort of the patient — rather than his cure — is the treatment goal, and this requires a continued regular and interested presence. Compassion need not interfere with competence, although it should always be clear that no one person should have to deal with all aspects of the dying process (Kavanaugh 1974). As suggested earlier, attentive listening helps the patient clarify feelings, express them, and become calmer, less depressed, and more restful. The patient and nurse can then search together for understanding that will be meaningful to the patient, to help him feel less alone. If the patient senses that someone else thinks his death is important, he can better grasp the importance of his approaching death. Returning to the patient to give care, to talk, to sit, and to listen tells the patient that he and his approaching death are indeed important.

One must first grant the individual autonomy to choose the specific path he feels he can take, as the nurse's presence is not therapeutic if the patient prefers her absence. As the relationship continues it is strengthened by the sense of support felt by the patient. Through this suppport the nurse validates over and over again the patient's sense of worth. This sense or worth can be aided by encouraging the patient to enumerate in detail those things that are valuable to him and to verbalize feelings of anger and frustration that diminish a sense of worth.

In a hospital environment most patients look to doctors and nurses to do the reaching out, to take the risk of caring. Instead, too many ill people find themselves ground down by detachment, by grim adherence to antiquated rules and procedures. Some judicious ignoring of the rules may be necessary for staff to carry out the somewhat tenuous therapy of "presence." Family and friends may be more therapeutic than staff, and should be encouraged to remain (if it is the wish of the patient) in spite of the rules. However, for many patients, staff are the only visitors. When this is the case, sufficient time should be spent with the dying patient to preserve his self-esteem and convey that staff members care and are available. It is not always necessary to spend 30 or 60 minutes at a time with him; indeed, 10 minutes focused completely on the patient and his concerns may actually better meet his needs, as he will feel less fatigued physically after the interaction. Frequent, short visits emphasize staff availability and concern, and indicate that he and his approaching death are important to them. During the short visits he should be given the opportunity to say as little or as much as he can for that time. Intense feelings cannot always come forth all at once. However, when the patient has much to say all at once, staff should be prepared to spend more time in one visit. Often listening can be combined with giving physical care. Planned, attentive listening helps the patient to clarify his feelings, and has the added virtue of usually reducing his demands or his manipulative, angry behavior (Wygant 1967).

While ideally activities with dying patients should *not* be postponed, when staff cannot remain longer than 10 minutes because of the needs of other patients they may do one of several things. First, they must be honest with the patient and say why they cannot stay. They may offer to return later, telling him that they want to hear what he has to say if he can wait. An offer to call another team member to whom he also feels close can be made, or the offer to bring a tape recorder, so that staff may later listen and respond. The more verbal person, or one who is interested in machines, may not feel intimidated by talking into a machine and may appreciate the interest in having his thoughts and feelings saved. He may find recording and listening to the recording to be very therapeutic. Sometimes saying things aloud is enough to release tension, promote problem-solving, encourage decision-making, or foster self-acceptance. However, if staff are very important to the patient, or if he is intimidated by the taping equipment, he may choose to wait until the nurse can return.

The offer of the tape recorder may help the patient feel that his reminiscing, his words of counsel, or his life review are important enough to save — not only for later staff response but also for loved ones to keep. The patient who fears what his future may hold, who is concerned about what will happen to certain family members, who wants a memory of him to remain, or who does not believe in immortality may feel reassured by having the opportunity to say what is important, knowing that if the family did not really understand the first time, they can rehear it. Some persons may prefer writing or art work as the medium of communication rather than the tape recorder, but a therapeutic presence can be provided in the absence of family or staff.

Koenig (1973) suggests that broad encouragement or false, generalized reassurance do not help the patient. Current life problems may not be resolved, but they can be circumvented by the staff — if they know of them — to help him make the best of the present. Emotional support, which is time consuming, must be based on an understanding of past and current troubles so that specific needs of each patient can be met. If the nurse is unable to do this, she should get someone who can. However, the recurring conflicts in a patient's life are not usually obscure. With good rapport, and continued interaction the patient will reveal the basic issues of the conflict in a conversation. He probably does not need or want the painful, prolonged process of confrontation and insight psychotherapy. Techniques of positive reinforcement and support can be done by nurses and be more comforting than reiterating old crises or adding to feelings of disappointment and failure. The dying patient is especially receptive to overt affection and attentive ministrations.

The experience of being *cared for* may benefit the patient more than the direct effects of *medical care*. Additionally, the staff feel gratified because they feel they are doing something to help the patient feel better. The relationship is a soothing source of comfort to the patient and nurse; neither feel as hopeless and frustrated as if nothing can be done.

The nurse should approach the dying patient from the perspective of the current situation — today's routines, joys, and problems; dying is secondary. If the nurse believes the patient is troubled by the anxieties of annihilation, she can do nothing, for death will eventually come. If the nurse believes she can help the patient face the fears and anxieties of the moment, she can accept the chronic depression or anxiety typical of the terminally ill person, and remain with him to do what she can.

If hope is synonymous with cure, the patient and nurse will despair. If hope is related to the day-by-day feelings of promoting comfort and *being available* to the patient, then the nurse can structure the relationship accordingly (Koenig 1973).

Nurses must resist the temptation to take advantage of patient's kindness or their own denial through the fantasy of "we've done all we could." The patient's greatest need is the continuing relationship, and identification with staff leads to expectations by patients of a certain attention and continuity of care.

Benoliel (1972) has identified at least five types of contacts between nurses and patients facing death: (1) the patient is definitely in need of terminal nursing care and requires direct physical ministrations or assistance in matters of daily living; (2) the patient is facing death but is given life-prolonging and sometimes intensive care to promote recovery, so that comfort is relegated to a secondary position; (3) the patient may be given less dramatic intensive care because the period of dying tends to be slow, as with cancer or neurological diseases, and these patients are in and out of the hospital several times before they enter for the final time (these patients may be socially dead through partial or complete loss of brain activity but are kept biologically alive through life-prolonging machinery); (4) the patient needs immediate emergency care because of an accident, or mass or natural disaster, and the reality of unexpected and sudden death is present and families are in early stages of grief; (5) the patient has a chronic and life-threatening disease and is at various stages of incapacitation and thus needs help in coping with psychological and physical problems imposed by long-term illness. Adaptation to all chronic illness involves grieving in patient and family, so that the nurse is always in contact with this experience.

Because working with dying persons is emotionally taxing for nurses, withdrawal from personal involvement and frequent interaction with patients may function as a protective mechanism. For some personnel, the psychological strain comes from almost continuous exposure to the lingering process of dying. For others, the stress comes from conflicting demands of recovery care and comfort care in settings in which loss of the patient is sometimes tantamount to personal failure. Further stress comes from the threat to self-esteem posed by the behaviors of other people under stress — patients, families, doctors, other nurses. Stress is compounded when communication between medical and nursing staffs is strained or limited, when doctors withdraw, and when patient and family have not been told the truth. All of these conditions threaten the use of merely remaining with the patient as a technique of therapy.

In an effort to combat the multiple problems, Benoliel (1970) suggests that a systems-oriented approach must be used to provide personalized nursing care for patients facing death so that *continuity* of care is provided a large number of people. A systems approach would be concerned with the psychosocial environment of the institution as a whole and depends upon interdisciplinary cooperation. The group rather than one-to-one approach must be considered.

Personalized care means that each patient has: (1) continuity of contact with at least one person who is interested in him as a human being; (2) opportunity for active involvement in social living and to the extent he is able; and (3) confidence and trust in those who are providing his care.

The goals of such nursing care include: (1) to help the patient with activities he would carry out unaided if he were able to do so; (2) to reduce stresses for patient and family resulting from the illness; (3) to develop the nurse-patient relationship while giving intimate physical care in order to convey caring, dignity of person, importance of the person; (4) to carry out principles of crisis intervention with the grieving family and the patient; and (5) to give relief of pain and freedom from anxiety.

Benoliel (1970) believes that personalized care during terminal illness is the exception rather than the rule for many reasons:

1. Personalized care depends on *continuity* of contact with at least one concerned person; institutional care is given by groups of staff and work is organized to minimize emotional involvement that may be disruptive to the social order.

2. Systematic accountability for psychosocial components of patient care is lacking in most institutions. Some nurses on their own quietly help dying patients and their families cope with emotional and social problems, but they are not in the majority.

3. Lack of authority in institutions to carry out patient care frustrates or prevents the use of the nurse's knowledge and skill on behalf of the dying patient.

4. Work done in hospitals and nursing homes is a direct reflection of society. Social rewards go to nurses engaged in recovery care; the highest rewards go to nurses in intensive-care settings. Terminal care has low status and is often done by lower-echelon workers.

5. The patient suffers social deprivation and a fragmented experience because of the low value on and lack of organized approach to meeting psychosocial needs.

Meyerowitz (1974) maintains that the fear of dying is the fear of abandonment. Whether or not all of the goals of personalized nursing care can be met by staff caring for dying patients, that fear can be alleviated. The nurse can make herself available to the dying patient during physical care and at other times as well, and refrain from the rationalization that the patient wants to be left alone. The patient needs to know someone cares, is interested in him, and will listen if he wants to talk, or will remain quietly if he wishes only to have someone with him.

THERAPEUTIC USE OF FAMILIES

Appendix E (q.v.) outlines the many dimensions of a family's response to a loved one's death. In the context of strategies of care, families must themselves be supported through the dying and death of the patient and at the same time be encouraged to provide comfort and support to the patient. In the institution they are not at home; thus they cannot (or will not) carry out activities with the patient that are supportive to both unless they are encouraged by staff to do so. The presence of the nurse is at best a substitute for the presence of the family; patients are more likely to find comfort and hope in the inexpert ministrations of family members than in the most skilled nursing care. Nurses who specialize in the care of children have been aware of the fact that they must nurse the patient (the child) through the significant other (the parent) and are not uncomfortable doing so. Maternity nurses are more lately made aware of the need to support the patient (the woman in labor) through the significant other (mother or husband), but are beginning to be able to do this. The care of the dying, however, is carried out by nurses who identify with a medical-surgical nursing speciality, and the family has traditionally been excluded from rather than included in their activities.

Families, however, can be a major source of strength to the dying patient, and should be utilized as such by staff. This requires assessment of family relationships. If the patient was in a pivotal position — as a leader in the family, or as the main scapegoat for their problems — the balance of the family system is threatened. The change in role affects family work, leisure, interactions, and self-gratification now and in the future. If one family member is dying, some other family members may have to give up their own sick-role behaviors. Dependency needs are threatened because the emotional or financial support given by the dying person to the family is no longer available. The family may identify with the patient, or they may resent having to directly care for him and deal with the many emotional, physical, financial, and family stresses related to his illness. The patient's care needs, his immobility, his personality characteristics may evoke hostility and aggressive behavior. If he was hard to live with, the family may be eager for him to die, and feel a sense of triumph at his helplessness; they may even be abusive verbally or physically. If the patient does not cooperate, fails to adhere to treatment, was accustomed to and continues to demand indulgence, or complains constantly about neglect or unfulfilled ambitions, his family may refuse to care for him at home or to visit him in the institution. Aggressive family reactions, may, however, be redirected into the mechanism of reaction formation — that is, the family may show excessive concern for the patient because aggressive reactions may cause them to feel guilt. As the family care for the patient they may develop an emotional isolation, as the lack of emotional expression may help them to do the necessary but unpleasant tasks required.

While the patient may prefer to die at home, the family may not be willing or able to handle this. Hospitalization may be a function of family needs. Although an extended family may provide a wide network of support and may be willing to help, the members of the nuclear family may feel very alone, perceiving no real support from the extended family or community (Maddison and Raphael 1972).

In working with family members, nonverbal behavior and the general demeanor of the staff often give more support (or convey lack of support) than do words. If families are to help patients, *their* concerns must be addressed by staff. Superficial cheerfulness or suggestions that they try to forget and to think of something else are certainly to be avoided. A family is going to lose someone they care for, or are, at the least, used to. They need to be approached with kindness, respect, courtesy, and gentleness.

If the patient has many visitors, the family may need help in working out a visiting schedule so that neither family nor patient becomes fatigued. Obviously the family cannot become actively involved in the patient's therapy without the encouragement of the staff, and equally obviously such involvement is likely to be beneficial to both family and patient. However, staff must be cautioned against unrealistic expectations. No relative is able to provide daily devoted care for weeks and months without some relief, and family may become willing to leave the patient before he is willing to be left.

Staff must be willing, and find the time, to listen to family if they complain about the care or state positive or negative feelings about the patient. They should be allowed to express guilt if they wish. Staff should state honestly what helpful things they have accomplished, when they feel they should be doing more. Global reassurances are not helpful. If a family member expresses dislike of the patient, or eagerness for him to die, staff can listen without chastising, and acknowledge that his feelings are real to them and that blood relatives do not necessarily love each other.

Staff can give the family some idea about how to talk to the dying person, especially about death, if they express a wish to do so. Nurses who have worked through their own feelings can help the family through denial or avoidances.

His family is important to the patient's sense of identity and emotional health, and should not be hampered by rigid visiting hours. Families who wish to participate in care should be allowed to do so. They may help with feeding, or bathing the patient; fluffing the pillow, wiping his face, holding the arm with the intravenous tubing in it; this may allow them to show their love or compensate for their sense of frustration, helplessness, or guilt. Often the family can persuade the patient to eat when no one else can; they are willing and able to go slowly, to talk during the meal, or to bring in favorite foods. What the family says to or does with the patient may seem strange and nontherapeutic to the staff, but it may be a part of a comforting family pattern; thus staff should not interfere unless the family is doing something unsafe or obviously annoying to the patient.

It is necessary, however, that staff recognize when family members are fatigued or anxious, and relieve them from care activities at that point and encourage them to rest and meet their own needs for support and care. A lounge where the family can rest, and yet be near to the patient should be part of any hospital; it is particularly required when patients are dying. Out-of-town visitors may need, and should receive, special consideration or help in finding meals and lodging.

Staff should accept — and help the family to accept and understand — the mourning process, and the necessity to express their grief in whatever ways they can. In some cultures, the dying person is comforted by the family's expression of grief directly to him. For other families, privacy is sought for grieving, and should be provided in the institution.

Information should be provided daily of the patient's status and the family prepared for sudden changes in his condition or appearance so that they feel less shocked or overwhelmed when walking into his room.

News of impending or actual death is best conveyed to the family unit rather than to a lone individual, in order to allow the people involved to give each other mutual support. The message should be given in a private area so that they may express grief in whatever ways are appropriate to them. A staff member should stay with them as long as necessary, and, if required, help with decision-making, with initial plans with a mortician, or even arrange for transportation of the family members to the home of a neighbor or friend. Even when death is expected, an aging or lone family member may feel overwhelmed, be confused, or be unable to engage in logical thinking when the death actually occurs. The most beneficial aid that can be given at this time is help with immediate plans, and extending the advice that major decisions regarding lifestyle of the survivors be delayed for at least a month after the death of the family member (Clayton et al. 1971).

During the time when the patient is disengaging himself from them and the world, staff must be prepared to explain the process to the family and to give extra support, to help them remain in communication through short visits, touch, and caring silence.*

The crisis of the death may result in other life crises for the family. Living routines and arrangements may be hard to change. Role reversals, the assumption of extra responsibilities, fatigue from caring for a loved one for a long time, working with other family members without the guidance or support of the patient, change in responsibilities and leisure activities, or meeting financial obligations can seem overwhelming. Failure of relatives and friends to help, or their insistence upon helping or giving unneeded advice, are equally burdensome. The nursing responsibility extends to listening, to exploring with them how to cope with new demands, or encouraging them to seek help from other persons or agencies. Such behavior on the part of institutional staff may be enough to help the family mobilize their strengths to work together and cope with remaining problems (Hampe 1975).

Another point bears emphasis: isolation is experienced by the patient when family and friends relate differently to him because he is dying from a terminal illness. They may no longer share with him conversation about the near or distant future, crises or problems at home, current troubles on the job, or problems about the illness. Talk becomes superficial, stilted, narrow, and lacks spontaneity (Koenig 1973). Too, the patient who is facing physical and social dependency may reactivate unresolved problems in personal relationships with others. Tensions may increase between the patient and his family, causing quarrels or withdrawal. A breakdown in communication causes the patient to feel abandoned and to experience a sense of loss of personal control over the decisions about how daily living and dying will be managed. Institutionalization, of course, represents to the patient—and perhaps to the family—an extreme loss of control.

Problems Faced by Family Members

Family must cope with major changes in role responsibilities; they frequently are unprepared for how to behave with the dying. Often old established rituals between family members and between family and patient no longer exist as markers of social reality and personal confirmations. They may lack support systems to help them adapt to maintaining investment in the future of the sick person while at the same time preparing for his death through anticipatory mourning. The family must maintain a sense of mastery and control while coming to terms with the disease. The patient concurrently faces the task of integrating the losses and physical changes produced by his illness into a new definition of self while fulfilling his potentialities for life.

Prolonged illness can also make excessive demands on financial and social resources of the family. Vocational plans, educational ambitions, established

---

*Sometimes the patient has no surviving family members or friends, or they do not come to visit. In this situation, staff become family-surrogates.

marital and parent–child relationships, financial stability, and overall lifestyle are disrupted (Benoliel 1978).

Relatives' acceptance of a forthcoming death may relate to how advanced they are in their grieving. The family may have worked through their grief by the time the patient dies if the patient has lingered.

Staff may help families decide when and how long to visit and how much they can get involved in the patient's care. Staff must also become comfortable carrying out routine procedures in the presence of family members; they must remain tactful and calm even if the family are defensive, imply neglect of their loved one, appear overanxious, make many demands about the patient's care, or are expressive in their grief. Families should never be allowed to feel that they are in the way.

Just as staff may have problems with the family, the family may feel they have problems with the staff because they wish to remain with the patient, help with comfort measures, or say their final farewells or take a final look at him.

The patient, rather than the family, is more likely to be the center of the staff's attention, unless he is comatose, or nearly so; but nurses often are the major listeners, supporters, and comforters of the relatives during the final days even though social workers and chaplains may also involve themselves with the family in their grief work. Emphasis on the mourning process has been so great in the past few years that the professional may deliberately pace the family through the process according to all the stages described in the literature, rather than letting the family proceed at their own pace. This "pushing through" the mourning process (according to preset theory) is probably as detrimental as giving no help at all with the grief work.

Hampe's (1975) study of the spouses of dying patients is a rich source of information. She found that spouses could recognize their own needs, but felt that their needs were not met because the nurses were too busy to help them. They felt that although the nurses' primary responsibility was to the dying patient, they also needed acceptance, comfort, and support from the caregivers. They identified needs to be with the patient, to be helpful to him, to be assured that he will be kept as comfortable as possible, to be kept informed of his condition, and to be made aware of impending death.

Because health professionals feel frustrated in the face of death, they may avoid the dying person and his family — so that less care may be given because the nurse is not with the patient long enough to assess his needs adequately. Family members may then attempt to take over care and comfort measures that may satisfy their need to care for the person — to *do* something for him — but in the process become emotionally drained.

The spouses in Hampe's study were likely to associate cleanliness and order in the patient's room with the comfort of the patient; good grooming and hygiene measures — along with an attractive environment — do help the dying person to maintain his body image, but this comfort was not provided to the majority of the dying patients.

Health professionals did not enter the room of the dying patient as often when the spouse was present as when the patient was alone, which could encourage the patient to turn to the spouse for emotional support and for help with physical comfort needs. This did allow the spouse to come to terms with the impending loss of the mate and preserved the husband-wife relationship. Most spouses (90 percent) had accepted the forthcoming death of their mates. Family members communicated differently with nurses than with physicians, expecting the two groups to deal differently with health problems. Physicians were expected to inform the family about the patient's diagnosis, prognosis, and medical treatment plan. Nurses were expected to inform them of day-to-day progress.

The need to be kept informed of the mate's condition was not met adequately. When the family is aware of the patient's terminal condition, their need to be informed about his condition intensifies, and demands for information increase.

The grieving person is helped to begin to accept his loss when he can ventilate his feelings, but few of the spouses in Hampe's (1975) study were given an opportunity to express feelings. The hospital environment and the staff offered little opportunity for privacy to express or explore feelings. In addition, physicians and nurses were perceived as too busy to be concerned with the spouse's difficulties. They did, however, report appreciation of the health professionals who did become involved.

The family remained central to the patient, and the function of the family members appeared to be to distract the spouse from his grief. Most family members encouraged stoic acceptance of the forthcoming death. As both spouse and the dying patient have needs to share feelings with another person to alleviate loneliness and isolation, it is not surprising that 10 out of the 26 couples shared in both giving and receiving emotional support.

Spouses in Hampe's study could not differentiate a registered nurse from a licensed practical nurse—as was common in our own study. They appeared to look the same and to do the same things. Personalized nursing care is considered by many nurses to be a function that distinguishes nursing from medical care, yet from the viewpoint of the grieving spouse personalized nursing care of the mate was the exception rather than the rule. Nurses were perceived as helpful and concerned about the spouses and were considered to be the ones to do the technical tasks prescribed by the doctor. The nurses were expected to be courteous and efficient. Emotional support for the spouse or his mate was not expected, nor was it perceived as given.

In another report of family support of the dying patient, Driver (1978) explains how she and her husband tried to humanize the hospital environment during his many admissions because of leukemia. Their actions included initiating friendly conversation with the medical and nursing staff (reaching out emotionally until they responded with open conversation and empathy) and bringing in posters for the walls, rugs for the floor, an FM set, and an electric skillet and dishes to cook their own food at times. The wife remained with the husband in his room throughout each hospitalization, sleeping on a cot, bathing and caring for him, and cleaning the room to reduce the number of personnel coming into the room. She brought the children in to visit periodically — although hospital rules forbade visiting — because she felt her husband should die as he lived, surrounded by his loved ones. Most significantly her presence often prevented errors in treatment, such as placing him in a ward with pneumonia patients when chemotherapy had reduced his white blood count, and stopping an interne from giving an intramuscular medication intravenously.

Two things are clear; families can be therapeutic for dying patients, and in order for families to be utilized as therapeutic influences, changes in priorities of nursing care within hospitals are imperative. Traditionally organized work routines must be reorganized. Nurses must be freed to care for emotional and physical needs of patients and emotional support needs of family members as well as the patient's immediate environment.

Nurses

The nurses in the institution who are caring for dying persons seem — in order to function — to develop a psychic closing off, a distance between the experiences of the death of others and their own personal relationship to death. There is evidence to suggest that most dying patients want to share their dying experience with others, but staff are likely to become distraught at this suggestion and denounce as inhumane those who talk with the dying about their death. To try to understand and to work with those who are dying invokes intense personal feelings. It is unrealistic for family or staff to expect only positive attitudes in themselves or in others toward the dying person. The stress of dying does not automatically make people pleasant. Some dying individuals are likeable, and some are not. Staff wish to relate to some patients, and not to others; the death of some patients causes feelings of sorrow, and there is only relief at the death of others. It is important to recognize and accept the range of feelings as they may affect interactions with family members. Similarly, professional caregivers must also recognize the phenomenon of death saturation; they can work with the dying for only so long and invest themselves only to a given intensity before reaching a personal limit of tolerance. Helping the dying patient and his family is a demanding task and periodically staff must leave the situation and rest from the demands.

The dying individual is ultimately alone in the problems of coping with the process of dying. One patient who felt violated by both her disease and its treatment reported that the only way she could adapt to her situation was to teach herself how to identify and solve her own emotional problems. She reported that no one else was really able to help. To find quality in life, she found it necessary to use her own inner resources, and to concentrate on living within herself (Daly 1974). Quality in dying can be provided only by the dying individual — the privilege and responsibility of the nurse is to provide physical comfort and a caring acceptance of the dying individual. If nurses can do this much, then surely there is little else that can be expected.

References

Ashby N: The will to live. Family Health 7 (2):47, 1975

Beland I, Passos J: Clinical Nursing: Pathophysiological and psychological approaches, 3rd edition. New York, Macmillan, 1975, pp. 887-894

Belleville JW, Forrest W, Miller E, Brown B: Influence of age on pain relief from an analgesic. JAMA 217 (13):1835, 1971

Benoliel JQ: Care, communication and human dignity. In Garfield C (ed), Psychosocial Care of the Dying Patient. New York, McGraw-Hill, 1978, pp. 34-35

——: Nursing care for the terminal patient: a psychosocial approach. In Schoenberg B, Carr A, Peretz D, Kutscher A (eds), Psychosocial Aspects of Terminal Care. New York, Columbia University Press, 1972, pp. 145-161

——: Talking to patients about death. Nurs Forum 9 (3):254, 1970

Benson H: Your innate asset for combating stress. Nurs Dig 5 (3):38, 1975

Billars K: You have pain? I think this will help. Am J Nurs 70 (10):2143, 1970

Birrin J: Psychology of Aging. Englewood Cliffs, N.J., Prentice-Hall, 1964

Braden W: Long-livers find death frightening. St. Louis Post-Dispatch, Dec. 14, 1975, p. 9H

Brunner L, Emerson C, Ferguson LK, Suddarth D: Textbook of Medical Surgical Nursing, 2nd edition. Philadelphia, Lippincott, 1970

Buehler J: What contributes to hope in the cancer patient? Am J Nurs 75 (8): 1353, 1975

Carini E, Owens G: Neurological and Neurosurgical Nursing, 6th edition. St. Louis, Mosby, 1974

Cashatt B: Pain: A patient's point of view. Am J Nurs 72:2, 281

Cassini N: Care of the dying person. In Grollman E (ed), Concerning Death: A Practical Guide for the Living. Boston, Beacon, 1974, pp. 13-48

Clayton P, Halik SJ, William M: The bereavement of the widowed. Dis Nerv Syst 32 (9):594, 1971

Copp L: The spectrum of suffering. Am J Nurs 74 (3):491, 1974

Daly K: Don't wave goodbye. Am J Nurs 74 (9):1641, 1974

Driver C: What a dying man taught doctors about caring. In Garfield C (ed), Psychosocial Care of the Dying Patient. New York, McGraw-Hill, 1978, pp. 72-77

Evans J: Living with a Man Who Is Dying. New York, Vaplinger, 1971

Frankl V: Man's Search for Meaning. New York, Pocket Books, 1971

Fuerst E, Weitzel M: Fundamentals of Nursing, 5th edition. Philadelphia, Lippincott, 1974, pp. 483-496.

Gliedman L, Gantt WH, Teitelbaum H: Some implications of conditioned reflex studies for placebo research. Am J Psychiatry 113:1103, 1957

Gottheil E, McGurn W, Pollak O: Is it right to joke with a dying man? Prism 2 (12):16, 1974

Hampe S: Needs of the grieving spouse in a hospital setting. Nurs Res 24 (2): 113, 1975

Hannan J: Talking is treatment too. Am J Nurs 74 (11):1991, 1974

Harmer B, Henderson V: Textbook of the Principles and Practice of Nursing, 5th edition. New York, Macmillan, 1958

Hogshead H: The art of delivering bad news. In Garfield C (ed), Psychosocial Care of the Dying Patient. New York, McGraw-Hill, 1978

Kavanaugh R: Facing Death. Baltimore, Penguin, 1974

Koenig R: Dying vs. well-being. Omega 4 (3):181, 1973

Kozier B: DuGas' Introduction to Patient Care, 2nd edition. Philadelphia, Saunders, 1972, pp. 440-447

Kübler-Ross E: On Death and Dying. London, Collier-Macmillan, 1969

Kutscher A: The psychosocial aspects of the oral care of the dying patient. In Schoenberg B, Carr A, Peretz D, Kutscher A (eds), Psychosocial Aspects of Terminal Care. New York, Columbia University Press, 1972, pp. 126-140

Maddison D, Raphael B: The family of the dying patient. In Schoenberg B, Carr A, Peretz D, Kutscher A (eds), Psychosocial Aspects of Terminal Care. New York, Columbia University Press, 1972, pp. 185-200

Matheny R, Nolan B, Hofan A, Griffin G: Fundamentals of Patient Centered Nursing, 3rd edition. St. Louis, Mosby, 1972

McCaffery M, Hart L: Undertreatment of acute pain with narcotics. Am J Nurs 76 (10):1586, 1976

Melzack R, Ofilsh J, Mount B: The Bromptom Mixture: effects on pain in cancer patients. In Garfield C (ed), Psychosocial Care of the Dying Patient. New York, McGraw-Hill, 1978, pp. 386-395

Meyerowitz J: Dying: Dromenon versus drama. In Schoenberg B, et al (eds), Anticipatory Grief, New York, Columbia University Press, 1974, pp. 79-93

Moss F, Meyer B: Effects of nursing interaction upon pain relief in patients. Nurs Res 15:303, 1966

Mount B, Ajemian I, Scott J: Use of Bromptom Mixture in treating malignant disease. In Garfield C (ed), Psychosocial Care of the Dying Patient. New York, McGraw-Hill, 1978, pp. 396-402

Murray R, Zentner J: Nursing Concepts for Health Promotion, 2nd edition. Englewood Cliffs, N.J., Prentice-Hall, 1979

Reeves R: Reflections on two false expectations. In Schoenberg B, et al. (eds), Anticipatory Grief. New York, Columbia University Press, 1974, pp. 280-284

Saunders C: Caring for the dying. In Lack S, Lamerton R (eds), The Hour of Our Death. London, Geoffrey Chapman, 1974, pp. 18-27

Schmalz A, Patterson W: Comfort care only — treatment guidelines for the terminal patient. In Garfield C (ed), Psychosocial Care of the Dying Patient. New York, McGraw-Hill, 1978, pp. 13-21

Schneidman E: Some aspects of psychotherapy with dying persons. In Garfield C (ed), Psychosocial Care of the Dying Patient. New York, McGraw-Hill, 1978, pp. 201-218

Stackman J: Some patients prefer silence. Am J Nurs 73 (6):1058, 1973

Stewart E: To lessen pain: relaxation and rhythmic breathing. Am J Nurs 76 (6):958, 1976

Straus R: Hospital organization from the viewpoint of patient centered goals. In Georgopoulous B (ed), Organization Research on Health Institutions. Ann Arbor, Institute for Social Research, University of Michigan, 1972

Strauss A, Fagerbaugh Y, Glaser B: Pain: An organizational-work-interactional perspective. Nurs Outlook 22 (9):560, 1974

Verwoerdt A, Wilson R: Communication with fatally ill patients: Tacit or explicit. Am J Nurs 67 (11):2307, 1967

Volicer B, Bohannon M: A hospital stress rating scale. Nurs Res 24 (5):352, 1975

Walker M: The last hour before death. Am J Nurs 73 (9):1228, 1973

Weisman AD: Psychosocial considerations in terminal care. In Schoenberg B, Carr A, Peretz A, Kutscher A (eds), Psychosocial Aspects of Terminal Care. New York, Columbia University Press, 1972, pp. 162-172

Woodward K: Life after death? Newsweek (12 July 1976), p. 41

Worcester A: The Care of the Aged, the Dying and Dead, 2nd edition. Springfield, Ill., Thomas, 1961, pp. 33-66

Wygant W: Dying, but not alone. Am J Nurs 67 (3):547, 1967

Appendix A

Research Design and Data Analysis

RESEARCH DESIGN

Over a two-year period, 126 interviews were obtained with institutionalized terminal patients and the nurses employed in the institutions.

The general research questions explored were: What are the expectations held by nurses and by patients concerning how patients in an institution should die? What is the nursing role in facilitating patient performance to meet the expectations? What does the terminal patient perceive as the most important nursing function? When the patient is institutionalized with a terminal prognosis, are the nurses' perceptions of the role of the patient and the role of the nurse congruent with the patients' perceptions of those roles? What institutional constraints (for instance, institutional goals, staffing patterns, and medical directives) are generally operative in the care of the institutionalized terminal patient? How do these constraints affect nursing behaviors and patient behaviors?

The specific aims of the study were to establish if there is congruence of perception between patients institutionalized with terminal prognoses and the nurses caring for them as regards the parameters of: expected and observed behaviors of terminal patients; expected and observed behaviors of persons caring for terminal patients; and kinds of nursing interventions facilitating preferred behaviors in patients.

Semistructured interview schedules were utilized to elicit responses from: a selection of terminal patients in institutions in which cure is the primary goal; a random selection of nursing personnel caring for patients in those institutions; a selection of terminal patients in institutions in which limited treatment objec-

277

tives make palliation the primary goal; a random selection of nursing personnel caring for patients in those institutions. Patient demographic data were obtained from the charts, and information concerning organization structure and goals was obtained by means of investigator observation and from appropriate administrative personnel.

The nurse interview schedule and the patient interview schedule were used as frameworks for discussion with nurses and patients. Interviews were tape recorded and transcribed.

For purposes of this study, respondents are defined as either terminal patients or nurses as follows:

> *Terminal patient:* A terminal patient is a patient who, in the opinion of the professional nurse in charge of his care, is manifesting irreversible symptoms of a progressive disease.

> *Professional nurse:* A professional nurse is employed by the department of nursing service; has a baccalaureate degree in nursing; has a state license to practice nursing; is involved in patient-care activities.

> *Technical nurse:* A technical nurse is employed by the department of nursing service; has a diploma in nursing or has an associate arts degree in nursing; has a state license to practice nursing; is involved in patient-care activities.

> *Licensed practical nurse:* A licensed practical nurse is employed by the department of nursing service; has completed a licensed practical nurse program or passed an equivalence examination; has a state license to practice nursing; is involved in patient-care activities.

> *Nursing assistant:* A nursing assistant is employed by the department of nursing service; has completed the institution's in-service training program; is involved in patient-care activities.

Sampling

Data were collected in six institutions. With the exception of one institution, sampling was carried out as described below. In one institution that was visited for a longer period of time, random selection from all patients and all nurses was made.

Taped interviews were conducted with patients and nurses during a 2½ day period in each institution. Patient interviews generally lasted from 20 to 40 minutes; nurse interviews generally lasted from 30 to 50 minutes. Patients were interviewed during the day and into the early evening. Nurses were interviewed at any time staff considered convenient and as was assigned by their supervisors.

Patients interviewed were those whom the professional nurses in charge of their care designated as manifesting irreversible symptoms of a progressive disease. They were conscious, alert, English-speaking, and able to sustain 20 to 40 minutes of conversation. Interviews were obtained at the bedside. At least four patients from long-term care divisions and four patients from acute-care divisions of the institution were selected into the sample, although they did not all participate. Frequently terminal patients are not interested in participating in research; therefore, as many names as possible were selected in order to obtain a desirable number of interviews. None of the institutions yielded eight patients who both fit the criteria and agreed to be interviewed; however, a larger number of patient interviews were obtained during the longer stay.

The nurses interviewed were selected at random from a roster of all nursing-service personnel involved in patient-care activities. The roster included nursing assistants, orderlies, licensed practical nurses, staff nurses, team leaders, and head nurses; it excluded supervisors and nursing administrators. In the situation in which there was only one registered nurse on duty — as is sometimes the situation on the evening and night shifts — that person's name was included in the roster even if she carried the title of supervisor.

Three personnel rosters (as described above) were developed in each institution, consisting of nurses who usually work the day shift, the evening shift, and the night shift. Three persons were randomly selected from each list and assigned to interview times as their work allowed, at all hours of the day and night. All interviews were obtained by the investigator, following training sessions to develop interview skills.

Human-subjects committees would not allow the use of the expressions "terminal patients" or "dying patients" in the patient interviews. Therefore, the medical diagnosis for which the patient was hospitalized was obtained with the first question, and all references in the interview after that were to "patients like you."

Patient-Interview Schedule

Introduction to patient before activating tape recorder: "Good morning (afternoon, evening) Mr. (Ms.) _____. My name is [Mary Castles]. I would like to ask you some questions about nurses and how you think they can be helpful to patients in the hospital. The information you give me will be used in a study, but your name will not be used in the study results. I wonder if you will share some of your thoughts and feelings with me."

If the patient states or indicates "no," accept his wishes as follows: "I understand feelings can be difficult to share. I would like to stop in again to see you and see how you are doing. May I?"

If patient agrees to a later return, ask him when and return. If the patient states or indicates "yes," ask him for permission to tape the conversation. If the patient refuses permission to tape the conversation, thank him for his time, and leave when it seems appropriate to do so.

If the patient agrees to taping the conversation, activate the tape recorder and proceed as follows: "As I said earlier, Mr. (Ms.) _____, I am carrying out a study of what patients think nurses can do for them in the hospital; that is, what you think patients need from nurses. Now in any kind of study in which human subjects are involved, even if you are only answering questions, the investigator must provide certain information, and ask you to consent to be part of the study. I would like to give you that information now.

"I have about 25 or 30 questions I would like you to answer; it shouldn't take more than 45 minutes. As far as I can tell, there is no risk to you in answering them, and they shouldn't make you uncomfortable. If you should become uncomfortable about answering them, or if for any reason you want to stop the interview, you are free to do so, and need only to say so. Certainly you don't have to take part in this study if you would rather not, and you may withdraw at any time. And I do want to tell you that what you say will not get back to the people who take care of you, and your name will not be used when I write up the material.

"I am doing this study because I think that obtaining information from many patients about what nurses can best do for them is a good way to begin to improve nursing care.

"I'm also interested in how you think patients should act when they are in the hospital, and there will be a few questions about that. Later, when all this information is analyzed, we can make some statements to nurses about what patients need. I will be glad to answer any questions you have about the study, now or any time after we are finished. I expect to be around the hospital for a few days.

"Are you willing to talk to me, and answer my questions? First, I would like to talk a little about you:

Can you tell me why you are in the hospital?

Have you been hospitalized before with this condition?

How long have you been in the hospital now?

What aspect of your illness is the most distressful to you?

Can you share some of the things you think about now?

Would you like to talk to anyone in particular about yourself, your illness, or anything?

Can you tell me what the nurses do for you?

What do you want the nurses to do for you?

What could they be doing that they are not doing to make you more comfortable?

What do you look for most of all in the nurses who care for you here?

What have they done in the past that you consider most meaningful or important to you?

What do you consider the most annoying things nurses do or say?

How often do the nurses come in to see you?

Would you prefer that they come more often? Less often?

Do the nurses sit and talk with you? Do you want them to?

Are there specific things any nurse here does for you that you find particularly helpful?

If you could make an anonymous suggestion to improve the care provided by the nursing staff, what would you suggest?

How do you think patients with [diagnosis or symptom patient presents in answer to first question] should behave when they are in the hospital?

Is it all right for patients with [this ailment] to yell or complain when they feel like it?

Should patients with [this ailment] appear to be sad?

Should patients with [this ailment] appear to be angry?

How do patients with [this ailment] generally behave?

"I would like to ask you a few more questions — about pain, and about the things that help you most now that you are sick:

Do you have much pain? Do you take medicine for it?

Do you get something for pain soon enough when you ask?

Do the nurses ever offer you pain medicine before the pain starts? Would you like them to?

What's the most helpful to you now? Or, what has been helpful to you in trying to keep you spirits up? [Probe.] Your family? Your religion?

How is [whatever patient identifies in about question] helpful to you?

"Thank you, Mr. (Ms.) _____. Your answers have been very helpful to me. Are there any questions you would like to ask me? I have enjoyed talking with you, and I appreciate your giving me all this time. I hope you have a pleasant hospital stay."

Nurse-Interview Schedule

INTRODUCTION
Ask for permission to record the conversation. Give name, institutional affiliation, and a candid statement of the general thrust of the research — as follows.

RESEARCH QUESTIONS
What are nurses' perceptions of the death scene in terms of normative expectations about how patients should die? What is the nurse's role in

facilitating patient performance to that norm? What does the terminal patient need from the nurse? Are the nurses' perceptions of the role of the patient and the role of the nurse congruent with the patient's perceptions of the role of the patient and the role of the nurse when the patient is institutionalized with a terminal prognosis?

EXPLANATION OF INFORMED CONSENT PROCEDURE

Any investigation involving human subjects requires the informed consent of the subject. Elements of informed consent are as follows.

1. An explanation of the procedures to be followed must be offered: The procedure in this study is a semistructured interview.

2. An explanation of the possible risks must be offered: There are no identifiable risks to you in this study.

3. An explanation of the benefits expected must be offered: The benefits to be expected from this study are to be found in the provision of bases for nursing interventions in the care of the terminal patient.

4. An offer to answer questions concerning the procedure is required: I will be glad to answer any questions about the study now, or during the interview, or at anytime during my stay here.

5. An explanation must be given that participation in the study is voluntary: You may choose not to participate, or you may withdraw at any time during the interview; your name will not be used in the final report; your answers will not be seen by your colleagues or supervisors — only the investigators will have access to the data.

Are you willing to participate in this study? If so, I must ask you not to discuss the content of the interview with your colleagues.

How old are you? (If male nurse, state sex.)

Where did you go to school?

What is your nursing experience?
Years?
Kind?

How do you think patients should behave when they are dying?

How do you think patients do behave when they are dying?

Do you think patients know when they are dying?
Why do you think so?

What do you do for the dying patient?

What is the most important thing you do for the dying patient?

What do you think the dying patient needs most from you?

Do you spend much time with patients who are terminal?
Doing what?

What do you like most about caring for a patient with a terminal prognosis?

What do you like least about caring for a patient with a terminal prognosis?

Do you talk with patients about the fact that they are dying?
If yes, what kinds of things do you say?
If no, why not?

How do you feel when a patient you have taken care of dies?

Would it be useful to you to meet once in a while with your colleagues to talk about some of your feelings about caring for terminal patients?

Is there anything you would like to discuss with me about the care of the dying patient, or any other subject?

Do you have any questions to ask me, or anything to tell me?

Thank you for your time.

DATA ANALYSIS

Categories of Response

PATIENT RESPONSE

A coder panel consisting of three nurses and one non-nurse assessed the responses independently. There was coder agreement that four patient behavior categories can be identified from the responses. Affective components are also described by subjects for the identified behaviors. Behavior categories are summarized in Table 2.

NURSE RESPONSE

The same panel assigned nurses' behaviors to categories of *instrumental, expressive,* or a combination of the two. The combination instrumental–expressive indicates that instrumental is the primary component, but that expressive factors are present; the combination expressive–instrumental indicates predominantly expressive factors, accompanied by some instrumental component. The categories of nurse behavior are adopted from Lavin's development of an expressive–instrumental orientation scale (1969); the Johnson and Martin work (1958) was also consulted. The nurse behavior categories are presented in Table 3.

Findings

As can be seen in Table 4, both nurse and patient samples are rural (92 rural subjects; 34 urban subjects), and are not young. Most of the respondents work

TABLE 2. CATEGORIES OF PATIENT BEHAVIOR AND DESCRIPTIVE TERMS

BEHAVIOR	DESCRIPTIVE TERMS
Idiosyncratic	
Condition-dependent — e.g., on disease, amount of pain, etc.	Individual changes in affect — every individual behaves differ-
Personality-dependent — e.g., patient is fearful, religious, or a fighter	ently than every other individual, and every individual behaves dif-
Organization-dependent — e.g., does what regulations require or allow	ferently during each hospitaliza- tion
Cooperative	
Courteous to staff and family	Trusting
Complies with requirements of treatment	Peaceful
	Open
Does not call "unnecessarily"	Sharing
Verbalizes plans for future, even if this is inappropriate	Easy-going
	Cheerful
	Hopeful
	Dignified
	Prepared
	Accepting
	Tranquil
Dependent	
Demanding	Apprehensive
Turns on light frequently	Angry
Turns on light unnecessarily	Afraid
Cannot be pleased	Rebellious
	Bitter
	Denying
	Aggressive
	Passive
	Irritable
	Lonely
Disengaged	
Sleeps a lot	Depressed
Does not eat	Moody
Does not talk	Withdrawn
	Not caring

TABLE 3. CATEGORIES OF NURSE BEHAVIOR AND DESCRIPTIVE TERMS

BEHAVIOR	NURSE ROLE	DESCRIPTIVE TERMS
Instrumental	Doing for Doing to	Behavior is directed to the future attainment of a functionally specific goal — actions are directly related to moving a system toward its goal
Expressive	Being with Being to	Behavior is not directed to a functionally specific goal–the behavior organizes the flow of emotional gratification, wards off threatened deprivations; actions are related to maintaining emotional equilibrium
Instrumental–expressive		Behavior is directed toward both functions, but is primarily instrumental in nature
Expressive–instrumental		Behavior is directed toward both functions, but is primarily expressive in nature

(57 of 83) and are cared for (35 of 43) in institutions in which cure is the identified goal. Men are underrepresented (12 of 83) in the nurse sample. Nurses tend to have more than five years of experience. The nurse sample is heavily loaded with personnel who are not registered nurses (52 of 83), and only 4 of the 31 registered nurses meet the study criteria for assignment to the category of professional nurse. However, there is no doubt that the sample is representative of the population of nursing personnel presently caring for terminal patients. In fact, if nursing homes were to be included as housing terminal patients, this sample would underrepresent technical nurses, licensed practical nurses, and nursing assistants because the number of professional nurses in such settings is likely to be small. In any case, the sample was randomly selected from nurses caring for terminal patients in the acute-care- and long-term-care institutions visited.

The sample of patients is not representative of a general population of institutionalized ill persons, but may describe a terminal population in that most of the subjects (32 of 43) had some form of malignancy, and a portion of the remainder (8 of 11) had degenerative diseases. Most of the patients (28 of 43) were freely ambulatory, and only 2 were entirely bedfast. This is considered to impose a systematic bias on the findings, as freedom of movement allows subjects to be independent of nurse behavior in relevant ways (Table 4).

The study has been reported elsewhere (Castles, 1971; Castles and Keith, 1979), and only a few tables are presented here.* Table 5 indicates that nurses

*Numbers vary in Tables 5–8 because not all respondents answered all questions.

TABLE 4. CHARACTERISTICS OF THE SAMPLE

	NURSES	PATIENTS
Setting		
Rural	56	36
Urban	27	7
Age		
Mean	36.8	55.7
Standard deviation	13.8	19
Organization goal		
Palliation	26	8
Cure	57	35
Sex		
Men	12	24
Women	71	19
NURSES		
Years of experience		
Mean	7.6	
Standard deviation	7	
Level of education		
Nursing assistant	35	
Licensed practical nurse	17	
Registered Nurse		
Diploma	1	
Associate degree	26	
Baccalaureate	4	
Clinical specialty		
Maternal–child care	3	
Medical–surgical nursing	69	
Psychiatric nursing	1	
Combined specialty	10	
PATIENTS		
Medical diagnosis		
Tumor		32
Cardiovascular disease		2
Degenerative diseases		8
No diagnosis		1
Mobility		
Ambulatory		28
Limited		13
Bedfast		2

TABLE 5. EXPECTED PATIENT BEHAVIOR BY STATUS

| STATUS | BEHAVIOR | | |
	Idiosyncratic	*Cooperative*	*Total*
Nurse	37	43	80
Patient	6	36	42
Total	43	79	122

$\chi^2 = 10.83; p < .001$

TABLE 6. OBSERVED PATIENT BEHAVIOR BY STATUS

| STATUS | BEHAVIOR | | | |
	Idiosyncratic	*Cooperative*	*Dependent-disengaged*	*Total*
Nurse	45	11	24	80
Patient	6	27	0	33
Total	51	38	24	113

$\chi^2 = 50.16; p < .001; d.f. = 2$

and patients have significantly different norms for patients' behavior — with nurses more willing than patients to condone idiosyncratic behaviors (37 of 80 as opposed to 6 of 42). However, it is of interest to note that more than half of the nurses believe that patients should behave in cooperative ways.

Comparison of Table 5 with Table 6 suggests that either nurses are missing cues, or patients are misperceiving the meaning of what they do. Patients not only believe they should cooperate (36 of 42, Table 5) but they also believe that they *do* cooperate (27 of 33, Table 6). Nurses, on the other hand, are willing to allow patients not to cooperate, and perceive that they do not. However, the behavior category (dependent or disengaged) identified by more than a quarter of the nurses (Table 6) and by none of the patients is accompanied by somewhat negative feeling tones in the responses. When patients believe they are fully cooperative with staff and with treatments and staff perceive that they are not cooperative, both parties to interactions are likely to be bewildered by the behavior of others.

Patient subjects are likely to describe normative nurse behaviors in instrumental terms, while the nurses believed that their behaviors should be expressive or some combination of expressive and instrumental (Table 7). However, there is no significant difference in perceptions of actual nurse behaviors, with the majority in both samples reporting instrumental behaviors in nurses (Table 8).

TABLE 7.   EXPECTED NURSE BEHAVIOR BY STATUS

STATUS	BEHAVIOR			
	Instrumental	Expressive	Combined	Total
Nurse	25	43	12	80
Patient	19	5	7	31
Total	44	48	19	111

χ^2 = 13.13; $p <.01$; d.f. = 2

TABLE 8.   OBSERVED NURSE BEHAVIOR BY STATUS

STATUS	BEHAVIOR				
	Instrumental	Expressive	Instrumental–expressive*	Expressive–instrumental†	Total
Nurse	34	18	22	9	83
Patient	26	3	10	4	43
Total	60	21	32	13	126

χ^2 = 6.07; n.s.; d.f. = 3

*Instrumental, primary behavior; expressive also identified.

†Expressive, primary behavior; instrumental also identified.

References

Castles M: Dying: Taxonomy and correlates. *The Missouri Nurse.* Missouri State Nurses Association, 1971

Castles M, Keith P: Patient concerns, emotional resources and perceptions of nurse and patient roles. Omega 10, 1979

Johnson MM, Martin HW: A sociological analysis of the nurse role. Am J Nurs 58:373, 1958

Lavin MA: Development of an expressive-instrumental orientation scale in nursing. Unpublished manuscript, 1969.

Appendix B

Documents of Ethical Statements

THE NIGHTINGALE PLEDGE

For many years The Nightingale Pledge* was considered the nursing equivalent of the Hippocratic Oath, and generations of nurses memorized it to repeat in unison at capping and graduation ceremonies. Of late years, it has fallen into disuse, but on reexamination one sees that it remains a strong ethical statement:

> *I solemnly pledge myself before God and in the presence of this assembly to pass my life in purity and to practice my profession faithfully.*
>
> *I will abstain from whatever is deleterious and mischievous, and will not take or knowingly administer any harmful drug.*
>
> *I will do all in my power to maintain and elevate the standards of my profession and will hold in confidence all personal matters committed to my keeping and all family affairs coming to my knowledge in the practice of my profession.*
>
> *With loyalty will I endeavor to aid the physician in his work, and devote myself to the welfare of those committed to my care.*

---

*Formulated in 1893 by Lystra E. Gretter, R.N., Harper Hospital, Detroit, Michigan.

CODE FOR NURSES WITH INTERPRETIVE STATEMENTS*

Whatever the merits of the Nightingale Pledge, a more sophisticated, more independent, and more legally accountable professional group requires the expanded ethical declaration of the ANA Code.

INTRODUCTION
The development of a code of ethics is an essential characteristic of a profession and provides one means for the exercise of professional self-regulation. A code indicates a profession's acceptance of the responsibility and trust with which it has been invested by society. Upon entering the profession of nursing, each person inherits a measure of the responsibility and trust that has accrued to nursing over the years and the corresponding obligation to adhere to the profession's code of conduct and relationships for ethical practice.

The Code of Nurses, adopted by the American Nurses' Association in 1950 and periodically revised, serves to inform both the nurse and society of the profession's expectations and requirements in ethical matters. The Code and the Interpretive Statements together provide a framework for the nurse to make ethical decisions and discharge responsibilities to the public, to other members of the health team, and to the profession. While it is impossible to anticipate in a code every type of situation that may be encountered in professional practice, the direction and suggestions provided here are widely applicable.

The Code for Nurses and the Interpretive Statements are both directed toward present-day practice. Previous Codes have been more prescriptive, identifying codes of both personal and professional behavior, describing appropriate relationships with physicians and other health professionals, and identifying certain responsibilities of the nurse as a citizen, an employee, and a person. The present Code, while remaining prescriptive, depends more on the nurse's accountability to the client, and, in that sense, represents a change to an ethical code.

The requirements of the Code may often exceed, but are never less than those of the law. While violations of the law may subject the nurse to civil or criminal liability, the constituent associations may reprimand, censure, suspend, or expel ANA members from the Association for violaations of the Code. The possible loss of the respect and confidence of society and one's colleagues are serious sanctions which may result from violation of the Code. Each nurse has a personal obligation to uphold and adhere to the Code and to insure that nursing colleagues do likewise. Guidance and assistance in implementing the Code in local situations may be obtained from the American Nurses' Association or its state constituents.

PREAMBLE

The Code for Nurses is based on belief about the nature of individuals, nursing, health, and society. Recipients and providers of nursing services are viewed as individuals and groups who possess basic rights and responsibilities, and whose values and circumstances command respect at all times. Nursing encompasses the promotion and restoration of health, the prevention of illness, and the alleviation of suffering. The statements of the Code and their interpretation provide guidance for conduct and relationships in carrying out nursing responsibilities consistent with the ethical obligations of the profession and quality in nursing care.

CODE FOR NURSES

1. The nurse provides services with respect for human dignity and the uniqueness of the client unrestricted by considerations of social or economic status, personal attributes, or the nature of health problems.

2. The nurse safeguards the client's right to privacy by judiciously protecting information of a confidential nature.

3. The nurse acts to safeguard the client and the public when health care and safety are affected by the incompetent, unethical, or illegal practice of any person.

4. The nurse assumes responsibility and accountability for individual nursing judgments and actions.

5. The nurse maintains competence in nursing.

6. The nurse exercises informed judgment and uses individual competence and qualifications as criteria in seeking consultation, accepting responsibilities, and delegating nursing activities to others.

7. The nurse participates in activities that contribute to the ongoing development of the profession's body of knowledge.

8. The nurse participates in the profession's efforts to implement and improve standards of nursing.

9. The nurse participates in the profession's efforts to establish and maintain conditions of employment conducive to high quality nursing care.

10. The nurse participates in the profession's effort to protect the public from misinformation and misrepresentation and to maintain the integrity of nursing.

11. The nurse collaborates with members of the health professions and other citizens in promoting community and national efforts to meet the health needs of the public.

CODE FOR NURSES WITH INTERPRETIVE STATEMENTS

1.   *The nurse provides services with respect for human dignity and the uniqueness of the client unrestricted by considerations of social or economic status, personal attributes, or the nature of health problems.*

1.1. *Self-determination of clients:*
      Whenever possible, clients should be fully involved in the planning and implementation of their own health care. Each client has the moral right to determine what will be done with his/her person; to be given the information necessary for making informed judgments; to be told the possible effects of care; and to accept, refuse, or terminate treatment. These same rights apply to minors and others not legally qualified and must be respected to the fullest degree permissible under the law. The law in these areas may differ from state to state; each nurse has an obligation to be knowledgeable about and to protect and support the moral and legal rights of all clients under state laws and applicable federal laws, such as the 1974 Privacy Act.
      The nurse must also recognize those situations in which individual rights to self-determination in health care may temporarily be altered for the common good. The many variables involved make it imperative that each case be considered with full awareness of the need to provide for informed judgments while preserving the rights of clients.

1.2. *Social and economic status of clients:*
      The need for nursing care is universal, cutting across all national, ethnic, religious, cultural, political, and economic differences, as does nursing's responses to this fundamental need. Nursing care should be determined solely by human need, irrespective of background, circumstances, or other indices of individual social and economic status.

1.3. *Personal attributes of clients:*
      Age, sex, race, color, personality, or other personal attributes, as well as individual differences in background, customs, attitudes, and beliefs, influence nursing practice only insofar as they represent factors the nurse must understand, consider, and respect in tailoring care to personal needs and in maintaining the individual's self-respect and dignity. Consideration of individual value systems and life-styles should be included in the planning of health care for each client.

1.4. *The nature of health problems:*
      The nurse's respect for the worth and dignity of the individual human being applies irrespective of the nature of the health problem. It is reflected in the care given the person who is disabled as

well as the normal; the patient with the long-term illness as well as the one with the acute illness, or the recovering patient as well as the one who is terminally ill or dying. It extends to all who require the services of the nurse for the promotion of health, the prevention of illness, the restoration of health, and the alleviation of suffering.

The nurse's concern for human dignity and the provision of quality nursing care is not limited by personal attitudes or beliefs. If personally opposed to the delivery of care in a particular case because of the nature of the health problem or the procedures to be used, the nurse is justified in refusing to participate. Such refusal should be made known in advance and in time for other appropriate arrangements to be made for the client's nursing care. If the nurse must knowingly enter such a case under emergency circumstances or enters unknowingly, the obligation to provide the best possible care is observed. The nurse withdraws from this type of situation only when assured that alternative sources of nursing care are available to the client. If a client requests information or counsel in an area that is legally sanctioned but contrary to the nurse's personal beliefs, the nurse may refuse to provide these services but must advise the client of sources where such service is available.

1.5. The setting for health care:
The nurse adheres to the principle of non-discriminatory, non-prejudicial care in every employment setting or situation and endeavors to promote its acceptance by others. The nurse's readiness to accord respect to clients and to render or obtain needed services should not be limited by the setting, whether nursing care is given in an acute care hospital, nursing home, drug or alcoholic treatment center, prison, patient's home, or other setting.

1.6. The dying person:
As the concept of death and ways of dealing with it changes, the basic human values remain. The ethical problems posed, however, and the decision-making responsibilities of the patient, family, and professional are increased.

The nurse seeks ways to protect these values while working with the client and others to arrive at the best decisions dictated by the circumstances, the client's rights and wishes, and the highest standards of care. The measures used to provide assistance should enable the client to live with as much comfort, dignity, and freedom from anxiety and pain as possible. The client's nursing care will determine to a great degree how this final human experience is lived and the peace and dignity with which death is approached.

2. The nurse safeguards the client's right to privacy by judiciously protecting information of a confidential nature.

2.1. *Disclosure to the health team:*
It is an accepted standard of nursing practice that data about the health status of clients be accessible, communicated, and recorded. Provision of quality health services requires that such data be available to all members of the health team. When knowledge gained in confidence is relevant or essential to others involved in planning or implementing the client's care, professional judgment is used in sharing it. Only information pertinent to a client's treatment and welfare is disclosed and only to those directly concerned with the client's care. The rights, well-being, and safety of the individual client should be the determining factors in arriving at this decision.

2.2. *Disclosure for quality assurance purposes:*
Patient information required to document the appropriateness, necessity, and quality of care that is required for peer review, third party payment, and other quality assurance mechanisms must be disclosed only under rigidly defined policies, mandates, or protocols. These guidelines must assure that the confidentiality of client information is maintained.

2.3. *Disclosure to others not involved in the client's care:*
The right of privacy is an inalienable right of all persons, and the nurse has a clear obligation to safeguard any confidential information about the client acquired from any source. The nurse-client relationship is built on trust. This relationship could be destroyed and the clients' welfare and reputation jeopardized by injudicious disclosure of information provided in confidence. Since the concept of confidentiality has legal as well as ethical implications, an inappropriate breach of confidentiality may also expose the nurse to liability.

2.4. *Disclosure in a court of law:*
Occasionally, the nurse may be obligated to give testimony in a court of law in relation to confidential information about a client. This should be done only under proper authorization or legal compulsion. Privilege in relation to the disclosure of such information is a legal right that only the patient or his representative may claim or waive. The statutes governing privilege and the exceptions to them vary from state to state, and the nurse may wish to consult legal counsel before testifying in court to be fully informed about professional rights and responsibilities.

2.5. *Access to records:*
If, in the course of providing care, there is need for access to the records of persons not under the nurse's care, as may be the case in relation to the records of the mother of a newborn, the person should be notified and permission first obtained whenever possible. Although records belong to the agency where collected, the indi-

vidual maintains the right of control over the information provided by him, his family, and his environment. Similarly, professionals may exercise the right of control over information generated by them in the course of health care.

If the nurse wishes to use a client's treatment record for research or nonclinical purposes in which confidential information may be identified, the client's consent must first be obtained. Ethically, this insures the client's right to privacy; legally, it serves to protect the client against unlawful invasion of privacy and the nurse against liability for such action.

3. *The nurse acts to safeguard the client and the public when health care and safety are affected by incompetent, unethical, or illegal practice of any person.*

3.1. *Role of advocate:*
The nurse's primary commitment is to the client's care and safety. Hence, in the role of client advocate, the nurse must be alert to and take appropriate action regarding any instances of incompetent, unethical, or illegal practice(s) by any member of the health care team or the health care system itself, or any action on the part of others that is prejudicial to the client's best interests. To function effectively in the role, the nurse should be fully aware of the state laws governing practice in the health care field and the employing institution's policies and procedures in relation to incompetent, unethical, or illegal practice.

3.2. *Initial action:*
When the nurse is aware of inappropriate or questionable conduct in the provision of health care, concern should be expressed to the person carrying out the questionable practice and attention called to the possible detrimental effect upon the client's welfare. When factors in the health care delivery system threaten the welfare of the client, similar action should be directed to the responsible administrative person. If indicated, the practice should then be reported to the appropriate authority within the institution, agency, or larger system. There should be an established mechanism for the reporting and handling of incompetent, unethical, or illegal practice within the employment setting so that such reporting can go through official channels and be done without fear of reprisal. The nurse should be knowledgeable about the mechanism and be prepared to utilize it if necessary. When questions are raised about the appropriateness of behaviors of individual practitioners or practices of health care systems, documentation of the observed behavior or practice must be provided in writing to the appropriate authorities. Local units of the professional association should be prepared to provide assistance and support in reporting procedures.

3.3. Follow-up action:
When incompetent, unethical, or illegal practice on the part of any-
one concerned with the client's care is not corrected within the em-
ployment setting and continues to jeopardize the client's care and
safety, additional steps need to be taken. The problem should be
reported to other appropriate authorities such as the practice com-
mittees of the appropriate professional organizations or the legally
constituted bodies concerned with licensing of specific categories of
health workers or professional practitioners. Some situations may
warrant the concern and involvement of all these groups. Reporting
should be both factual and objective.

3.4. Peer review:
In addition to the role of advocate, the nurse should participate in
the planning, establishment, and implementation of other activi-
ties or procedures which serve to safeguard clients. Duly consti-
tuted peer review activities in employment agencies directed toward
the improvement of practice are one example. This ongoing method
of review is based on objective criteria, it includes a mechanism for
making recommendations to administrators for correction of defi-
ciencies, it facilitates the improvement of delivery services, and it
promotes the health, welfare, and safety of clients.

4.   The nurse assumes responsibility and accountability for individual
nursing judgments and actions.

4.1. Acceptance of responsibility and accountability:
The recipients of professional nursing services are entitled to high
quality nursing care. Individual professional licensure is the protec-
tive mechanism legislated by the public to ensure basic and mini-
mum competencies of the professional nurse. Beyond that, society
has accorded to the nursing profession the right to regulate its own
practice. The regulation and control of nursing practice by nurses
demands that individual professional practitioners of nursing bear
primary responsibility for the nursing care clients receive and be in-
dividually accountable for their practice.

4.2. Responsibility:
Responsibility refers to the scope of functions and duties associated
with a particular role assumed by the nurse. As nursing assumes
functions, these functions become part of the responsibilities of ex-
pectations of performance of nurses. Areas of responsibilities ex-
pected of nurses include: data collection and assessment of the
health status of the client; determination of the nursing care plan
directed toward designated goals; evaluation of the effectiveness of
nursing care in achieving the goals of care; and subsequent reassess-
ment and revision of the nursing care plan as defined in the ANA
Standards of Nursing Practice. By assuming these responsibilities,
the nurse is held accountable for them.

4.3. *Accountability:*
Accountability refers to being answerable to someone for some-thing one has done. It means providing an explanation to self, to the client, to the employing agency, and to the nursing profession. Over and above the obligations such accountability imposes on the individual nurse, there is also a liability dimension to accountability. The nurse may be called to account to be held legally responsible for judgments exercised and actions taken in the course of nursing practice. Neither physician's prescriptions nor the employing agency's policies relieve the nurse of ethical or legal accountability for actions taken and judgments made. Accountability, therefore, requires evaluation of the effectiveness of one's performance of nursing responsibilities.

4.4. *Evaluation of performance:*
Self-evaluation. The nurse engages in ongoing evaluation of indi-vidual clinical competence, decision-making abilities, and profes-sional judgments. The nurse also engages in activities that will improve current practice. Self-evaluation carries with it the respon-sibility for the continuous improvement of one's nursing practice.
Evaluation by peers. Evaluation of one's performance by peers is a hallmark of professionalism, and it is primarily through this mechanism that the profession is held accountable to society. The nurse must be willing to have practice reviewed and evaluated by peers. Guidelines for evaluating the appropriateness, effectiveness, and efficiency of nursing practice are emerging in the form of re-vised and updated nurse practice acts, ANA's Standards of Nursing Practice, and other quality assurance mechanisms. Participation in the development of objective criteria for evaluation that provide valid and reliable data is the responsibility of each nurse.

5.   *The nurse maintains competence in nursing.*

5.1. *Personal responsibility for competence:*
Nursing is concerned with the welfare of human beings, and the nature of nursing is such that inadequate or incompetent practice may jeopardize the client. Therefore, it is the personal responsi-bility and must be the personal commitment of each individual nurse to maintain competence in practice throughout a professional career. This represents one way in which the nurse fulfills accounta-bility to clients.

5.2. *Measurement of competence in nursing practice:*
Competence is a relative term, and an individual's competence in any field may be diminished or otherwise affected by the passage of time and the emergence of new knowledge. This means that for the client's optimum well-being and for the nurse's own professional development, nursing care should reflect and incorporate new tech-

niques and knowledge in health care as these develop and especially as they relate to the nurse's particular field of practice.

Measures of competence are developing; they include peer review criteria, outcome criteria, and ANA's program for certification.

5.3. *Continuing education for continuing competence:*
Nursing knowledge, like that in the other health disciplines, is rendered rapidly obsolete by mounting technological advances and scientific discoveries, changing concepts and patterns in the provision of health services, and the increasing complexity of nursing responsibilities. The nurse, therefore, should be aware of the need for continuous updating and expansion of the body of knowledge on which practice is based and should keep knowledge and skills current. The nurse should assess personal learning needs, should be active in finding appropriate resources, and should be skilled in self-directed learning. Such continuing education is the key to maintenance of individual competence.

5.4. *Intraprofessional responsibility for competence in nursing care:*
All nurses, be they practitioners, educators, administrators, or researchers, share responsibility for quality nursing care. Therefore all nurses need thorough knowledge of the current scope of professional nursing practice. Advances in theory and practice made by one professional must be disseminated to colleagues. Since individual competencies vary in relation to educational preparation, experience, client population and setting, when necessary, nurses should refer clients to and/or consult with other nurses with expertise and recognized competencies, e.g., certified nurses and clinical specialists.

6. *The nurse exercises informed judgment and uses individual competence and qualifications as criteria in seeking consultation, accepting responsibilities, and delegating nursing activities to others.*

6.1. *Changing functions:*
Because of the increased complexity of health care, changing patterns in the delivery of health services, continuing shortages in skilled health manpower, and the development [sic] acceptance of evolving nursing roles, nurses are being requested or expected to carry out functions that have formerly been performed by physicians. In turn, nurses are assigning some nursing functions to variously prepared ancillary personnel. In this gradual shift of functions, as the scope of practice of each profession changes, the nurse must exercise judgment in seeking consultation, accepting responsibilities, and assigning responsibilities to others to ensure that clients receive quality care at all times.

6.2. *Joint policy statements:*
Nurse practice acts are usually expressed in broad and general lan-

guage in order to provide the necessary freedom for interpretation of the law so that future developments, new knowledge, and changing roles will not necessitate constant revision of the law. The nurse must not engage in practice prohibited by law or delegate to others activities prohibited by practice acts of other health care personnel or by other laws. Recognition by nurses of the need of a more definitive delineation of roles and responsibilities, however, has resulted in collaborative efforts to develop joint policy statements. These statements may involve other health care providers or associations and usually specify the functions that are agreed upon as appropriate and proper for the nurse to perform. Such statements represent a body of expert judgment that can be used as authority where responsibilities are not definitively outlined by legal statute.

6.3. *Seeking consultation:*
The provision of health and illness care to clients is a complex process that requires a wide range of knowledge and skills. Interdisciplinary team effort with shared responsibility is the most effective approach to provision of total health services. Nurses, whether practicing in clearly defined or new and emerging roles, must be aware of their own individual competencies. When the needs of the client are beyond the qualifications and competencies of the nurse, consultation must be sought from qualified nurses or other appropriate sources.

Discretion must be exercised by the nurse before intervening in diagnostic or therapeutic matters that are not recognized by the nursing profession as established nursing practice. Such discretion should be based on education, experience, legal parameters, and professional guidelines and policies.

6.4. *Accepting responsibilities or delegating activities:*
The nurse should look to mutually agreed upon policy statements for guidance and direction; but even where such statements exist, personal competence should be carefully assessed before accepting responsibility or delegating activities. Decisions in this area call for knowledge of and adherence to joint policy statements and the laws regulating medical and nursing practice as well as for the exercise of informed nursing judgments.

6.5. *Accepting responsibility:*
If the nurse does not feel personally competent or adequately prepared to carry out a specific function, the nurse has the right and responsibility to refuse. In so doing, both the client and the nurse are protected. The reverse is also true. The nurse should not accept delegated responsibilities that do not utilize nursing skill or competencies or that prevent the provision of needed nursing care to clients. Inasmuch as the nurse is responsible for the client's total

nursing care, the nurse must also assess individual competence in assigning selected components of that care to other nursing service personnel. The nurse should not delegate to any member of the nursing team a function for which that person is not prepared or qualified to perform.

7.   The nurse participates in activities that contribute to the ongoing development of the profession's body of knowledge.

7.1.   The nurse and research:
Every profession must engage in systematic inquiry to identify, verify, and continually enlarge the body of knowledge which forms the foundations for its practice. A unique body of verified knowledge provides both framework and direction for the profession in all of its activities and for the practitioner in the provision of nursing care. The accrual of knowledge promotes the advancement of practice and with it the well-being of the profession's clients. Ongoing research is thus indispensable to the full discharge of a profession's obligations to society. Each nurse has a role in this area of professional activity, whether involved as an investigator in the furthering of knowledge, as a participant in research, or as a user of research results.

7.2.   General guidelines for participating in research:
Before participating in research the nurse has an obligation:

1.   To ascertain that the study design has been approved by an appropriate body.

2.   To obtain information about the intent and the nature of the research.

3.   To determine whether the research is consistent with professional goals.

Research involving human subjects should be conducted only by scientifically qualified persons or under such supervision. The nurse who participates in research in any capacity should be fully informed about both nurse and client rights and responsibilities as set forth in the publication Human Rights Guidelines for Nurses in Clinical and Other Research prepared by the ANA Commission on Nursing Research.

7.3.   The protection of human rights in research:
The individual rights valued by society and by the nursing profession have been fully outlined and discussed in Human Rights Guidelines for Nurses in Clinical and Other Research; namely, the right to freedom from intrinsic risks of injury and the rights of privacy and dignity. Inherent in these rights is respect for each individual to exercise self-determination, to choose to participate, to have full information, to terminate participation without penalty.

*It is the duty of both the investigator and the nurse partici-
pating in research to maintain vigilance in protecting the life, health,
and privacy of human subjects from unanticipated as well as anticipated risks. The subjects' integrity, privacy, and rights must be
especially safeguarded if they are unable to protect themselves because of incapacity or because they are in a dependent relationship
to the investigator. The investigation should be discontinued if its
continuance might be harmful to the subject.*

7.4. *The practitioner's rights and responsibilities in research:*
      *Practitioners of nursing providing care to clients who serve as
      human subjects for research have a special need to clearly under-
      stand in advance how the research can be expected to affect treat-
      ment and their own moral and legal responsibilities to clients. Here,
      as in other problematic situations, the practitioner has the right not
      to participate or to withdraw under the circumstances described in
      paragraph 1.4 of this document. More detailed guidance about the
      rights and responsibilities of nurses in relation to research activities
      may be found in* Human Rights Guidelines for Nurses in Clinical
      and Other Research.

8.   *The nurse participates in the profession's efforts to implement and
      improve standards of nursing.*

8.1. *Responsibility to the public:*
      *Nursing has the responsibility to admit to the profession only those
      who have demonstrated a capacity for those competencies believed
      essential to the practice of nursing. Areas of concern for nursing
      competence should include adequate performance of nursing skills,
      academic achievement, humanitarian concern for others, accep-
      tance of responsibility for individual actions, and the desire to
      improve nursing practice. Nurses involved in the evaluation of
      student attainment carry a primary responsibility for ensuring that
      the profession's obligation to the public relative to entry qualifica-
      tions for practice are met.*
          *The nursing profession exists to give assistance to those persons
      needing nursing care. Standards of nursing practice provide guid-
      ance for the delivery of quality nursing care and are a means for
      evaluating that care received by clients. The nurse has a responsi-
      bility to the public for personally implementing and maintaining
      optimal standards.*

8.2. *Responsibility to the discipline:*
      *The professional practice of nursing is founded on an understanding
      and application of a body of knowledge reflected in its standards.
      As the profession's organization for nurses, ANA has adopted
      standards for nursing practice, nursing service, and nursing educa-
      tion. The nurse has the responsibility to monitor these standards in*

everyday practice and through voluntary participation in the profession's ongoing efforts to implement and improve standards at the national, state, and local levels.

8.3. *Responsibility to nursing students:*
The future of nursing rests with new recruits to the profession. Nursing has a responsibility to maintain optimal standards of nursing practice and education in schools of nursing and/or wherever students engage in learning activity. This places a particular responsibility on all nurses whose services are concerned with the educational process.

9.   *The nurse participates in the profession's efforts to establish and maintain conditions of employment conducive to high quality nursing care.*

9.1. *Responsibility for conditions of employment:*
The nurse must be concerned with conditions of economic and general welfare within the profession. These are important determinants in the recruitment and retention of well-qualified personnel and in assuring that each practitioner has the opportunity to function optimally.

  The provision of high quality nursing care is the responsibility of both the individual nurse and the nursing profession. Professional autonomy and self-regulation in the control of conditions of practice are necessary to implement standards of practice as established by organized nursing.

9.2. *Collective action:*
Defining and controlling the quality of nursing care provided to the client is most effectively accomplished through collective action. Collective action may include assistance and representation from the professional association in negotiations with employers to achieve employment conditions in which the professional standards of practice can be implemented and which are commensurate with the qualifications, functions, and responsibilities of the nurse. The Economic and General Welfare program of the professional association is the appropriate channel through which the nurse can work constructively, ethically, and with professional dignity. This program, encompassing commitment to the principle of collective bargaining, promotes the right and responsibility of the individual nurse to participate in determining the terms and conditions of employment conducive to high quality nursing practice.

9.3. *Individual action:*
A nurse may enter into an agreement with individuals or organizations to provide health care, provided that the agreement is in accordance with the Standards of Nursing Practice of the American Nurses' Association and the nurse practice law of the state and pro-

vided that the agreement does not permit or compel practices which are in violation of this Code.

10.   *The nurse participates in the profession's effort to protect the public from misinformation and misrepresentation and to maintain the integrity of nursing.*

10.1. *Advertising services:*

A nurse may make factual statements that indicate availability of services through means that are in dignified form, such as:

A professional card identifying the nurse by name and title, giving address, telephone number, and other pertinent data.

Listing name, title, and brief biography in reputable directories and reputable professional publications. Such published data may include the following: Name, address, phone, field of practice or concentrates; date and place of birth; schools attended, with dates of graduation, degrees, and other scholastic distinctions; offices held; public or professional honors; teaching positions; publications; memberships and activities in professional societies; licenses; names and addresses of references.

A nurse shall not use any form of public or professional communication to make self-laudatory statements or claims that are false, fraudulent, misleading, deceptive, or unfair.

10.2. *Uses of titles and symbols:*

The right to use the title "Registered Nurse" is granted by state governments through licensure by examination for the protection of the public. Use of that title carries with it the responsibility to act in the public interest. The nurse may use the title "R.N." and symbols of academic degrees or other earned or honorary professional symbols of recognition in all ways that are legal and appropriate. The title and other symbols of the profession should not be used, however, for personal benefit by the nurse or by those who may seek to exploit them for other purposes.

10.3. *Endorsement of commercial products or services:*

The nurse does not give or imply endorsement to advertising, promotion, or sale of commercial products or services because this may be interpreted as reflecting the opinion or judgment of the profession as a whole. Since it is a nursing responsibility to engage in health teaching and to advise clients on matters relating to their health, it is not unethical for the nurse to utilize knowledge of specific services and/or products in advising individual clients. In the course of providing information or education to clients or other practitioners about commercial products or services, however, a variety of similar products or services should be offered or de-

scribed so that the client or practitioner can make an informed choice.

10.4. *Protecting the client from harmful products:*
It is the responsibility of the nurse to advise clients against the use of dangerous products. This is seen as discharge of nursing functions when undertaken in the best interest of the client.

10.5. *Reporting infractions:*
Not only should the nurse personally adhere to the above principles, but alertness to any instances of their violation by others should be maintained. The nurse should report promptly, through appropriate channels, any advertisement or commercial which involves a nurse, implies involvement, or in any way suggests nursing endorsement of a commercial product, service, or enterprise. The nurse who knowingly becomes involved in such unethical activities negates professional responsibility for personal gain, and jeopardizes the public confidence and trust in the nursing profession that have been created by generations of nurses working together in the public interest.

11. *The nurse collaborates with members of the health professions and other citizens in promoting community and national efforts to meet the health needs of the public.*

11.1. *Quality health care as a right:*
Quality health care is mandated as a right to all citizens. Availability and accessibility to quality health services for all citizens require collaborative planning by health providers and consumers at both the local and national level. Nursing care is an integral part of quality health care, and nurses have a responsibility to help ensure that citizens' rights to health care are met.

11.2. *Responsibility to the consumer of health care:*
The nurse is a member of the largest group of health providers, and therefore the philosophies and goals of the nursing profession should have a significant impact on the consumer of health care. An effective way of ensuring that nurses' views regarding health care and nursing service are properly represented is by involvement of nurses in political decision making.

11.3. *Relationships with other disciplines:*
The complexity of the delivery of health care service demands an interdisciplinary approach to delivery of health services as well as strong support from allied health occupations. The nurse should actively seek to promote collaboration needed for ensuring the quality of health services to all persons.

11.4. *Relationship with medicine:*
The interdependent relationship of the nursing and medical pro-

fessions requires collaboration around the need of the client. The evolving role of the nurse in the health delivery system requires joint practice as colleagues, deliberations in determining functional relationships, and differentiating areas of practice between the two professions.

11.5. *Conflict of interest:*
Nurses who provide public service and who have financial or other interests in health care facilities or services should avoid a conflict of interest by refraining from casting a vote on any deliberation affecting the public's health care needs in those areas.

THE NUREMBERG CODE

The Nuremberg Code* consists of ten standards that medical practitioners are required to meet when they utilize human subjects in medical experimentation. It was developed as a judgment of one of the Nuremberg Military Tribunals (August 1947) during the post-World War II trials at Nuremberg. This is the first code to provide specific guidelines for human experiments, although professional codes are as old as the professions and human experiments had been previously mentioned in medical oaths. The Nuremberg Code was promulgated in a judgment condemning the behavior of German physicians involved in human experimentation during the Nazi regime in Germany.

THE NUREMBERG CODE
The great weight of the evidence before us is to the effect that certain types of medical experiments on human beings, when kept within reasonably well-defined bounds, conform to the ethics of the medical profession generally. The protagonists of the practice of human experimentation justify their views on the basis that such experiments yield results for the good of society that are unprocurable by other methods or means of study. All agree, however, that certain basic principles must be observed in order to satisfy moral, ethical and legal concepts:

1. *The voluntary consent of the human subject is absolutely essential. This means that the person involved should have legal capacity to give consent; should be so situated as to be able to exercise free power of choice, without the intervention of any element of force, fraud, deceit, duress, overreaching, or other ulterior form of constraint or coercion; and should have sufficient knowledge and comprehension of the elements of the subject matter involved as to enable him to make an understanding and enlightened decision. This latter element*

*From Frenkel D: Human experimentation: code of ethics. Legal Med Q 1(1):7, 1977. By permission of Legal Medical Quarterly, 620 Sheppard Ave. West, Downsview, Ontario, Canada M3H 2S1.

requires that before the acceptance of an affirmative decision by the experimental subject there should be made known to him the nature, duration and purpose of the experiment; the method and means by which it is to be conducted; all inconveniences and hazards reasonably to be expected; and the effects upon his health or person which may possibly come from his participation in the experiment.

The duty and responsibility for ascertaining the quality of the consent rests upon each individual who initiates, directs, or engages in the experiment. It is a personal duty and responsibility which may not be delegated to another with impunity.

2. *The experiment should be such as to yield fruitful results for the good of society, unprocurable by other methods or means of study, and not random and unnecessary in nature.*

3. *The experiment should be so designed and based on the results of animal experimentation and a knowledge of the natural history of the disease or other problem under study that the anticipated results justify the performance of the experiment.*

4. *The experiment should be so conducted as to avoid all unnecessary physical and mental suffering and injury.*

5. *No experiment should be conducted where there is an* a priori *reason to believe that death or disabling injury will occur; except, perhaps, in those experiments where the experimental physicians also serve as subjects.*

6. *The degree of risk to be taken should never exceed that determined by the humanitarian importance of the problem to be solved by the experiment.*

7. *Proper preparations should be made and adequate facilities provided to protect the experimental subject against even remote possibilities of injury, disability, or death.*

8. *The experiment should be conducted only by scientifically qualified persons. The highest degree of skill and care should be required through all stages of the experiment of those who conduct or engage in the experiment.*

9. *During the course of the experiment the human subject should be at liberty to bring the experiment to an end if he has reached the physical or mental state where continuation of the experiment seems to him to be impossible.*

10. *During the course of the experiment the scientist in charge must be prepared to terminate the experiment at any stage, if he has probable cause to believe, in the exercise of the good faith, superior skill, and careful judgment required of him, that a continuation of the experiment is likely to result in injury, disability, or death to the experimental subject.*

THE HELSINKI DECLARATION

The most recent statement on human experimentation by medical practitioners is to be found in The Declaration of Helsinki, adopted by the World Medical Association in 1964.* This document distinguishes between clinical research that is combined with patient care, and nontherapeutic clinical research. Item 2 in the section "Clinical Research Combined with Professional Care" is of particular concern to nurses who care for patients with terminal malignancies, as there is some question as to the therapeutic value of the chemotherapies to the individual patient–subject.

INTRODUCTION
It is the mission of the doctor to safeguard the health of the people. His knowledge and conscience are dedicated to the fulfillment of this mission.

The Declaration of Geneva of the World Medical Association binds the doctor with the words: "The health of my patient will be my first consideration" and the International Code of Medical Ethics declares that "Any act or advice which could weaken physical or mental resistance of a human being may be used only in his interest."

Because it is essential that the results of laboratory experiments be applied to human beings to further scientific knowledge and to help suffering humanity, the World Medical Association has prepared the following recommendations as a guide to each doctor in clinical research. It must be stressed that the standards as drafted are only a guide to physicians all over the world. Doctors are not relieved from criminal, civil and ethical responsibilities under the laws of their own countries.

In the field of clinical research a fundamental distinction must be recognized between clinical research in which the aim is essentially therapeutic for a patient, and clinical research the essential object of which is purely scientific and without therapeutic value to the person subjected to the research.

I. Basic Principles

1. *Clinical research must conform to the moral and scientific principles that justify medical research and should be based on laboratory and animal experiments or other scientifically established facts.*

2. *Clinical research should be conducted only by scientifically qualified persons and under the supervision of a qualified medical man.*

3. *Clinical research cannot legitimately be carried out unless the importance of the objective is in proportion to the inherent risk to the subject.*

---

*From Frenkel D: Human experimentation: code of ethics. Legal Med Q 1(1):7, 1977. By permission of Legal Medical Quarterly, 620 Sheppard Ave. West, Downsview, Ontario, Canada M3H 2S1.

4. *Every clinical research project should be preceded by careful assessment of inherent risks in comparison to foreseeable benefits to the subject or to others.*

5. *Special caution should be exercised by the doctor in performing clinical research in which the personality of the subject is liable to be altered by drugs or experimental procedure.*

II. *Clinical Research Combined with Professional Care*

1. *In the treatment of the sick person, the doctor must be free to use a new therapeutic measure if in his judgment it offers hope of saving life, reestablishing health, or alleviating suffering.*

    If at all possible, consistent with patient psychology, the doctor should obtain the patient's freely given consent after the patient has been given a full explanation. In case of legal incapacity consent should also be procured from the legal guardian; in case of physical incapacity the permission of the legal guardian replaces that of the patient.

2. *The doctor can combine clinical research with professional care, the objective being the acquisition of new medical knowledge, only to the extent that clinical research is justified by its therapeutic value for the patient.*

III. *Non-therapeutic Clinical Research*

1. *In the purely scientific application of clinical research carried out on a human being, it is the duty of the doctor to remain the protector of the life and health of that person on whom clinical research is being carried out.*

2. *The nature, the purpose and the risk of clinical research must be explained to the subject by the doctor.*

3a. *Clinical research on a human being cannot be undertaken without his free consent after he has been fully informed; if he is legally incompetent, the consent of the legal guardian should be procured.*

3b. *The subject of clinical research should be in such a mental, physical and legal state as to be able to exercise fully his power of choice.*

3c. *Consent should, as a rule, be obtained in writing. However, the responsibility for clinical research always remains with the research worker; it never falls on the subject, even after consent is obtained.*

4a. *The investigator must respect the right of each individual to safeguard his personal integrity, especially if the subject is in a dependent relationship to the investigator.*

4b. *At any time during the course of clinical research the subject or his guardian should be free to withdraw permission for research to be continued. The investigator or the investigating team should discon-*

tinue the research if in his or their judgment it may, if continued, be harmful to the individual.

THE DECLARATION OF GENEVA

The Declaration of Geneva* was adopted by the general Assembly of the World Medical Association in 1948. It is the modern version of the Hippocratic Oath, which has, like the Nightingale Pledge, fallen into disuse.

THE DECLARATION OF GENEVA
At the time of being admitted as a member of the medical profession I solemnly pledge myself to consecrate my life to the service of humanity;
I will give to my teachers the respect and gratitude which is their due;
I will practice my profession with conscience and dignity;
The health of my patient will be my first consideration;
I will respect the secrets which are confided in me;
I will maintain by all the means in my power the honour and noble traditions of the medical profession;
My colleagues will be my brothers;
I will not permit consideration of religion, nationality, race, party politics or social standing to intervene between my duty and my patient;
I will maintain the utmost respect for human life, from the time of conception; even under threat, I will not use my medical knowledge contrary to the laws of humanity.
I make these promises solemnly, freely and upon my honour.

---

*From Frenkel D: Human experimentation: code of ethics. Legal Med Q 1(1):7, 1977. By permission of Legal Medical Quarterly, 620 Sheppard Ave. West, Downsview, Ontario, Canada M3H 2S1.

Appendix C

Legal Concerns

MEDICARE

The following summary of the provisions of the original Medicare legislation* is presented for the information of a professional group that explicitly states it deals with holistic man. The constraints imposed on the identification and treatment of illness by the legislation — which indicates clearly which illnesses can be supported through insurance payments, where the patient must be housed for payment, and which practitioners can receive payment from the insurance source — are not always explicit in the treatment situation.

SUMMARY OF MAJOR BENEFIT AND CONTRIBUTION PROVISIONS, P.L. 89–97, TITLE XVIII (MEDICARE)
Two health insurance programs are established for persons aged 65 and over: Part A — a hospital insurance plan providing protection against the costs of hospital and related care; Part B — a voluntary medical insurance plan covering payments for physician services and certain other medical and health services.

Part A: Hospital Insurance and Related Benefits

There are four categories of care provided under this plan:

---

*From Somers HM, Somers AR: Medicare and the Hospitals: Issues and Prospects. Washington, D.C., Brookings Institute, 1967.

1. *Inpatient hospital services. Up to 90 days in each "spell of illness". A "spell of illness" begins with the first day that the patient is furnished inpatient services and ends on the last day of a 60 consecutive-day period during which he is not an inpatient in a hospital nor an extended care facility.*

    The patient pays the first $40 of charges (the deductible) and $10 a day for the 61st–90th day (coinsurance). Covered services include room and board, ordinary nursing care, drugs, supplies, and most other services customarily furnished by a hospital. They do not include private-duty nursing or the services of physicians except those provided by interns and residents under an approved teaching program. Inpatient psychiatric hospital services are covered, but with a lifetime limit of 190 days. The cost of any blood, after the first three pints furnished to a patient during a given spell of illness, is covered.

2. *Post-hospital care in an extended care facility. Up to 100 days in each spell of illness following a hospital stay of at least three days. An extended care facility is defined as an institution engaged in providing skilled nursing care or rehabilitation services to inpatients, with certain approved medical care facilities and having an arrangement with a hospital for the transfer of patients. After the first 20 days, the patient pays $5 a day for the remaining 80 days of such care (coinsurance).*

3. *Outpatient hospital diagnostic services. The patient pays the first $20 of cost (deductible) of such services received during a 20-day period in the same hospital, plus 20 percent of the remainder of the bill (coinsurance). Deductibles paid for such service count as incurred expenses under Part B.*

4. *Post-hospital home health services. Up to 100 visits during the year following discharge from a hospital, after at least a 3-day stay, or after a covered stay in an extended care facility. The person must be under the care of a physician and under a plan, calling for such services, that was established by a physician within 14 days of the patient's discharge. The service must be provided by an approved home health agency. The covered services include those of visiting nurses, physical therapists, and other health workers, but not the physician. The patient must be homebound.*

Deductibles and coinsurance will be increased if necessary to keep pace with hospital costs, but no increase will be made before 1969.

Part A is financed through a distinct social security earnings tax, and the revenues are deposited in a separate trust fund, except that benefits for persons currently aged 65 and over, who are not insured under the social security or railroad retirement systems, are financed out of federal general revenues. This is a transitional provision for almost all non-insured persons who are now or will reach age 65 before 1968. Excluded are federal employees and their spouses who are covered or could be covered under the Federal Employees Health Benefits Act of 1959, and aliens who have been U.S. residents for less than 5 years.

Contribution rates, which apply equally to employees, employers, and self-employed persons, are the following percentages of the first $6,600 of earnings in a calendar year:

1966	*0.35%*
1967–72	*0.50%*
1973–75	*0.55%*
1976–79	*0.60%*
1980–86	*0.70%*
1987 and thereafter	*0.80%*

Part B: Supplementary Medical Insurance

The services covered are:

1. *Physicians' and surgeons' services, whether furnished in a hospital, clinic, office, home, or elsewhere. This includes services and supplies furnished as an incident to provision of a physician's service, if commonly furnished in a physician's office without separate charge, and hospital services incident to physician's services rendered to outpatients, such as drugs and biologicals which cannot be self-administered.*

2. *Home health services under an approved plan (with no requirement of earlier hospitalization) for a maximum of 100 visits during each calendar year.*

3. *Diagnostic x-ray and laboratory tests, and other diagnostic tests.*

4. *X-ray, radium and radioactive isotope therapy.*

5. *Ambulance services.*

6. *Surgical dressings and splints, casts, and other devices for reduction of fractures and dislocations; rental of durable medical equipment for use in the patient's home, such as hospital beds; prosthetic devices (other than dental) that replace all or part of an internal body organ; and braces and artificial legs, arms, and eyes.*

Payment for outside-the-hospital treatment of mental, psychoneurotic and personality disorders is limited. No more than 62½ percent or $500 of such charges in one calendar year are considered. In effect, this means that the maximum benefit for these services is $250 a year, or 50 percent of the charges, whichever is less.

The program will not pay for custodial care, routine physical check-ups, dentures, eyeglasses, hearing aids, orthopedic shoes, cosmetic surgery, and personal comfort items.

Initially, enrollees pay $3 a month, deducted, where possible, from social security, railroad retirement, or civil service retirement benefits. The *government matches the payment. The premium is subject to increase as medical costs go up, but not more often than every two years. The payments will be placed in a separate trust fund from which all benefit and administrative expenses will be paid.*

The enrollee is responsible for payment of the first $50 of expenses incurred in a calendar year (the deductible). However, any expenses incurred in the last three months of a calendar year, including any expenses for outpatient hospital diagnostic services, and applied toward the deductible in such year can also be credited toward the deductible for the following year. The amount of any deductible imposed for outpatient hospital diagnostic services under Part A in any year will be credited as an incurred expense under Part B for such year.

After the $50 deductible requirement has been satisfied, payment will be made to the enrollee, or to the physician or provider of services in the case of a mutually agreed "assignment", for 80 percent of the "reasonable charges" for the services rendered (20 percent coinsurance).

A person who was 65 on or before May 31, 1966, had to sign up for the plan by May 31 to begin coverage on July 1. As a general rule, those reaching 65 in the future are allowed seven months to enroll, beginning three months before their 65th birthday. Thereafter, they can enroll only during general enrollment periods which will run from October 1 to December 31 in each odd year (1967, 1969, etc.) but no one may enroll more than three years after the close of the first period in which he could have enrolled.

Persons who are in the plan but drop out will have a chance to reenroll in a general enrollment period within three years of termination of the previous enrollment. The premium rate for a person who enrolls after the first period when enrollment was open to him or for one who terminates and then enrolls again will be increased by 10 percent for each 12-month period he stayed out of the program.

NATURAL DEATH LEGISLATION

The increased number of judicial and legislative actions related to death and dying has resulted in a growing body of law concerned both with the rights of dying patients (usually considered as the right to get on with dying), and the criteria for determining whether death has occurred, which is overwhelming even to attorneys. However, because nurses care for the dying and death is more likely than not to occur in an institution, nurses must have some deeper awareness of the legal activities than can be found in headlines such as those reporting the Quinlan decision.

There is some need that nurses be able to differentiate among definitions of standards for determining human death and standards for exercising the right to die. The two concepts are not well separated in the various legislative efforts. Pronouncing that death has occurred is the prerogative and the responsibility of the physician; the treatment of the dying preceding the event of death is the responsibility — although not always the sole prerogative — of the nurse.

A good many of the states have enacted or are considering enactment of legislation that will establish statutory definition of death. The model proposal presented below* follows a critical review of early legislation passed in Kansas:

> *A person will be considered dead if in the announced opinion of a physician, based on ordinary standards of medical practice, he has experienced an irreversible cessation of spontaneous respiratory and circulatory functions. In the event that artificial means of support preclude a determination that these functions have ceased, a person will be considered dead if in the announced opinion of a physician, based on ordinary standards of medical practice, he has experienced an irreversible cessation of spontaneous brain functions. Death will have occurred at the time when the relevant functions ceased.*

Capron and Kass maintain that this proposed statute provides a definition of death at the level of general physiological standards and that it speaks of the death of a person (a human being as a whole), thus correctly disregarding the sequential cessation of function of various organs and cells. It does not establish a separate kind of death (i.e., brain death) but rather specifies the circumstances under which the establishment of brain death rather than irreversible cessation of spontaneous function is appropriate. According to Capron and Kass, statement of the definition in terms of the cessation of bodily functions — but not in terms of the specific criteria or tests of measurement of functions — allows physicians to change their procedures as technology provides them with new ones. In fact, the proposal speaks merely to when death has occurred, leaving to other than legislative forums discussions concerning rights to refuse treatment, or to demand treatment in the presence or absence of certain medical conditions. These factors are certainly relevant to decisions about care; they are just as certainly peripheral and confounding to a legal statement, and should be left to technical and ethical forums.

MODEL DEATH BILL

The Society for the Right to Die, Inc., published a Legislative Manual (1976 edition) which presents the text of the right-to-die death-with-dignity statutes introduced in state legislatures since 1975, analyzing their content in relation to specific issues requiring resolution. The issues include who can elect to take formal action resulting in death, how one can elect to do so, and how one can revoke such a decision. Immunity for and objections by physicians and others,

---

*From Capron AM, Kass LR: A statutory definition of the standards for determining human death: an appraisal and a proposal. University of Pennsylvania Law Review 121:87, 1972

and violations and sanctions for violations are considered as these are addressed in the various statutes which have been introduced. The Manual also includes a model bill drafted by the Society.*

> AN ACT to amend the Public Health law in order to permit an individual to execute a document directing discontinuance of maintenance medical treatment in the event of terminal illness.
>
> The Public Health law is hereby amended by inserting a new Article to read as follows:

> Article _____. Termination of Medical Treatment.
> I. As used in this Act, unless the context requires otherwise:
> (a) "Maintenance medical treatment" means medical treatment designed solely to sustain the life processes.
> (b) "Physician" means an individual licensed by the Board of Medical Examiners for the State of _____.
> (c) "Terminal illness" means an illness that will result in natural expiration of life, regardless of the use or discontinuance of maintenance medical treatment.
> II. (a) An individual of sound mind and 18 years of age or older may execute a document directing that no maintenance medical treatment be utilized for the prolongation of his life at such time as he is suffering from a terminal illness.
> (b) A document described in subsection (a) of this section is not valid unless it has been executed with the same formalities as a will under Article _____.
> III. (a) For purposes of this Act, certification of a terminal illness may be rendered only by the physician or physicians in charge of the individual who is terminally ill. A copy of any such certification shall be maintained in the records of the medical facility where the patient is being maintained. If the patient is not being maintained in a medical facility, a copy shall be retained by the physician in his own case records.
> (b) A physician who certifies a terminal illness under this section is presumed to be acting in good faith. Unless it is alleged and proved that his action violated that standard of reasonable professional care and judgment under the circumstances, he is immune from civil or criminal liability for such action.
> IV. An individual who has executed a document under this Act may, at any time thereafter, revoke such document. Revocation may be accomplished by destroying such document, or by contrary indication expressed in the presence of two witnesses 18 years of age or older.

---

*By permission of the Society for the Right to Die, Inc., 250 West 57th Street, New York, NY 10019

V. (a) A physician who relies on a document executed under this Act,
        of which he has no actual notice of revocation or contrary indi-
        cation, is presumed to be acting in good faith in withholding
        maintenance medical treatment from an individual who exe-
        cuted such document. A physician is immune from civil or
        criminal liability when, in reliance upon such document, he has
        withheld medical treatment, unless it is alleged and proved that
        his actions violated the standard of reasonable professional care
        and judgment under the circumstances.

   (b) For purposes of this Act, a physician may presume that an indi-
        vidual who executed a document under this Act was of sound
        mind when it was executed, in the absence of actual notice to
        the contrary.

MODEL BILL FOR DECISION MAKING

In a comprehensive analysis of legislative proposals related to euthanasia and
treatment refusal, Veatch has considered more than 85 bills that would apparently legalize "mercy killing" or clarify either the rights of competent patients
to refuse treatment or the decision-making authority for noncompetent patients.
He identifies as the critical variables in the bills related to euthanasia the following: whether the request of the individual is required; who may make such a
request or otherwise be a candidate for euthanasia; what are the penalties for
abuse; and what other provisions are included. Bills that would clarify the rights
of competent patients are criticized for ambiguities. They do not make clear
(1) that the wishes expressed by a competent person remain valid when he
becomes incompetent; (2) who should have the authority to interpret the instructions written while the individual was competent; (3) what penalties are
applied if instructions are not followed; and (4) whether refusal of life-saving
treatment in itself indicates incompetency.

In any case the competent patient now has the right to refuse treatment,
and as a general rule this right is not explicitly violated. Veatch is primarily
concerned with the clarification of who has decision-making authority for
patients who either are not now and never have been competent, or who are
not now competent and have not expressed their wishes while they were competent. Following a review of the several bills that have been introduced into
state legislatures, Veatch proposed a model bill summarized as follows.*

The bill begins with the recognition of the continuing right of the legally
competent patient to refuse any specific medical treatment and specifies that
such refusal, in itself, should not be taken as evidence of incompetency. It then
provides that if a person is not competent, authority should go to one he may
have designated while competent to be his agent for such purposes. If no such

---

*After Veatch RM: Death and dying: the legislative options—an analysis of
three types of bills. Hastings Cent Rep 7:5, 1977.

person has been designated, the authority should go to the next of kin. If there are no relatives, the authority would go to [a] guardian appointed by the court for the purpose.

It then provides that in determining the authority of the patient's agent in case of incompetency, the court shall honor any document of the patient executed to state grounds for which he would want an agent disqualified. It provides that patients entering into medical care arrangements must be told of their right to be treated and to refuse treatment; that no medical personnel shall be guilty of any offense while acting in good faith without negligence according to the law; and that no medical personnel shall be required to participate in any medical treatment they find morally objectionable, provided that they withdraw from the case and inform the patient and other medical personnel of their withdrawal.

THE LIVING WILL

The Living Will is a prototype of the documents related to treatment in case no recovery from physical or mental disability is expected and the individual can no longer make or communicate his own decision to refuse treatment. Currently such documents do not have the legal status of wills or other documents that take effect only after death has occurred. However, the documents clearly must impinge on nursing-care plans, as they are explicit statements of the wishes of the patient. When nurses are aware that the patient has signed such a document, nursing decisions about the execution of the role of patient advocate must be made.

A LIVING WILL

prepared by

Euthanasia Educational Council
250 West 57th Street
New York, N.Y. 10019

TO MY FAMILY, MY PHYSICIAN, MY LAWYER, MY CLERGYMAN
TO ANY MEDICAL FACILITY IN WHOSE CARE I HAPPEN TO BE
TO ANY INDIVIDUAL WHO MAY BECOME RESPONSIBLE FOR MY
HEALTH, WELFARE OR AFFAIRS

Death is as much a reality as birth, growth, maturity and old age — it is the one certainty of life. If the time comes when I, _____, can no longer take part in decisions for my own future, let this statement stand as an expression of my wishes, while I am still of sound mind.

If the situation should arise in which there is no reasonable expectation of my recovery from physical or mental disability, I request that I be allowed to die and not be kept alive by artificial means or "heroic measures." I do not fear death itself as much as the indignities of deterioration, depen-

dence and hopeless pain. I, therefore, ask that medication be mercifully administered to me to alleviate suffering even though this may hasten the moment of death.

This request is made after careful consideration. I hope you who care for me will feel morally bound to follow its mandate. I recognize that this appears to place a heavy responsibility upon you, but it is with the intention of relieving you of such responsibility and of placing it upon myself in accordance with my strong convictions, that this statement is made.

Signed   _____

Date   _____
Witness   _____
Witness   _____

Copies of this request have been given to:

_____
_____
_____
_____

Appendix D

The Hospice Movement

The current hospice movement developed as an effort to meet the needs of patients suffering from chronic degenerative diseases with no known cure, and who had a limited life span. Care of such patients in institutions where the major emphasis is on life-saving procedures and acute-care situations is neither economical nor humane. Because they cannot meet institutional and professional goals for cure and discharge, such patients are perceived by staff as misplaced and they perceive themselves as mistreated in the acute-care setting. Their needs are subordinated to the more usual curative techniques and activities.

In spite of a growing number of structured efforts to care for chronically and terminally ill persons in their homes, institutions remain the most commonly utilized care setting. Special institutions for the care of the dying are beginning to be considered, and a few are in operation. Probably the best known of these is St. Christopher's Hospice in Great Britain, and it serves as an example of the major differences in hospital and hospice care.

Ingles (1974) states that in the hospice care must be given by nurses who are able to accept their own feelings about death in order that they are able to listen compassionately and constructively to the fears of others. They provide physical and psychological support that enables the patient to make the transition from life to death peacefully, and continue to support the grieving family. This comprehensive and utopian care is reported to be given at St. Christopher's. The hospice is defined as a place for the dying, where the needs of individuals who no longer benefit from curative treatment are considered. Death in this setting is seen as a legitimate and normal event and in the hospice no last-stand measures to prolong life are used. The provision of comfort is considered the most important nursing function.

The organization of work in the hospice is flexible in order to accommodate the unique and individual needs of each person living there. The patient does what he wants and is able to do; he makes decisions regarding his treatment and care plan — with help from his physician, nurses, clergyman, and family. In St. Christopher's the hospice personnel are not concerned with medical diagnosis or with various types of specialized treatment. Without the focus on medical specialization, fragmentation of services and rigid routines are avoided. Care and comfort, relief from pain, and concern for the well-being and happiness of the individual are general goals. Hope is encouraged but techniques of care rather than techniques of cure are paramount. The intent is that the care given is that which would be given at home if the family were able to offer it. Visitors are welcome — children as well as adults. The patient is given enough medication on a regular schedule to reduce his pain, but the combination and dosage of drugs are such that he remains alert with the capacity to enjoy his family and friends, his food, and whatever activities are possible for him (Hendin 1973).

Dying patients are given relief from the distressing symptoms of their diseases, the security of a caring environment, sustained expert nursing, and the assurance that they and their families will not be abandoned by staff when cure is no longer expected.

Symptom control, emotional support, and spiritual care are given by an interdisciplinary team. Each patient is seen as part of a family unit whose total well-being and life-style affect and are affected by care. Staff responsibility does not cease with the death of the patient; survivors are supported in the mourning process.

In the nursing plan, symptom management is considered essential. Craven and Wald (1975) state if the patient is preoccupied with pain, such concepts as self-respect, self-control, freedom, independence, and dignity may be sacrificed. When pain is controlled, the patient may stay alert and capable of participating in life as fully as possible. Other symptoms that must be alleviated include depression, anorexia, weakness, lethargy, breathlessness, and gastrointestinal difficulties. Such symptoms — especially the nagging, chronic pain — are distressing physically but also emotionally because they provide a constant reminder to the patient of his condition. However, management of pain must be handled with consideration for possible fears of addiction, or feelings of lack of control or of helplessness. Some patients place a high value on stoicism and control.

At St. Christopher's the patients are not disturbed for routine vital signs. Comfort is promoted by frequent changes of position (not the every two- to four-hour schedule seen in other institutions), back rubs, baths, mouth care, and attention to other small details. Patient rooms are filled with flowers; handmade afghans, a television set, radio, and other personal items of the patient remain part of his environment.

The nurses work in pairs, so that there is an interchange with and support to one another emotionally and physically as they lift, move, and care for the patient. The atmosphere is informal; however, although the nurses are affectionate and informal, the patients are always called by title and last name unless the patient initiates a request to be called by his first name. There are few institutional rules, and no age or time limits for visitors. Children and pets are welcome. Monday is identified as the family's/visitor's day off. Patients do not expect visitors on this day, in recognition of the family's need for a free day to do normal and essential things in the home. The staff and volunteers plan Monday's activities so that patients do not feel neglected.

Patients in hospice care have many freedoms that some institutions do not allow. They mark menus to control diet, smoking and cocktails are permitted, and the family can bring beverages and food of choice. The questions of the patient and family are answered honestly, with kindness. Teaching is done about the disease and prognosis; however, if no questions are asked, the need for privacy of patients and families is maintained. If the patient or family are demanding, the staff accept and try to understand the meaning of the behavior. Extra time is spent talking with the patient, explaining his care and treatment. Religion is considered a private affair, and the patients may or may not attend chapel. The nurses work closely with the chaplain to meet the patient's needs, but avoid trying to push the patient into religious behaviors. If they wish, patients are helped with life review and reminiscing, as helps to self-acceptance and a sense of ego integrity. When the patient dies, the bed curtains are drawn, and staff and family kneel around the bed as the head nurse reads a prayer. Ingles reports that both nurses and family have found this activity to be helpful in acknowledging death. The patient is placed in normal alignment, left in bed, and his face is left uncovered. For one hour the relatives may sit with the deceased patient if they wish. The nurse may also stay if it is appropriate. At the end of the hour, the patient is moved to a private room, bathed, and taken in the bed to the chapel where the family may be joined by their spiritual advisor. The dead body is then taken to the mortuary.

Resolution of the crisis of death is accomplished in part through the Pilgrim Club. Family and friends of the deceased are invited to join the club. Meetings are held one evening each month to help family members work through the loss, separation, grief, and loneliness; help is also available for practical problems.

Time and effort of the staff is devoted to symptom control for patient comfort and the relief of pain, and to support of the family group through the dying process and the death.

In this country the hospice concept of care of the terminally ill is gaining momentum; however, while there are a good number of out-patient facilities giving care within the framework of the hospice philosophy, there are no operating institutions of the St. Christopher's type. Dobihal has identified 58 groups in 28 states working within the hospice framework, but as of June 1977 there were no in-service facilities. The New Haven group that Dobihal directs offers the following hospice-service categories: nursing, medical, and other care in the home for the patient and the family (in the New Haven area only); relative consultation, to family members only (statewide); medical consultation — hospice physicians to other physicians (statewide); and nursing consultation — hospice nurses to other nurses (statewide). He describes the goals of the hospice as: to keep the patient home as long as possible; to supplement but not to duplicate existing services; to educate health-care professionals and the public; to support the entire family as the unit of care; to help the patient live as fully as possible and to keep costs down.

A somewhat different institutional implementation of the hospice philosophy is found in the Palliative Care Service, a hospice-type unit in the Royal Victoria Hospital, McGill University, Montreal. The project is reported here in some detail* because the apparently successful incorporation of a palliative care unit into a general hospital provides another institutional option for care of the terminal patient.

The Palliative Care Services [PCS] comprise three areas of care (plus research, teaching, and administration): these are the Palliative Care Unit [PCU] itself, the Domiciliary Service, and Consultation Service. The PCU is a 12-bed unit, opened in the hospital in January 1975. It is staffed by an especially trained interdisciplinary team. The team approach is strongly emphasized. The team includes physicians, nurses, a psychiatrist, a social worker, a physiotherapist, a dietician, a unit coordinator, chaplains and a large group of volunteers. Many of the volunteers are families of patients who have died in the unit, and the cadre of volunteers is an extremely important component of the team. The emphasis of the team is to improve the quality of the life remaining to the patient by specialized nursing care, expert treatment of pain and other medical problems, attention to the patient's psychological and spiritual needs and concern for the family as well as the patient.

The Domiciliary Service was established in February 1975. This service facilitates comprehensive home care of selected RVH patients with advanced malignancy by working in concert with visiting nurses and other community resources.

The Consultation Service is provided by the PCS. Physicians visit patients in other parts of the hospital in consultation for evaluation regarding the admission of patients to the PCU, to Domiciliary care, or to symptomatic palliative care. In cases where admission to the PCU or to the domiciliary service is not possible or advisable, the patient may be followed on his original service by members of the PCU team.

The patient pool for the 12-bed PCU consists of individuals previously treated in the hospital for a diagnosed malignant disease; they must be in the phase of the disease where the only appropriate therapy is palliative care. Two goals of palliation are described in the treatment of cancer; palliation aimed at increasing the length of the survival (active treatment) and palliation aimed at increasing the quality of survival (symptomatic control only). The second goal is met in PCU care.

Before all else, palliative care is considered to mean excellent symptom control. This is achieved by a team skilled in clinical pharmacology. Since pain control is the key to good palliative care for this patient population, the team

---

*The following information is taken from Palliative Care Service: Pilot Project. Montreal, Royal Victoria Hospital, McGill University, 1975.

approach is to attack total pain in the context of a supportive milieu. The grounding in clinical pharmacology is required because of the need for the most appropriate choice of a variety of pharmaceuticals, and careful dosage and titration. In the PCU, as at St. Christopher's, administration is oral when possible, and on a round the clock basis, so that patients never suffer, and become afraid of suffering. The PCU also utilizes the Bromptom Mixture described earlier.

The team approach to care is considered essential. In general hospitals individual disciplines tend to emphasize their own importance at the expense of the others, and of the patient. In the PCU the concept that no one discipline or person has all the answers is paramount. Total care is made easier and more efficient by a variety of personnel with a variety of resources working together. Such a team approach is not easy, and members must guard against interprofessional rivalries and defensive attitudes.

In such a situation of interdependence, it is impossible to avoid pressures, and these are identified in this publication as external and internal in nature. Externally induced pressures include: the serious nature of the disease process; the frequent staff involvement with distraught relatives; a greater than usual nursing role in medical decision making, and the constant awareness by nurses that the attitudes of the rest of the hospital are ambivalent toward the activities on the PCU. Internally induced pressures arise from methods of resolution of discrepancies among the differing expectations imposed on nurses by patients, families, other nurses and the hospital administrators. Due to the nature of special care units in general hospitals expectations for staff are likely to be comprehensive, and implicit rather than explicit. Implicit expectations are less amenable to open discussion, and generate anxiety and confusion as the individual attempts to reconcile them.

The initiation of group meetings to allow ventilation and to deal with the pressures was not immediately successful.

> While early group meetings did aspire to some of the envisaged goals, and some feelings did manage to reach expression, uneasiness and frustration soon predominated. This was reflected by dwindling attendance, a serious questioning of the groups utility and determined rejection of one of the PCU leaders whose stance was psychologically interpretive. The group was clearly resentful of headshrinking sessions and felt threatened by any attempt to analyze them. . . . [When] emphasis was shifted from staff oriented to patient and family oriented discussion, debating problems of clinical management facilitated a more overtly task oriented group and at the same time a more acceptable vehicle for the sharing of work related affective experiences. Restraints [were] placed on group membership, with only nursing, medical and para-medical staff involved with direct patient care participating . . . in this format, significant stabilization developed, and ongoing flexibility. (PCS 1975, p. 107)

The weekly meetings now lead to enhanced staff communication, and consequently more integrated and consistent staff response to perceived patient need. Staff also benefit from the more cohesive peer group and the decreased likelihood of becoming emotionally isolated.

The unit psychiatrist provides consultation to staff for their own as well as their patients' problems. In a setting in which involvement with the dying is a therapeutic requirement, such consultation is a necessary support. The psychiatrist (PCS 1975, p. 473) reports that "In providing the emotional climate that would fulfill the PCS credo of 'death with dignity' the staff were perpetually in the dilemma of forming a relationship and preparing for the termination of that relationship simultaneously. The resulting ambivalence, never easily resolved, constituted an exhausting exercise." He suggests that staff stress is a significant factor affecting the quality and effectiveness of the care given in the PCS; that continued development and refinement of staff support systems is a priority task; that phase specific and situation specific stress can be anticipated in similar health care systems; and that frequent exposure to patient loss appears to represent a primary cause of staff stress.

The nursing care is planned around the primary need of the patient for physical comfort and relief from suffering, and the emotional and psychological needs of the patient and his family. The description of the admission procedure emphasizes courteous attention to the problems of both patient and family. Nursing care is a major factor in symptom control.

> *Palliative care nursing can challenge the skills of any nurse and offers proportionately greater personal reward. It is obvious however that the potential can only be achieved if there is time to listen, to understand and to provide care. The number of nurses must be sufficient, and must be supplemented with volunteers and para-medical personnel. (PCS 1975, p. 76)*

While there is no doubt that terminal patients need not be subjected to the same procedures — oriented toward life-saving or cure — which are appropriate for patients who will recover if such measures are taken, there is some question whether society will provide for the development of special institutions or even special units for the care of the dying. There is also some question whether the care is or should be so very different. Most of the nursing and medical activities described as occurring at St. Christopher's, at the hospice at New Haven, and at the PCS in Montreal are activities to which *all* patients are entitled. It does not seem correct that a terminal prognosis is required for patients to receive courteous and individualized attention and time, or to have the benefit of visits from family members whenever they desire. The goals of palliative and curative care may differ, but for nursing at least the care need not be that different. The needs of the patients and the interventions planned to meet these needs are not so different in terminal and nonterminal patients, although the attitudes and needs of the staff appear to be quite divergent. Nurses would do well to remember the statement by Barbara McNulty of St. Christopher's, quoted in the PCS Manual (PCS 1975, p. 73):

> *The art of caring for the dying is the same as that for all good nursing;*

*what is needed is an acute power of observation, an exquisite sensitivity
to the patients' needs, and an infinite capacity for taking pains.*

References

Craven J, Wald F: Hospice care for dying patients. Am J Nurs, 75 (10):1816,
    1975
Dobihal E: Paper presented at the Hastings Center Workshop on Death, Dying
    and Bereavement, Sarah Lawrence College, New York, 25 June 1977
Hendin D: Death as a Fact of Life. New York, Warner, 1973
Ingles T: St. Christopher's hospice. Nurs Outlook, 22 (12):759, 1974
Palliative Care Service. Pilot Project. Montreal, Royal Victoria Hospital, McGill
    University, Montreal, 1975

Appendix E

Families of the Dying

Initially, when the family is told of the patient's condition, some hope within the realm of truth should be stated when the diagnosis is a terminal disease. The possibility that treatment might lengthen the patient's life or palliate symptoms of the disease must be outlined.

PSYCHOLOGICAL RESPONSES

When the patient's physical condition deteriorates, the family begins to feel more helpless. Each member of the family must purge himself of guilt; guilt feelings may be alleviated by directing anger toward medical personnel for failure in care, and sometimes staff are blamed for the disease state. If the patient demonstrates emotional stability, the family are likely to respond similarly. However, the opposite is also true. An upset patient and an upset family are usually found in conjunction.

The burdens of the family increase if the dying patient leaves the hospital to return home and they may be so busy giving care and covering feelings in the patient's presence that little grief is expressed. The slow progression of the disease, the increase of pain and debility, the inability to eat, and, finally, loss of consciousness in the patient all cause the family to be grateful for the death and termination of suffering. Mourning has occurred in anticipation of death (Heimlich and Kutscher 1970).

However, there may be family conflicts with the dying patient in the presence of emotional dependency needs that are threatened: overidentification with the dying person, or emotional and financial dependency on the dying person

326

may generate needs that can no longer be met. Maddison and Raphael suggest (1972) that when such dependent needs are not met, family members become aggressive and subject to feelings of triumph over the dying person. Magical and omnipotent hostile or revengeful fantasies occur. Hostility can arise because of the necessity for constant care being given to the dying person, and because of his lack of mobility. The patient's personality may evoke aggression or hostility in others. His lack of cooperation, failure to adhere to treatment regimens, past indulgence, and disappointment over unfulfilled ambitions may cause resentment in his family. In the family members, aggressive reactions may be displaced into phobia or paranoid delusions — internalized into depression, or overcompensated by reaction formation — so that excessive concern is shown for the patient. Guilt may arise from aggressive responses and from feeling responsible for the illness. Sadomasochistic problems may arise if nursing measures by the family member cause the patient much pain. Sexual conflicts may also occur. Identification with the patient may highlight previous sexual inadequacies or activate castration anxiety if the illness involves sexual organs or if the disease is mutilating. Isolation of affect, denial, and motor activity may be healthy defenses in some cases.

Denial and Other Defense Mechanisms

Denial is a major defense and is often used excessively if guilt is marked or the diagnosis is delayed. It is maintained longer by more distant relatives, who are not directly involved with problems of care.

Isolation of affect may appear as a coping device that enables the family member to perform the necessary practical functions for the terminal patient; however, this may also cause withdrawal from the patient, with the family behaving as if the patient were already dead. Less isolation of affect may enable a family member to become a confidant to the patient, thereby lessening the speed of his deterioration.

Sublimation may also occur, enabling the family to deal more appropriately with practical problems. Repression and reaction formation may be excessive in the presence of major problems, with aggressive wishes and the frustration of dependency needs. Displacement of hostility may be made to other family members or to medical personnel, and sexual and dependent needs may also be displaced. Projection of hostile and dependent wishes onto the patient or other family members is common. Introjection of aspects of the patient may occur with family members taking on the patient's illness or personality characteristics as a defense against the imminent loss. Hysterical identification with the patient's symptoms may occur.

Reactions of the Family Group

Disturbance of balances and interactions within the family system and family integration develops, especially if the patient was in a pivotal position as an expressive or instrumental family leader, or as the family scapegoat. The necessary changes in role behavior affect work, leisure, interactions, and self-gratification of the family group, both currently and in the future. Caring for the dying patient at home may mean further role adjustment, and often family members must enact multiple roles. All of the financial and emotional resources of the family may become concentrated on the ill person.

Sick-role behavior may have to be given up by other family members. Communication patterns are modified, decreased, or may become pathological. Silence about the prognosis prevents honest talk among family members about their feelings; they are unable to work through their anxieties or share their problems and pleasures. This results in withdrawal from the dying person, so that hospitalization as a function of family needs, rather than the demand of the illness, can result. Patients prefer to die at home, but hospitalization may be necessary to help the family survive as a unit. Transfer of the patient to a nursing home may cause such guilt that denial cannot be maintained.

Although an extended family unit may provide a network of support, the nuclear family often perceives these people as unsupportive. In fact, the community may isolate the dying patient and his family.

GRIEVING

Healthy adults generally consider death more tragic for the person left behind than for the one who dies. Only a small percentage think of death as suffering; many think of it as a blessing (Riley 1970). Death is considered as something that occurs at the end of the life cycle — to old people who are no longer in the work world. At the same time, even if death comes early, there is little disruption in the work world because work is organized in a way so that our major institutions are relatively independent of the persons who carry out the roles within them (Blauner 1966). Death is upsetting primarily if it occurs prematurely or is accompanied by suffering or violence. In other cultures, open expression of grief is acceptable; professional mourners may be hired to help the family grieve loudly and openly. Places for the recently dead individual are set at the table, food is placed at the grave, or the deceased person's room is kept the same. In the United States, restraint and composure are perceived as models in happiness and grief alike, which is contrary to human needs and may produce lifelong stress (Marks 1976). Quint (1971) points out that when any form of important relationship is gone, life organization is damaged and a concomitant sense of distress and trauma follows. A deficit in the person's life results because of a continuing absence of functions provided by the previous relationship; often that deficit cannot be filled by new relationships.

Nurses can help the family recognize the importance and normality of the grief experience and the reality of the death. If a family member does not grieve when the other members do, he should be given support and the family should be helped to understand the possible reasons. Otherwise, later he may grieve alone because the family are angered by his earlier lack of grieving. Because guilt is such a prominent part of the mourning process, the patient and family need help in expressing and working through guilt through reinforcement of reality factors. Nurses may facilitate the grieving process by listening and encouraging rather than inhibiting emotional expression; by being nonpunitive, nonjudgmental, and nonauthoritarian; and by helping in concrete ways. Reality should be gently reinforced. Most importantly, the nurse must be in touch with personal feelings about dying and grief (Glaser and Strauss 1968).

Readiness to grieve a loss does not appear during the stages of shock and defensive retreat, but only as family members become aware of the loss of former life patterns. Individuals cannot be pushed to grieve. Grief work takes time, so that changes can be assimilated into a definition of reality. This occurs only if the emotional impact of each stage of grief can be experienced in a nonjudgmental way and with support from others (Quint 1971).

Types of Grief

Types of grief states include: anticipatory grief; normal grief; inhibited, delayed, or absent grief; chronic grief; emotional or physical grief reactions — depression, hypochondriasis, exacerbation of preexisting somatic conditions, development of medical symptoms and illness, psychophysiologic reactions, acting out; and specific neurotic and psychotic states (Peretz et al. 1970). The first two will be discussed here; the other (less adaptive) types will be discussed under *Mourning*.

ANTICIPATORY GRIEF

Anticipatory grief occurs prior to loss, as the person faces his own or a loved one's declining health, serious illness, impending surgery, or death. Anticipatory grief reactions may range from quiet periods of sadness and tears to symptoms associated with normal grief. If anticipatory grief is prolonged or thorough, the relationship between the dying person and the potentially bereaved family member may be emotionally terminated before it is physically over. The more hopeless is the future, the more intense is the anticipatory grief. Individuals who are usually pessimistic and disposed to hopelessness, guilt, or self-punishment will also be likely to do anticipatory grieving early, before the loss is imminent. When the actual loss occurs, such persons will not show the usual grief reaction, although they may manifest depression (Peretz et al. 1970).

NORMAL GRIEF

Normal grief is characterized by intense mental suffering and distress, deep sorrow, and painful regret (Peretz et al. 1970). Following the death of a family member the initial response is shock — with a feeling of numbness and bewilderment, weeping, disbelief, and despairing acknowledgement of the loss. Somatic symptoms accompany the altered sensorium, and include shortness of breath, choking, sighing, dyspnea, hyperventilation, a lump or tightness in the throat, chills, tremors, weakness, anorexia, tightness or emptiness in the abdomen, insomnia, and exhaustion. Somatic symptoms may last from 20 minutes to several days. Anxiety, tension, restlessness, confusion, agitation in the form of hand-wringing or pacing may occur during the shock stage (Engel 1962; Lindeman 1944).

Disbelief and denial are expressed, and the grieving person may reject discussion of the loss or comforting from others. Feelings of unreality, emotional distance from people, intense preoccupation with the image or occasional hallucination of the lost object (person), painful loneliness, tearless weeping, and a sense of emptiness, helplessness, and disorganization are common manifestiations in early grief. In spite of apparent intellectual and verbalized acceptance of the loss, the implications are not understood. The bereaved person may overtly behave as if nothing happened or he may be unable to carry out ordinary activities of living, lacking the energy, organization, and initiative to do ordinary daily tasks.

As the reality of the loss penetrates awareness, the person feels despair and anguish and fears that emotional control and mental faculties are being lost; many people are frightened by the intensity and unusual quality of their feelings. Terrifying nightmares — and, later, pleasant dreams about the deceased — are common (Engel 1962; Lindeman 1944).

The loss is first felt as a defect in the psychic self as the mourner becomes increasingly aware of the many ways in which he was dependent on the lost person as a source of gratification, for a feeling of well-being, for effective functioning, and for his sense of self. Increased preoccupation with and yearning for the lost person, a heightened desire to talk about the loss, a search for evidence of failure "to do right," verbal self-accusation, and ambivalence toward the lost person is manifested as a part of acknowledgement of the loss (Lindeman 1944).

The greater the ambivalence felt toward the lost person, the greater the feelings of guilt and shame. With any love relationship, the person will at times feel anger or dislike toward (or desire to be rid of) the person, along with feelings of love toward him. The bereaved will recall ways in which he failed the deceased: quarrels, disappointments, infidelities in thoughts or deeds, negligence, impatience, or anger. If the deceased suffered a prolonged and painful illness, his family may feel both relief at his death and guilt over their relief. Expressions of guilt in relation to small, inconsequential acts may be a screen for more profound guilt about being the survivor. Additionally, the grieving person may feel angry at the dead person for having left him. Guilt and anger are a normal part of grieving, and are frequently displaced onto others: the doctor, the nurse, the employer, another family member, or God. If guilt is not resolved, self-blame for the loss and preoccupation with it and with future losses or with his own death will occur. Unsuccessful attempts at expiating guilt and anger may be made by blindly identifying with the dead person, by quickly seeking a substitute relationship or object, by absorbing himself in work, by compulsive behavior or overzealous religious activity, by overindulgence in alcohol or drugs, or by literally fleeing from the situation. At this stage, the griever is not ready to accept a new object in place of the old one, although passively and transiently he may accept a more dependent relationship with remaining objects, roles, or persons. He may fear he is going crazy because of his felt despair, loneliness, helplessness, hopelessness, and guilt (Engel 1962; Lindeman 1944). In an effort to reduce the intensity of such reactions, nurses may apply early crisis therapy, including granting acceptance, being available, giving assurance in relation to the normality of the feelings and past behavior, and listening.

Crying — the intensity of which depends largely on the culture — helps to express some of the anguish and is a form of communication that engenders support from others. In America, loss through death is one situation in which adult tears, even in the male, are acceptable and cause no loss of respect. However, bereaved persons are often embarrassed about crying in front of others and may be irritable toward those who try to be supportive or who encourage crying (Peretz et al. 1970).

Jackson (1974) is in agreement with the above observations concerning grief. He maintains that we grieve not so much for the person who has just died but rather for ourselves, our sense of loss and deprivation, and our own eventual death. Mixed with the sadness is a joy that we are still alive.

He identified the following manifestations of grief:

1. *Immediate and overwhelming discomfort.*

2. *Muscular weakness and tremors that last for a few minutes or a few hours.*

3. *Glandular response, with tears, dry mouth, disturbed digestion and sexual activity, and proneness to infections and viral illness.*

4. *Cardiovascular response, with hypertension, tachycardia, and arrhythmias.*

5. *Respiratory response, with rapid, shallow or gasping breaths, or deep sighing.*

6. *Gastrointestinal response, with dysphagia, anorexia, indigestion, diarrhea, or constipation.*

7. *Dermal response, with perspiration, cold and clammy sensation; flush, paresthesias.*

8. *Feelings of sorrow, fear, anxiety about the future, guilt, anger, disinterest in daily routines.*

9. *Withdrawal, doubt in religious faith. (Jackson 1974)*

Jackson describes grief as manifested by extremes: an inability to react emotionally at all, or prolonged emotional overreaction; excessive withdrawal from, anger at, or suspicion of another; and inappropriate elation or deep depression. He states that guilt is always a part of grief and takes many forms, including (1) unreasonable accusations against others, in order to protect the self; (2) anger at at others as a substitute for anger against oneself; and (3) memorial gifts as a symbolic restitution, a self-punishing fine, or a form of immortality to the dead person's memory.

Nichols and Nichols (1975) believe that the ultimate goal of grief work is to remember without emotional pain, and to reinvest emotional energy. Growth occurs in the presence of defeat, suffering, struggle, and loss, and to find a way out of these depths enriches and fulfills life. The integration of the loss of a loved one into the life of the bereaved ensures that the *capacity* to love is not also lost.

Jackson (1974) presents several strategies that may be used by families for coping with grief. They include: (1) facing the full reality of what has happened; (2) recognizing that reactions are a normal response to loss and that death is a part of life; (3) developing new interests, new acquaintances, new relationships, new challenges; (4) breaking the bonds emotionally with the deceased by investing emotionally in another living being; (5) treasuring memories, but not living only with memories; (6) allowing time to resolve the loss; and (7) using ceremonies and rituals to help resolve loss, if they are meaningful and not excessive or inappropriate.

Institution-based nurses may have little effect on the family grieving process after the initial shock of the death of a family member, but there is no doubt as to the need for nonjudgmental and open acceptance of whatever behavior is manifested by the family in the time immediately after death.

MOURNING

Mourners become increasingly aware of their own bodies. In addition to developing symptoms that are a normal part of grieving, they may develop symptoms similar to those suffered by a deceased loved person. This identification process maintains a tie with that person and appeases some of the guilt felt for harboring earlier angry feelings toward him. How such symptoms are expressed depends on constitutional factors as well as on past learning about which symptoms are most likely to get attention or to be defined as illness by the self and others. The mourner is preoccupied with the dead person and wishes to have a continuing experience with him. Feelings of helplessness and death wishes are common, and he frequently talks about the dead person and the pleasant memories and events associated with him. Constantly talking about the loss and its meaning is one way of reinforcing reality as well as of expiating guilt through repeated self-assurance that all possible action was taken to prevent the loss. This repetitious talking continues until the mourner forms an image in his mind almost completely devoid of the negative characteristics of the dead person, to replace that which no longer exists in the real world. This process of idealization follows the difficult and painful experience of alternating guilt, remorse, fear, and regret for real or fantasied past acts of hositility, neglect, and lack of appreciation, or even for personal responsibility for the loss incurred by death (Engel 1962; Lindeman 1944).

Through identification following idealization, the mourner may consciously or unconsciously adopt some of the behavior and admired qualities of the dead person. He changes his interests in the direction of activities formerly enjoyed by the lost loved one, adopts that person's goals and ideals, or even takes on certain mannerisms of the deceased. As this final identification is accomplished, preoccupation with the deceased, ambivalence, guilt, and sadness decrease, and thoughts return to life. However, when strong guilt is present, the person is more likely to take on undesirable characteristics, including the last disease symptoms, of the deceased. This negative identity may lead later to psychopathology. Feelings are gradually withdrawn from the lost object. A yearning to be with the lost person is replaced by a wish to renew life. The person gradually unlearns old ways of living and learns new life patterns. The lost object becomes detached from the person and is enshrined in the form of a memory, memorial, or monument. At first, the person's renewed concern for others may be directed toward other mourners or other persons in crisis. It is easier to feel closeness with someone who has experienced a similar loss (Lindeman 1944).

Finally, interest in new objects, relationships, pleasures, and enjoyments is expressed. At first the replacements must be very much like the former object, but eventually new relationships are formed and objects acquired that are equally (or even more) satisfying.

This process may take 6 to 12 months. Complete resolution of or adaptation to the crisis of loss is indicated by the ability to remember comfortably and realistically both the pleasures and disappointments of the lost relationship. When the mourning process is adaptive or successful, the person is capable of carrying on his life with new relationships and without mental or physical illness. This syndrome of feelings, thoughts, and behavior, although varying somewhat in sequence or intensity from person to person, is characteristic of grief and mourning (Lindeman 1944; Engel 1962; Peretz et al. 1970).

Factors Influencing Outcome

Braden (1970) and Lindeman (1944) identify additional factors that affect the resolution of any crisis, the duration of the reaction, and the manner in which adjustment to the changed social environment after loss is made:

1. The degree of dependency for support from the dead person — the greater the dependence, the more difficult is emancipation and resolution of loss.

2. The degree of ambivalence toward the dead person — because ambivalence in a relationship determines the amount of felt guilt, this emotion slows the processes of idealization, identification, and reinvestment of emotional energy in new objects.

3. The preparation for the loss (anticipatory grieving) — whether the loss was expected or had only been briefly thought of some time in the past.

4. The number and nature of other relationships — if prior to his loss the person derived satisfaction from a variety of other objects, persons, or

roles, he now has more bases of support and can more readily form new relationships.

5. The age of the mourner or of the deceased person — the death of a young person generally has a more profound effect on mourners than the death of an aged person in American culture. There is the feeling of great social loss for the young person who has had inadequate time to fulfill himself. Among mourners, children generally have less capacity for resolving loss than adults because of their relative inexperience with crisis and with abstract thinking.

6. The changes in the pattern of living necessitated by the loss.

7. The social and cultural roles of the mourner as defined by society — in American culture, mourning dress, fasting, and sacrifice are indefinitely prescribed. The role of mourner may also conflict with other roles — for example, with masculine or wage-earner roles. Society makes little provision for replacement of the loss or for discharge of hostility and guilt created by loss.

In general, obstacles to the normal progression of grieving arise when the person tries to avoid the intense distress connected with the grief experience and the expression of related emotions. Peretz (1970) describes a variety of reactions to loss.

ABSENT, DELAYED, OR INHIBITED GRIEF

The development of a bereavement state may not occur until days, weeks, or months after the loss has been experienced. If the relationship between the bereaved and the deceased was no longer very close — because of increased independence, separation, or establishment of and investment in new relationships — there may be little or no sign of grief. Absence of emotion immediately following loss may represent shock, denial, or postponement because of a felt obligation to remain strong in order to attend to certain funeral details, business responsibilities, or care of other survivors. Often grief is expressed only when it cannot be avoided — at the funeral service or burial in the cemetery. The person who appears not to grieve may actually grieve intensely in the privacy of his own room or home. This limits the degree to which he can receive support, however; nor can he resolve feelings about the embarrassment of feeling deeply about the deceased person. Sometimes such a survivor appears unfeeling and cold; he is not aware of feeling grief and may unconsciously fear that his grief will reveal the hostility as well as love inherent in the ambivalence of the relationship. Individuals who delay grief are vulnerable to "anniversary reactions," intensely experiencing loss on an important date associated with the deceased, at the anniversary of the death, or when the survivor reaches the age of the deceased at death. Subsequent losses, symbolic of the first loss, frequently reactivate remaining unresolved feelings of loss.

CHRONIC GRIEF

Persistent mourning is indicated when the home must remain the same as before the death. The survivor attempts to make no changes in life pattern, and pretends the deceased is still living or will return. Such a response represents prolonged denial and aims to protect against the anguish of grief and mourning and against anticipated guilt and depression, by denying the loss.

EMOTIONAL OR PHYSICAL GRIEF REACTIONS

Depression may occur as a dominant feature of mourning and may last for months during mourning or even after apparent recovery from grief. Transient depressive affects which are a normal part of mourning can be distinguished from severe depressive reactions by the depth of mood and change in motor behavior and thought processes. Depression is marked by sadness, often with inability to weep, tension, a sense of depletion, slowed movements and mental processes, despair, suicidal thoughts, anorexia with weight loss, constipation, decreased sexual interest, hypochondriasis, and self-preoccupation. Verbal communication is diminished and characterized by self-reproach and criticism, rather than being related to the deceased. The depressed person is persistently pessimistic, sad, hopeless, gloomy, and, if his mood lifts at all, this will occur toward evening. The mildly depressed individual responds to pressure and urging; the severely depressed individual is relatively unresponsive to any approach. The grief-stricken person not in a depressed state will show shifts of mood from sadness to a more normal state within one day and will, after a time, be able to laugh a little; he responds to warmth and reassurance. Friends and relatives tend to feel empathy for the grieving person in contrast to a growing irritation with the depressed person.

Hypochondriasis in the bereaved person is usually expressed by symptoms of a severe nature which are misconstrued by the sufferer. These include constipation (indicating malignancy) and arthritic pain (indicating heart disease). The complaint is frequently the same as or similar to the one causing death in the loved one. Medical consultation is necessary to rule out serious disease, to treat the presenting disease, and to clarify and resolve the emotional aspects of the disease and the underlying feelings. However, treatment may cause the emergence of underlying anxiety, guilt, grief, or depression, a shift to another hypochondriacal complaint, or a persistent conviction that the doctor was incompetent or inaccurate in his examination. Dynamics underlying hypochondriasis include intense feelings of anxiety, hostility, and guilt over a variety of aggressive fantasies. The body is used to expiate and gratify unacceptable wishes. Attention and physical care is gained, but at the price of agitation and worry. These symptoms must be respected by others without giving them undue attention — reassurance about the physical condition is necessary; understanding and patience are essential; and interpretation or confrontation should be avoided.

Psychophysiological reactions may occur, in that serious, life-threatening physical illness often has its onset during, or in lieu of, the mourning process. Activity, either compulsive or destructive, may be used to handle strong feelings rather than facing the emotional pain of the loss. Often the bereaved person

quickly finds a substitute for the deceased, behaves promiscuously, rapidly re-
marries, travels, uses drugs or alcohol, or immerses himself in work or hobbies.
A few people manage grief reactions by manifesting neurotic anxiety, phobic,
hysteric, depressive, or schizophrenic reactions.

Futterman et al (1972) have described the following desirable sequence of
anticipatory mourning for families of dying persons.

1. Acknowledgement that recognizes death is inevitable.

2. Grieving, in which the family experience and express the sadness and
    anger related to the anticipated loss and the physical, emotional, and
    interpersonal turmoil associated with such loss.

3. Reconciliation in which the family develop a perspective on the
    anticipated death which preserves confidence in the worth of the
    dying person's life and life in general.

4. Detachment in which the family withdraw emotional investment
    from the dying person as a growing, living being with a future.

5. Memorialization in which the family develop a fixed, conscious mental
    image of the dying person which will endure beyond death.

If this sequence occurs during the dying process, the bitterness and shock of
the death of a loved family member may be mitigated into a gentler and more
bearable grief.

References

Blauner R: Death and social structure. Psychiatry 29:378, 1966
Braden A: Reaction to loss in the aged. In Schoenberg B, Carr A, Peretz D,
    Kutscher A (eds), Loss and Grief: Psychological Management in Medical
    Practice. New York, Columbia University Press, 1970, pp. 199-217
Engel G: Psychological Development in Health and Disease. Philadelphia, Saun-
    ders, 1962
Futterman E, Hoffman I, Sabskin M: Parental anticipatory mourning. In Schoen-
    berg B, Carr A, Peretz D, Kutscher A (eds), Psychosocial Aspects of
    Terminal Care. New York, Columbia University Press, 1972, pp. 243-272
Glaser B, Strauss A: Time for Dying. Chicago, Aldine, 1968, pp. 5-6, 30
Heimlich H, Kutscher A: The family's reaction to terminal illness. In Schoenberg
    B, Carr A, Peretz D, Kutscher A (eds), Loss and Grief: Psychological Man-
    agement in Medical Practice. New York, Columbia University Press, 1970,
    pp. 270-279
Jackson E: Grief. In Grollman E (ed), Concerning Death: a Practical Guide for
    the Living. Boston, Beacon, 1974, pp. 1-12
Lindeman E: Symptomatology and management of acute grief. Am J Psychiatry
    101:257, 1944

Maddison D, Raphael B: The family of the dying patient. In Schoenberg B, Carr A, Peretz D, Kutscher A (eds), Psychosocial Aspects of Terminal Care. New York, Columbia University Press, 1972, pp. 185-200

Marks M: The grieving patient and family. Am J Nurs 76(9):1488, 1976

Nichols R, Nichols J: Funerals: a time for grief and growth. In Kübler-Ross E (ed), Death: The Final Stage of Growth. Englewood Cliffs, N.J., Prentice-Hall, 1975, pp. 87-96

Peretz D: Reaction to loss. In Schoenberg B, Carr A, Peretz D, Kutscher A (eds), Loss and Grief: Psychological Management in Medical Practice. New York, Columbia University Press, 1970, pp. 20-35.

Quint JQ: Assessments of loss and grief. J Thanatol 1(3):182, 1971

Riley J: What people think about death. In Brim O, Freeman H, Levine S, Scotch N (eds), The Dying Patient. New York, Russell Sage, 1970

Appendix F

Rituals
Surrounding Death

Throughout this book, we have emphasized how cultural and technological changes have removed most Westernized people from death as a customary aspect of life. Thus most Americans are poorly prepared to cope with the death of a loved one, and a variety of psychological defenses may be employed. Similarly, physical arrangements — e.g., immediate burial followed by a later memorial service versus participation in a more direct mourning process often facilitated by funeral-homes rituals — are frequently beyond the ken of survivors. Despite current trends to denigrate the funeral director, he is frequently the one most skilled at assisting a family through necessary arrangements.

Because the nurse is most commonly the professional who has the most intimate contact with the dying patient and his family — another emphasis of this book — we believe that nurses should be somewhat conversant with basic Judeo-Christian rituals that bereaved families may wish to observe when death comes, or that the nurse may wish personally to share.*

---

*The primary source for this material is the publication *Concerning Death: A Practical Guide for the Living*, edited by Earl Grollman (1974) and published by Beacon Press, Boston. Another useful source is *A Manual of Death Education and Simple Burial*, which is available for a small sum from The Celo Press, Burnsville, North Carolina, and provides useful information concerning memorial societies, simple burials, cremation, and various kinds of organ-donor procedures.

JEWISH RITUALS

To the person of traditional faith, death is not the end but a transition from one state of human existence to another. However, the process of dying is fraught with many anxieties not easily resolved, and the dying person who is taken to the regulated environment of the medical center is estranged from the emotional security provided by his family and a familiar environment.

The Jewish legal system (*Halacha*) provides a framework for informing the terminal patient of the severity of his illness, but allows the retention of some hope. The terminally ill are encouraged to put their temporal and spiritual affairs in order but not to fear death.

The deathbed confession, a statement of repentence, may be recited by the dying person according to the limits of his physical and mental condition.

The terminally ill person says a confession, puts his material affairs in order, blesses his family, gives ethical instruction to his children. These procedures enable the patient to express his fears and feelings, seek comfort in inner strength, and communicate meaningfully with those close to him.

In the Jewish legal system active euthanasia is viewed as murder; hastening death is forbidden. During the terminal illness all efforts must be made to support and prolong life. However, when the person is dying or near death, exterior forces extraneous to the patient himself which prevent death may be removed (Heller 1975).

Jewish mourning practices provide a total framework for the acceptance of death, mourning completely, and living again fully.

The dying person is considered the same as the living in every respect; the *Halacha* forbids a dishonest approach. The dying patient is treated as a complete person, capable of conducting his own affairs, and fully able to enter relationships.

Jewish tradition dictates that one is never to leave the bedside of the dying person — a practice of value both to the dying and to the mourners. The mourner is shielded from the guilt of knowing the patient was alone at the time of death and from feelings that more could have been done. The Jewish community provides reassurance that everything possible was done. At the same time every person is part of the community and is thus represented by whomever was present at the person's death.

Additionally, death is witnessed by those at the bedside, which reinforces reality. That, along with immediate burial and the sequential mourning process, helps the mourners to come to terms with death, so that life can then continue for them (Gordon 1975).

During the first period of grief, the mourner has an intense desire to do what he can for the dead. Jewish tradition meets this need by placing responsibility for all funeral arrangements on the mourner rather than employing a mortician to do the tasks that would shield the mourner. The mourner is released from the obligation to perform any religious commandment at this time so that he may devote himself to burial preparations and arrangements.

Reality and simplicity are characteristic of Jewish burial, which is in clear contrast to American funeral rituals that deny death. Valuable and healing grief work is built into the Jewish funeral. The passionate expression of grief is encouraged and the simplicity of the burial and religious prescriptions for a plain, unadorned, simple coffin and for avoiding ostentation in a funeral prevents the family from an irrational expenditure of money (Gordon 1975).

The most striking expression of grief is the rending of garments by the mourner prior to the funeral service. An opportunity for psychological relief, the rending allows the mourner to give vent to his pentup anger and anguish by means of a controlled, religiously sanctioned act of destruction.

Tearing of the clothes is a visual and dramatic symbol of the internal tearing-asunder that the mourner feels in his relationship with the deceased. Judaism opposes repression of emotion and encourages the mourner to express grief and sorrow openly. In the funeral itself there are several signals for a full outpouring of grief. The eulogy is intended to make the mourner aware of what he has lost, as are the familiar prayers.

The gaping hole in the earth, ready to receive the coffin, symbolizes the emptiness of the mourner at this moment of final separation. Burying the dead by actually doing some of the shoveling themselves helps mourners to ease the pain of parting by performing one last act of love and concern.

When the burial is completed, grief work intensifies as the focus of community concern shifts to the mourner. After burial, the mourner finds a mandatory meal of recuperation waiting. It is a resocializing and relearning experience, a visible sign of communal solidarity, reassuring the mourner that he is not alone. The meal also restates the theme of life: life must go on, even though he feels it has ended with the loss. Until this time, the mourner was allowed to withdraw in his pain, loss, and identification with the deceased; now the community reaches out to redirect him back to the path of complete living.

With that first meal begins the work of *Shivah*, through which tradition advances grief work for the mourner. Grief work begins with the initial release of feelings, expressed in recounting the events that led up to death and then to recounting of memories of life. The mourners get together to retell and relive their experience of the death and to share memories from the past when the family circle was whole. The condolence call provides the mourner with the opportunity to tell his story many times to many different people, and he is allowed to speak first so that his interests are the focus of the conversation. The visitor does not come to issue platitudes — only to listen, thus enabling the mourner to vent his feelings. If the mourner cannot find words to express his grief, the visitor comforts him with silence and his shared physical presence.

As will be detailed later, Judaism recognizes that there are levels and stages of grief and thus organizes a year of mourning into 3 days of deep grief, 7 days of mourning, 30 days of gradual readjustment, and 11 months of remembrance and healing. Thus the mourner is drawn from his temporary isolation to increasingly larger personal and communal responsibility and involvements so that by the end of the year he has been reintegrated into community and his loss accepted, though not forgotten (Lamna 1969).

Traditional Judaism is opposed to cremation as a denial of belief in bodily resurrection, although more liberal Jews accept it.

Ceremonies of death are significant to Jews because the Hebrew religion holds that rites aid in the grieving process. Bereaved persons must face the reality of the death and must fill the void in a constructive way. They are encouraged not to repress memories, even guilt-producing ones. A definite mourning period is assigned to the entire family. The rabbi is actively involved with the mourning family.

One is considered a "mourner" at the death of parents, spouse, children, or siblings. A child younger than 13 years, the age of religious adulthood, is not obliged to observe mourning rituals.

The funeral ceremony is performed standing to symbolize that sorrow should be met standing upright. The parent who is mourning wears a tear in his clothes for a week on the left side, over the heart; others wear the tear on the right side. The most intensive mourning occurs for the first 7 days (*Shivah*) after the funeral, excluding the Sabbath or Festivals. The bereaved individuals remain at home, receiving the continuous condolence calls. The *Shivah* begins immediately after the funeral, and during this time a candle remains burning. After *Shivah* comes *Sh-loshim*, a 30-day period when the mourners resume normal activity but avoid places of entertainment. Mourning ends after *Sh-loshim*, unless the deceased was a parent, in which case it continues for the entire year.

Jewish rituals are community rituals, and the traditions carry a sense of solidarity, belonging, and comfort. However, Judaism is strict in limiting mourning to the designated periods and rituals: excessive or prolonged mourning represents a lack of trust in God. After mourning is over, the person is not expected to be the same, but he is expected to take up his existence again. The garment that the pious mourner tore is mended and worn again — symbolic of the scar that remains, although life resumes its course.

Nursing personnel mourning a dead patient may pay their respects to the dead by attending the funeral service, following the procession to the Jewish cemetery, and visiting during the mourning period. Statements such as "How are you?" or "He lived to a ripe old age" should be avoided, as they show lack of sensitivity. Extra visits after the *Shivah* are especially appreciated, as the *Sh-loshim* is a particularaly lonely time when most visiting is concluded. Bringing food when one visits is acceptable. Flowers are usually not sent to the funeral, although a donation of money to worthy causes or to a charity is considered appropriate. A sympathy card or letter is also appropriate (Grollman 1975).

ROMAN CATHOLIC RITUALS

The Roman Catholic faith teaches that death is conquered by the resurrection of Christ, and of oneself. The victory over death comes not at the hour of death but in the final hour when Christ will come again. The sadness and suffering of death are not denied. Prior to death, or during any serious illness, the ritual of anointing of the sick is carried out. The priest does the anointing with oil at a specified time. Prayers are offered for forgiveness of sin and restoration of health. When possible, the family is present to join in the prayers and the patient is also encouraged to respond, if he is able. During the illness the priest will be invited regularly to visit and to bring communion to the sick person. At the hour of death, a final communion — called *viaticum* — is given to the dying person. In the event of a sudden death, the priest should be called and the anointing and *viaticum* should be administered, if possible. If the person is dead when the priest arrives, there is no anointing but the priest leads the family in prayers for the person who has just died.

The Roman Catholic funeral rite consists of three phases: the wake, the funeral mass, and the burial. Plans are made by the priest, the family, and the funeral director.

The wake is a vigil or period of waiting for the funeral and varies among ethnic groups and in sectional areas of the country. In the past the wake was held in the family home. The body was laid in an open casket after embalming, and friends and relatives would sit in an all-night vigil. The wake was an occasion for visiting — to sustain the family in the grief process, to pay respect to the deceased, and to join with others in an expression of faith. The primary expression was prayer. At present the wake is usually held in a funeral home at specified hours for one or two days. A wake service for the immediate family and friends — which includes scripture and meditative reading, or the saying of the rosary (a devotion centering on meditations of 15 mysteries of redemption and including a repetitive recitation of the "Hail Mary") — is held sometime during the wake. The wake is a preparation for the funeral and is kept simple so that the funeral is not anticlimactic.

The rituals used in the wake and funeral service were developed to support the family and friends of the bereaved, to define the grief experience, and to restate the faith that gives meaning to death.

The funeral is a prayer service incorporated into the celebration of mass. It begins with a procession from the funeral home to the church. After all are ushered to their seats, the priest meets the body of the dead person at the entrance. The casket is covered with a white cloth, symbolic of baptism. The priest wears white vestments, symbolic of the joy of faith that overcomes the sadness of death. A candle, the sign of Christ present through baptism, is placed at the casket. Scriptural passages are read, a homily is delivered, and prayers are said. The liturgy and prayers of the Eucharist follow, and communion is given to those wishing to partake. The Rite of Commendation ends the service. Throughout the service the congregation stands, sits, or kneels as indicated by the priest.

At the cemetery, the official rite is brief and includes a blessing of the grave, a Scripture reading, and several prayers. The family may or may not choose to stay for lowering of the casket into the grave.

Friends express condolence by attending the wake, funeral mass, and burial, by sending flowers or a memorial gift, or by obtaining a spiritual bouquet, a card announcing the celebration of mass for the deceased.

Although in the past cremation was not allowed because it implied the denial of resurrection of the dead, Catholics can now obtain permission for cremation.*

The bereaved persons continue to gain support from attending weekly celebrations of the mass, and a month after the death, a Month's Mind Mass may be celebrated (Butler 1975).

PROTESTANT RITUALS

Wide differences exist in Protestantism concerning the theology and rituals of death. A broad spectrum of belief and practices may exist even within the same denomination, although some few Protestant groups may insist that theirs is the only authentic Christian witness. Some Protestant theologies address the realities and meaning of life; others inhibit expression of grief, denying death and discouraging sadness as not becoming to a Christian.

Some Protestants view death as penalty and punishment for sins; others see death as a transition when the soul leaves the body for an eternal life. Others view death as an absolute end.

Rituals surrounding death vary widely. Some communicants believe the funeral service with a closed casket or memorial service with no casket present are more of a testimony to the joy and victory of Christian life than the open casket service. Others believe that viewing the dead person facilitates the grief process and that confronting the reality of death is a Christian context. The minister represents friendship, love, acceptance, forgiveness, and understanding, regardless of the Protestant faith represented.

Common elements with which all Protestants could agree include:

1. Death is a mystery that cannot be fully comprehended.

2. Death is a biological and spiritual event in the fellowship of believers.

3. Death is realized and experienced in the community of faith and calls forth the caring resources of the congregation to the bereaved.

4. Religious resources and rituals are significant to the bereaved in dealing with death.

The Protestant funeral may be conducted by the minister in the church sanctuary, a funeral home, or at a private home. The funeral is considered a service of worship, and is conducted according to the traditions of the denomination

---

*Cremation is seldom done in the United States (about 5 percent of deaths' although it is widely practiced in some countries with high population densit~ or where land is less available for use in cemeteries. Cremation is a mode of d position in which the dead body is quickly reduced to several pounds of its co ponent elements by intense heat; the ashes are then buried, scattered, or pl in an urn. A memorial or committal service may be held after cremation to the family complete the process of separation.

and local church, as well as the personal style of the minister. Reading of Scriptures, prayer, music, a eulogy of the deceased, and a brief meditation or sermon are usually a part of the funeral service. The committal service at the graveside is usually brief.

In Protestantism there is no absolute practice in relation to the condolence call before or after the funeral. A condolence call depends upon the local traditions and needs and wishes of the people involved. For those persons close to the deceased or the family, waiting until after the funeral to call may be experienced as disappointment, rejection, or hurt. It is considered more appropriate to call and stay briefly than to omit calling. On the afternoon and evening following the funeral some people want to have family and friends around them to share memories, break bread, and experience the supportive fellowship of a caring group.

The major attention is given to the bereaved in the first days following the death. However, attention should be sustained; loneliness becomes more intense with the passing of time. Visits by supportive friends and relatives are very welcome weeks and months following the funeral.

One's sorrow can be expressed to Protestant bereaved families in a variety of ways: sending a sympathy card or letter; condolence visits or phone calls; visits to the funeral home, if such are scheduled; attendance at the funeral service; memorial gifts to charity or to a cause designated by the deceased or the family, often instead of a flower gift; willingness to listen, to share, to continue to interact with the family; doing special tasks for the family, such as bringing food, caring for the children, or running errands; and manifesting a sustained concern for the family lasting through weeks and months.

It is important to consider the needs and wishes of the family rather than to express caring and love in ways which run counter to the wishes of the family. The family should have the right to express their sorrow in their own unique way without criticism and alienation (Jordan 1974).

A memorial or committal service may be held after cremation to help the family complete the process of separation.

References

Butler R: The Roman Catholic way in death and mourning. In Grollman E (ed), Concerning Death: A Practical Guide for the Living. Boston, Beacon, 1974, 101-118

Gordon A: The Jewish view of death: guidelines for mourning. In Kübler-Ross E (ed), Death, the Final Stage of Growth. Englewood Cliffs, N.J., Prentice-Hall, 1975, pp. 44-51

ɔllman E (ed): Concerning Death: A Practical Guide for the Living. Boston, Beacon, 1974, pp. x-xvii

r Z: The Jewish view of death: guidelines for dying. In Kübler-Ross E (ed), Death, the Final Stage of Growth. Englewood Cliffs, N.J., Prentice-Hall, 975, pp. 38-43

Jordan M: The Protestant way in death and mourning. In Grollman E (ed), Concerning Death: A Practical Guide for the Living. Boston, Beacon, 1974, pp. 81–100

Lamna M: The Jewish Way in Death and Mourning. New York, Jonathan David, 1969

Index